T0173226

Praise for *Osteopathy and Obstetrics* 2e

Stephen Sandler, who is one of the world's leading osteopaths in his field, has produced a book which should be a must-read for every osteopath (or any other manual therapist) who endeavors to treat the pregnant patient. The book is relevant to student, novice and experienced clinician alike. I guarantee that within its pages you will find useful gems of information and learn from the personal reflection and technical artistry of the author.

The book is laid out with simplicity – but it is a complex tour de force, complete with supporting evidence and background reading, describing the pathophysiological journey of the pregnant patient.

Dr Sandler's wide anatomical knowledge takes us beyond the exterior musculoskeletal realms, to the viscera, vascular, fascial and nervous systems within our patients. The aims and ambitions of the techniques he demonstrates allow us to interact and support the patient, making positive changes throughout pregnancy, and beyond. In the second edition of *Osteopathy and Obstetrics* Stephen Sandler defines osteopathy.

Stacey Bourne, DO, MSc(Ost), PgCAP, Senior Practice Educator, The University College of Osteopathy, London, UK

Stephen Sandler is a person with many osteopathic skills and talents:

- firstly, he is one of the most experienced osteopathic practitioners in the field of obstetrics,
- secondly, he is an experienced and very inspiring teacher,
- thirdly, he is an empathetic personality – which is important in general, but especially in this field,
- and fourthly, he is also a researcher.

All these competencies are demonstrated in the content of this second edition of *Osteopathy and Obstetrics* making it unique in what it has to offer. If you want to know how to deal with pregnancy from an osteopathic point of view, there is no better book to go to.

Torsten Liem, DO, MSc Ost, MSc Paed Ost. Joint Principal, German School of Osteopathy; lecturer in cranial, fascial and psychosomatic osteopathy; osteopathy practitioner, Hamburg, Germany

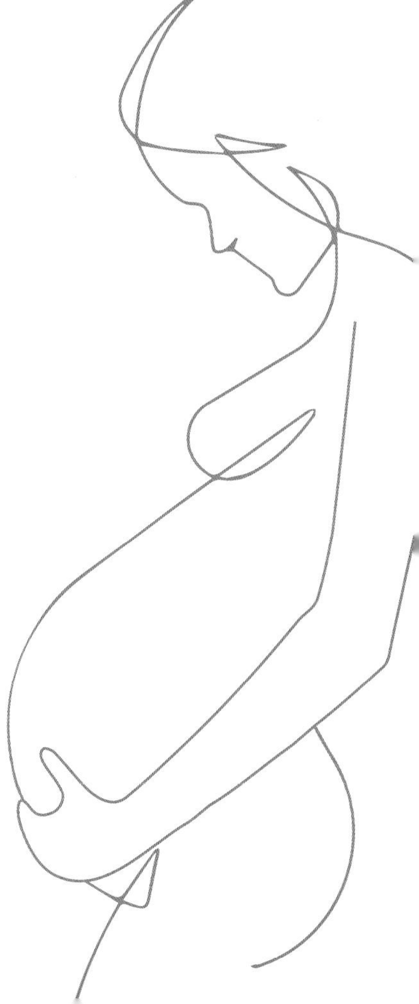

Osteopathy and Obstetrics

Osteopathy and Obstetrics

Second Edition

Stephen Sandler

Foreword

Eric Jauniaux

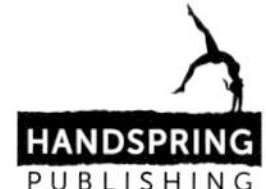

HANDSPRING PUBLISHING LIMITED
The Old Manse, Fountainhall,
Pencaitland, East Lothian
EH34 5EY, Scotland
Tel: +44 1875 341 859
Website: www.handspringpublishing.com

First edition published in 2012 Anshan Ltd
This edition first published in 2021 in the United Kingdom by Handspring Publishing Limited

ISBN 978-1-913426-23-1
ISBN (Kindle eBook) 978-1-913426-24-8

British Library Cataloguing in Publication Data
A catalogue record for this book is available from the British Library
Library of Congress Cataloguing in Publication Data
A catalog record for this book is available from the Library of Congress

Commissioning Editor Mary Law
Project Manager Morven Dean
Copy Editor Wendy Lee
Designer and Cover Design Kirsteen Wright
Indexer Aptara, India
Typesetter Amnet, India
Printer Finidr, Czech Republic

Book typeset in Minion Pro Regular 11/13.5

The
Publisher's
policy is to use
paper manufactured
from sustainable forests

CONTENTS

ABOUT THE AUTHOR

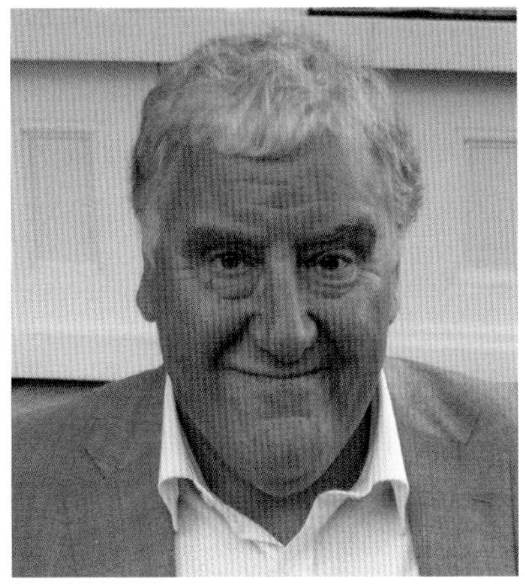

Dr Stephen Sandler PhD DO is a practicing osteopath. He graduated from the British School of Osteopathy (now the University College of Osteopathy) in 1975. He received his PhD in 2006 for his work exploring the relationships between the connective tissues and cyclic female hormones, in the normal menstrual cycle, pregnancy, the postpartum phase, and the menopause.

Over the past 45 years he has taught in osteopathic schools worldwide on various subjects relating to osteopathic practice and technique. Latterly, he has concentrated his teaching in the field of osteopathy and obstetrics. In 1982 he founded the Expectant Mother's Clinic at the British School of Osteopathy in London. This was the first clinic aimed at the treatment of the pregnant patient.

For more than 40 years he ran the Chingford Osteopathy Practice in northeast London, from where he has now retired. He spent 15 years in private practice at the Portland Hospital for Women and Children before moving to nearby Harley Street .

He is happily married and has three children and five grandchildren. Together with his interest in golf and tennis they keep him active and busy.

FOREWORD

Fifteen years ago, one of my pregnant patients who was treated by Dr Stephen Sandler came back to me and told me that this was the best birthday present she had ever had. Stephen and I were practicing in the same building at the time but we had never met. A few months down the line, I took my children for a trip to Disneyland Paris and came back to London with a frozen shoulder. I tried physiotherapy, which helped temporarily, but it was Dr Sandler who solved my problem after only two therapeutic sessions. At the same time he opened my eyes to the benefit of osteopathy and the science behind it.

I had the pleasure of reading the first edition of *Osteopathy and Obstetrics* but this second edition takes us to a new level of knowledge. It is practical and backed up by the latest scientific developments, which Dr Sandler, with his PhD and 45 years of experience in the pathophysiology of musculoskeletal disorders during pregnancy, is best placed to write about. These disorders are exacerbated in many pregnant women during the second half of gestation. Within this context, osteopathy has become one of the most efficient and safest alternative therapies for some common conditions such as lower back pain and symphopubic dysplasia. The nine chapters of the second edition of *Osteopathy and Obstetrics* cover the different aspects of the anatomy, physiology, pathology, and osteopathy treatments for musculoskeletal disorders during pregnancy. It is essential reading for osteopaths and for all those who provide care to pregnant women: midwives, physiotherapists, obstetricians, and family physicians/general practitioners.

Eric Jauniaux MD, PhD, FRCOG
Professor in Obstetrics and Fetal Medicine,
EGA Institute for Women's Health,
Faculty of Population Health Sciences,
University College London,
London, UK
July 2021

PREFACE

Many years ago, when I was a senior student at the British School of Osteopathy in London, I was faced with a pregnant patient for the first time in my limited clinical life. I remember it very clearly because I did not know where to start. Were pregnant patients the same as other clinic patients? Were there things I should look out for or that I should or should not do? My patient explained that she had been fine until, one day, for no reason at all, she developed sciatica. She was in her second trimester of pregnancy with her second child. Her GP had suggested paracetamol, which did not touch the pain, but he said it was unsafe to give her anything else. She was comfortable lying down but the midwife was concerned that she should be as mobile as possible in pregnancy. She rang one physiotherapist, who said he was not trained in women's health, and then another, who said that she was not trained in back problems and could only offer her exercises, which had not worked.

I eventually found a clinic tutor who had experience with pregnant patients and she was able to guide me as to the best possible way to proceed. To my surprise, this patient was very easy to treat, as her ligaments were already softening due to hormone changes. She came back the next week, very happy and much improved. This led me to do some research into the physiological changes of pregnancy and (in the days before internet searches) I spent a year after graduation looking for published work, especially on the risks of manipulation in pregnancy. From that day to this, I have yet to find one published article that shows manipulation has been linked with miscarriage or has had any other disastrous consequence. This enabled me to formulate a teaching program, and in 1980, the British School of Osteopathy opened the first clinic specifically offering osteopathic care to pregnant and postnatal patients.

I have spent the last 45 years teaching osteopathy and obstetrics all around the world, wherever osteopathy is practiced. The first edition of this book has now been upgraded with new information that is evidence-based, and with new photos and specifically commissioned illustrations, making it suitable for students, osteopaths, midwives, family physicians/GPs, and anyone that is confronted with pregnancy back pain in their daily lives.

Stephen Sandler
London, UK
July 2021

ACKNOWLEDGEMENTS

I would like to thank Ben James and Oli Sandler, the photographers; David Arbiser for his excellent drawings; and Mary Law and Andrew Stevenson of Handspring Publishing for their help during the project and for assistance in obtaining permission to use some of the illustrations.

I am also grateful to the models used in the photographs for their patience and understanding during the photo sessions.

I would especially like to thank the staff at Primal Pictures for their help and generosity in providing the 3D images, which I have been permitted to use at no charge. Likewise, I am grateful to the people at Elsevier for permission to use their illustrations, again generously supplied at no charge.

Every effort has been made to contact all the copyright holders of material used in this book. Any omissions will be rectified in subsequent printings if notice is given to the publishers.

Finally, I thank my long-suffering wife for her support and patience during the writing of this book.

Stephen Sandler
London, UK

1 Introduction

"Structure governs function" is often quoted as being one of the more important tenets of osteopathy. According to Caroline Stone, a leading lecturer and practitioner in the field of osteopathic obstetrics, it is better written as "Motion relates to physiology."[1]

As a philosophy, osteopathy shares this principle with many other natural or ancient therapies, including Ayurveda and traditional Chinese medicine. The concept is more easily understood if one thinks of a machine. If the machine is built correctly and regularly maintained, it will not break down. So it is with the human body, with its capacity for adaptation and autoregulation: we have the facility for enormous modification of our physiology according to the external circumstances or environment.

According to McKone,[2] the relationship between structure and function is one of the most basic of biological concepts. From insects to mammals, structure denotes an ability to function in a certain way, and function is limited or controlled by structure. McKone goes on to say that changes in the structure–function relationship can be influenced by the interaction of the external and internal environments acting individually or in combination.

Pregnancy and the immediate postpartum period are excellent examples of the capacity to change, and of the ability of a woman to change back to how things were physiologically before pregnancy once she has had her baby. Her body structure adapts to facilitate the physiological changes that she is undergoing. A "normal" pregnancy needs little medical intervention in what is essentially a physiological event. A "normal" pregnancy requires the services of the midwife, not the doctor.

However, if the patient has an underlying disease process to contend with during the pregnancy, then she may well need the attentions of the obstetric team, so that early anticipation of a medical problem that may adversely affect the pregnancy can be managed, leading to a successful outcome.

Examples include certain cardiac patients, people taking long-term medication for whatever reason, and those who are diabetic or have long-term thyroid disease. Likewise, from the obstetric point of view, for those women who demonstrate adverse changes to their structure – such as cephalopelvic disproportion, where the birth canal is too narrow to allow the presenting part to pass through – a planned elective cesarean section is always safer and better than an emergency operation.

Facilitating Change

One of the principal tenets of osteopathic medicine is that, given the correct set of circumstances, the body should be in a position to maintain health. If a patient has a bacterial infection, all an antibiotic drug will do is kill the bacteria and allow the body to heal. After a fracture, an orthopedic surgeon will pin plate or set broken bone, allowing a cast to be applied for structural stability, and then the healing takes place naturally.

In cases of neoplasia, normal growth is altered beyond normal physiology and metabolic demand, eventually leading to a situation where normal adaptation and physiological health become unattainable. The body is more likely to succumb to secondary disease processes, life becomes compromised, and death supervenes. Likewise, if the immune system is severely disturbed by diseases such as AIDS or any other immune-suppressing process, secondary infection can arise and the normal process of adaptation and defense will fail, leading to eventual death.

Chapter 1

When we treat a pregnant patient, she is in a physiological, not a pathological, state. We examine her and evaluate how she is undergoing that physiological change. We look principally at the musculoskeletal system because, being osteopaths, this is where we have been trained to place our emphasis. However, we do not do this exclusively. We question her about her general health and her pregnancy health because she may well be in a subclinical state where symptoms have not yet made themselves felt. Also, as we are primary care practitioners, many patients self-refer to us, and thus we have to be in a position to know if it is safe to treat them or whether we need to refer them for further care. Just because a patient has thoracolumbar pain, it does not mean that the pain is of mechanical origin. It might be, but it might not. Questioning her about her renal function and history might make you suspect that she has a kidney problem: for example, an infection that is giving her loin pain, and which needs to be referred to her family physician/GP or midwife.

We should examine each body system in turn and see how that system is dealing with the changing demands of pregnancy. The pregnant patient's cardiovascular system is changing, as are her cardiac output and peripheral resistance. How is her body coping with that change and the potential new demands? Is there something mechanical in the fascias, the respiratory mechanisms, or the rib cage which might be compromising these changes? How can the practitioner encourage her body to adapt by dealing with the factors that might impede that change?

Take a woman who, before pregnancy, had a short right leg, which gave her a minor organic scoliosis that changed direction at the thoracolumbar and cervicothoracic junctions. There may be rib crowding on the concavity of the curves as a result. What effect, if any, is this going to have on her ability to change during the pregnancy? Osteopathic evaluation will highlight these areas of altered structure, and the judicious use of techniques aimed at improving areas that need to change will facilitate it happening. If we can do this in advance of that change being needed, then when it does eventually become necessary, it will be easier and more likely to happen without adverse events. Thus, our ambition to improve the potential for change, so as to reduce or remove any compromise to it, will have been achieved.

The Importance of Motion to the Ability to Change

Every living thing, and every cell within every living thing, possess and display certain biological characteristics of life (Box 1.1), and no one of them is any more important to life than any other. However, the presence or absence of motion is often used as a defining characteristic within medicine, as, for example, when a pediatrician uses the APGAR score when a child is born. He assesses the heart rate via the pulse beat, the breathing rate and effort via motion in the chest, and the degree of activity or motion in the

BOX 1.1

The biological characteristics of life ("GRENRIM")

- Growth
- Reproduction
- Excretion
- Nutrition
- Respiration
- Irritability
- Movement

child in general, together with muscle tone. All of these factors use motion to define normality in that child.

We understand death to be the ultimate absence of motion at a macro and a micro level.

The process of autoregulation ensures that the organism minimizes cell damage by allowing motion only within preset physiological parameters. Using the example of a synovial joint, quality and quantity of motion are governed by the shape, plane, and integrity of the articular surfaces. The joint capsule and the intra- and extra-articular ligaments are designed to limit motion at the end of the joint's normal physiological range. The skeletal muscles and their accompanying tendons guide motion and control its speed, as well as providing postural stability and control. The force, speed, and direction of pull of the muscles all contribute to the control of motion. The central nervous system controls the whole, relating the postural and proprioceptive functions to the body's desire for motion. All of the factors above are controlled by a remarkable system of hormones, enzymes, and other biological and psychological factors which contribute towards motion control.

The qualitative assessment of motion – as it relates to the musculoskeletal system, for example – is further subdivided into hypomobility, normal mobility, and hypermobility.

In order to adapt and change, therefore, the tissue, and the organism that contains that tissue, have to able to move. In pregnancy, as a patient grows and changes shape, so her body has to adapt to that change in order for it to take place. If, for example, she had a cesarean section to deliver her first child, in second and subsequent pregnancies the scar tissue is going to have to soften and undergo change in order for the uterus to grow for the second time. As the organs below her diaphragm are squeezed and compressed, they will end up in a very different position from their pre-pregnant state. This means that the fascia and organs supporting that change in position will have to undergo change, too. And so it goes on. These changes are aided by alterations in hormones during pregnancy: notably, relaxin and estrogen. The function of these hormones is not just exerted on the structures related to her reproductive system; they effect global changes to every tissue in her body, aiding and facilitating their potential to change during the 40 weeks of normal gestation. It is our job to work with these changes and to encourage them with skillful techniques and an intelligent application of osteopathic concepts and principles. As osteopaths, we use the quality and quantity of motion throughout the body as the main tools in our diagnostic and therapeutic armory.

During the 40 weeks of normal pregnancy, the human body has to undergo reversible change throughout the many body systems. From the cardiorespiratory system to the neuromuscular and skeletal systems, from the digestive system to the urogenital and excretory systems, every part of the pregnant woman will change and adapt to her new physiological state to give the fetus nutrition for growth, and to give the mother the energy she needs to sustain this growth, both for labor and for lactation

When she comes to give birth, a woman undergoes the hardest physical day's work of her life. Her preparation for the day, in terms of physical and mental resources, is of paramount importance if she is to deliver her baby successfully. It would be unreasonable to expect a marathon runner to race without the best preparation possible to achieve the expected performance. So it is with osteopathic care during pregnancy.

The idea of the osteopath treating and caring for obstetric patents is not new. Andrew Taylor Still, MD, DO (August 6, 1828 to December 12, 1917), the founder of osteopathy and osteopathic medicine, was a physician and surgeon, and so treated obstetric cases as part of his normal practice. Also an author, inventor, and Kansas territorial and state legislator, he set up the American School of Osteopathy (now A.T. Still University), the world's first osteopathic medical school, in Kirksville, Missouri.

Unless they are medically qualified, the osteopaths of today are not involved in delivering the baby. This is restricted, quite rightly, to those who have the required training to practice legally in this way. However, the skills of an osteopath will ideally be available to encourage and prepare the pregnant woman for the physiological changes mentioned before. Structural, visceral, cranial, and myofascial techniques all have a safe and important part to play in this task.

Also, it is important to realize that low back pain and other types of musculoskeletal discomfort are extremely prevalent in pregnant women today, with some researchers citing more than two-thirds of patients who undergo some form of low back pain or pelvic pain during their pregnancy.[3] Osteopathy provides a safe and efficient way of dealing with these pains and thus allowing the pregnant patient to develop her energies for growing and dealing with the day-to-day physiological demands of being pregnant.[4]

This book will examine each of the important body systems, look at the changes needed in their physiology, and then explore the technical approaches that can be applied to enable the patient to better achieve those changes.

Another key tenet of Still's osteopathy explores the concept that all organs are interrelated when it comes to structure and function. No organ works alone but is part of an integrated whole, each element serving to aid all other parts. The interrelationships between the body systems allow osteopaths to use the links between the changing structural support systems and the changes in the organs when it comes to treating any dysfunction, or when working in anticipation of any change, as and before it happens. Likewise, the neurological and vascular changes taking place locally in the organs and globally throughout the whole body will mean that a thorough knowledge of the blood and nerve supply and drainage to the various changing structures allows the integrated use of osteopathic principles and techniques, again locally and globally throughout the body.

In this way, the osteopaths of today can rightly follow in the footsteps of their forebears in giving their pregnant patients the best osteopathic medicine available, so as to create optimum health for both prospective mothers and their children.

This book is set out in chapters that deal with changes above the diaphragm, below the diaphragm, and in the pelvis. Each chapter will begin with a review of the anatomy and physiology of the non-pregnant patient, and then the physiological and pathophysiological changes that can occur during pregnancy; it goes on to explore the various categories of osteopathic manual techniques that can be used to address those changes. Of necessity, it creates an artificiality by presenting each part alone, but in reality a multiplicity of factors leads the practitioner to a variety of approaches that will vary from patient to patient. In some cases there will be a predominance of musculoskeletal elements that need attention; in others it might be fascial elements that appear to be important. Each case will be individual, and therefore there can be no common approach to the treatment and resolution of these problems. Evaluation must be global, and the treatment specific and founded on the palpable findings in each case.

The book is not gender-specific where the text relates to the osteopath. For the sake of ease, only the male term has been used, but of course this is completely interchangeable with the female form.

Safety Issues and Osteopathic Treatment During Pregnancy

Osteopathy is a safe modality with which to treat patients who are pregnant. Before opening the Expectant Mother's Clinic at the British School of Osteopathy in 1982, the author spent many hours in medical school libraries researching papers linking manipulation to miscarriage and was not able to find a single published paper connecting the two. From that date to the present, using the facilities of Medline, Medsci, complementary and alternative medicine (CAM) journals and databases, and other peer-reviewed journal databases, the result is the same. There simply is no documented evidence to be found suggesting that the use of manipulation is in any way associated with damage to the fetus, the placenta, or the mother. Many articles suggest that manipulation in the first trimester should be avoided, but again these are not supported by any evidence.

Spontaneous Abortion

It has been estimated that 10–15% of first-trimester pregnancies will spontaneously abort but the figure could potentially be very much higher; we just do not know. The figure is not surprising, considering which tissues are being laid down in that first trimester, including the primitive nervous system and the primitive arterial system. Literally millions of cell divisions occur within the first month of life in the tissues of the developing central nervous system, and if a genetic or chromosomal defect results from just one of those cell divisions, it may well transpire that the damage is such that life cannot continue. In some cases the mother's body seems to recognize that damage and so it aborts the fetus, clears the uterus of its contents, and starts again.

It is true that, logically, a woman cannot know for sure that she has been pregnant unless she has had a positive pregnancy test. She may be convinced that she has conceived, but until the test is positive she has no proof. Therefore, when does she take the test? Normally, it is carried out after the first missed menstrual period, but if that period arrives a day or two early or late, and is maybe a little heavier than usual, does this constitute a spontaneous abortion? The answer is not unless she had a positive test. Millions of women conceive and lose a fetus every year without ever knowing they were pregnant.

There are many reasons why spontaneous abortions can occur.[5] They include parental structural chromosomal rearrangements, congenital and acquired anatomic faults in the fetus, endocrine disorders, and silent infection of the genital tract; each makes a contribution to the etiology of recurrent spontaneous abortion. In many patients a putative cause can be identified, but whether it really is the reason behind recurrent spontaneous abortion often remains elusive.

Another reason why some women spontaneously abort might be placental abnormalities such as anti-phospholipid syndrome causing thrombosis in the small blood vessels of the placenta, leading to subsequent fetal death. Once again, this has nothing to do with manipulation or any other manual technique.

Conception is an emotive subject. Couples pay thousands of pounds to assisted conception centers in attempts to get help to produce a much-wanted child. Every menstruation is a visible sign of the failure of the attempt to conceive. However, as stated before, spontaneous abortions are common, and in some cases they will occur very early on, within the first 4 weeks of life. Emotionally, this is a very difficult time for couples, who look for reasons as to why miscarriages occur and maybe blame themselves

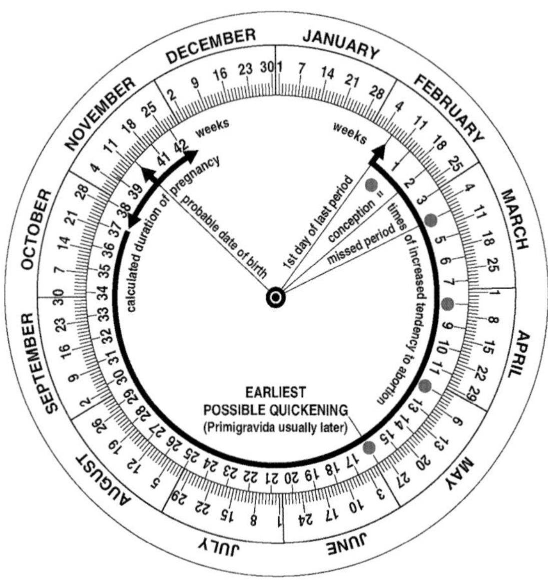

Fig 1.1
A pregnancy wheel.

for excessive physical activity or sports, but with no evidence to support these recriminations at all. Things happen spontaneously and that is it. We just do not know why and that is why we refer to them as spontaneous abortions.

Some midwives and obstetricians will use a menstrual calendar to predict the expected date of the child's birth (Fig 1.1). Others use a computer program. This is usually based on the date of the last menstrual period. Some of these calendars will show that weeks 4, 8, 12, and 16 are the commonest times for spontaneous abortions to occur. The reasons why abortions happen at these times is still not clear. The author's advice to his students is to avoid treating the patient around these specific dates and you are less likely to be associated with a disastrous event that is nothing to do with you. It is a way of protecting the student from unwanted feelings of guilt, and maybe avoiding the profession being associated with an event that is just a natural occurrence.

This is why it is essential to take a full and comprehensive obstetric history with all new patients, and to ask them about vaginal bleeding, cramping in the abdomen, or any other unwanted symptom every time you see them and before you treat them. If there is any doubt about safety issues, the patient must be referred back to the midwife or the doctor to ensure that the fetus is alive, well, and safe.

Safe Techniques and Treatment Positions

Pregnant patients should never be treated prone (face down), so as to avoid any undue pressure on the abdomen or the sensitive breast tissues. Treating your patient supine is also not without risk. Undue pressure of the gravid (pregnant) uterus on the inferior vena cava can reduce blood flow to the placenta.[6,7]

The best position to treat pregnant patients is lying on the left side or sitting (Figs 1.2 to 1.4). Soft tissue and myofascial techniques can be done above and below the diaphragm in the sitting position, as can techniques for the ribs and diaphragm. Osteopaths use sitting techniques more frequently during pregnancy, as they are safer and more comfortable for the patient .

If they are on their backs, they should be propped up at 45 degrees, with a pillow or a blanket under the knees and a small pillow in the lumbar lordosis.

Craniosacral techniques are easily performed in the side-lying position, with one hand cradling the occiput and the other the sacrum, thus allowing for easy assessment of the primary respiratory mechanism (Fig 1.5). Craniosacral techniques can be approached side-lying, instead of supine, to avoid the patient lying on her back for extended periods of time during pregnancy.

Cramp in the calf is a minor but common discomfort of pregnancy. Massage of the calf in

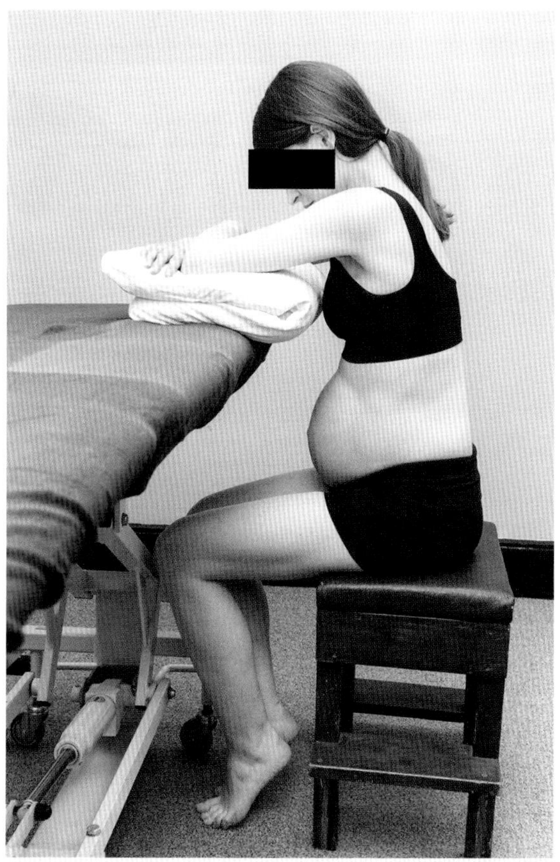

Fig 1.2
Patient sitting at the treatment table.

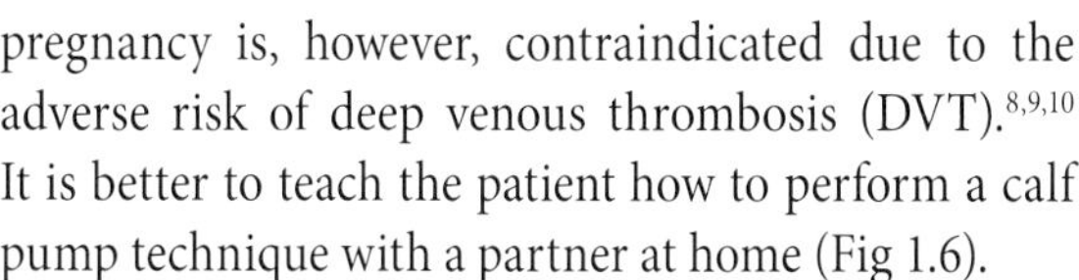

pregnancy is, however, contraindicated due to the adverse risk of deep venous thrombosis (DVT).[8,9,10] It is better to teach the patient how to perform a calf pump technique with a partner at home (Fig 1.6).

Sacroiliac pain is very common during pregnancy. Classic side-lying rotation techniques are best avoided, so as not to put any pressure on the abdomen. Instead, the techniques can be done with ease and safety from behind using a reverse sacroiliac joint manipulation (Fig 1.7).

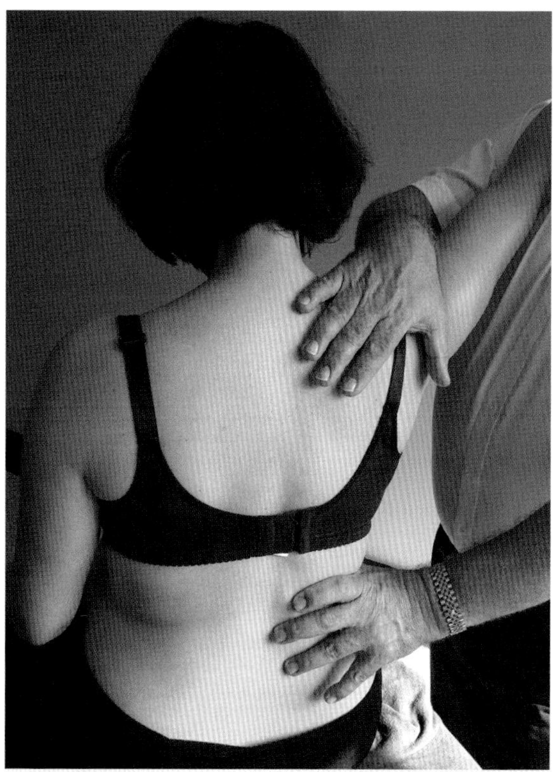

Fig 1.3
Patient sitting for a rib stretch technique.

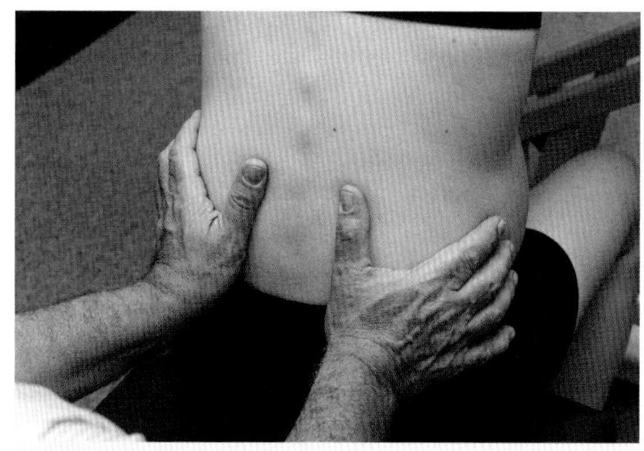

Fig 1.4
Patient sitting for a lumbar soft tissue technique.

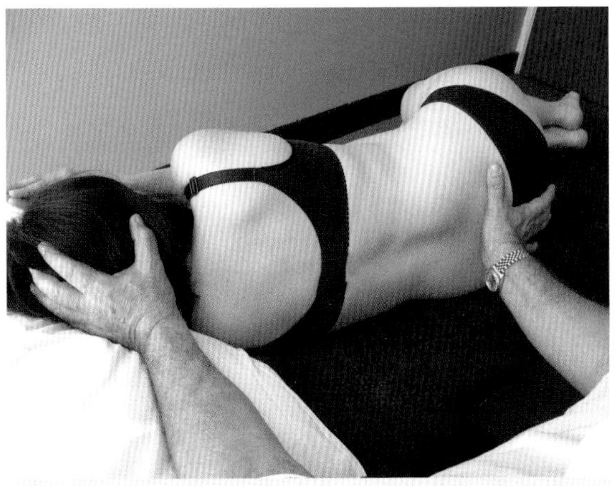

Fig 1.5
Patient lying on her side for craniosacral palpation.

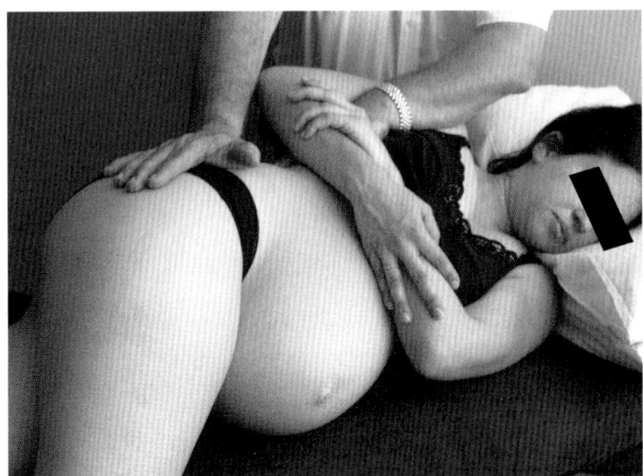

Fig 1.7
The "reverse" thrust for the sacroiliac joint during pregnancy.

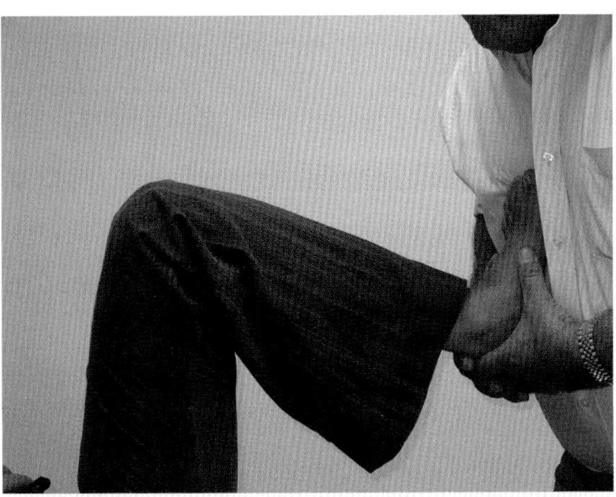

Fig 1.6
Safe use of the calf pump technique in pregnancy. Never massage the calf during pregnancy because of the increased risk of deep venous thrombosis (DVT). Instead, use a calf pump technique.

During pregnancy, two main hormones have an effect on the supporting muscles and ligaments. These are estrogen and relaxin. As the pregnancy progresses, the pregnant woman will become looser in her joints, and the muscles are more susceptible to fatigue.[11]

Your techniques need to be accurate and to use a minimum of leverage, so as not to stress the tissues. Short, repetitive techniques will be better than long levers that can overstrain the joints, leading to muscular fatigue. Myofascial unwinding techniques work really well, as they rely on feedback from the patient to guide your actions in releasing tensions.

In summary, if the practitioner takes a comprehensive case history, looking for "red flag" warning signs such as bleeding, hypertension, and abdominal cramping (which might indicate early labor in the late stages of pregnancy) (Box 1.2), and ensures that the patient is attending regular antenatal classes, then there is no reason why osteopathic treatment is not indicated.

With adaptation to avoid stress to the tissues, all types of maneuvers, including high-velocity, low-amplitude (HVLA) techniques (or high-velocity thrust (HVT) techniques), can be used safely and effectively to relieve symptoms or to prepare the tissues for further physiological changes.

BOX 1.2

Risk factors in pregnancy

- Focal movement patterns changed
- Low hemoglobin
- Weight loss or failure to gain weight
- Protein, glucose, or bacteria in the urine
- Blood pressure > 155 mmHg/90 mmHg
- Uterus large or small for dates
- Head not engaged in primiparous women (pregnant for the first time) by 38 weeks
- Vaginal bleeding
- Premature labor
- Vaginal infection

References

1. Stone C. *Science in the Art of Osteopathy*. Stanley Thornes, 1999.
2. McKone W. *Osteopathic Athletic Health Care*. Chapman and Hall, 1997.
3. Liddle SD, Pennick V. Interventions for preventing and treating low-back and pelvic pain during pregnancy, Cochrane Database Syst Rev. 2015(9):CD001139.
4. Sandler SE. The management of low back pain in pregnancy. Man Ther. 1996 Sep;1(4):178–185.
5. Tulppala M, Ylikorkala O. Current concepts in the pathogenesis of recurrent miscarriage. Curr Obstet Gynaecol. 1999 Mar;9(1):2–6.
6. Tamás P, Szilágyi A, Jeges S, Vizer M, Csermely T, Ifi Z, et al. Effects of maternal central hemodynamics on fetal heart rate patterns. Acta Obstet Gynecol Scand. 2007;86(6):711-14.
7. Gormus N, Ustun ME, Paksoy Y, Ogun TC, Solak H. Acute thrombosis of inferior vena cava in a pregnant woman presenting with sciatica: a case report. Ann Vasc Surg. 2005 Jan;19(1):120-2.
8. Ray JG, Chan WS. Deep vein thrombosis during pregnancy and the puerperium: a meta-analysis of the period of risk and the leg of presentation. Obstet Gynecol Surv. 1999 Apr;54(4):265-71.
9. Beers MH, Berkow R, eds. Normal pregnancy, labour, and delivery. In *The Merck Manual of Diagnosis and Therapy*, 17th edn. Merck Research Laboratories, 1999.
10. Callahan TL, Caughey AB, Heffner LJ. *Blueprints in Obstetrics and Gynecology*, 2nd edn. Blackwell, 2001.
11. Sandler SE. The Association Between Joint Laxity and Female Hormones: Changes in Joint Laxity Associated with the Menstrual Cycle, with Pregnancy, with the Postpartum Period, and with the Menopause. PhD thesis. Published by VDM, 2008.

Evaluation of the Pregnant Patient 2

Evaluation of the pregnant patient from an osteopathic point of view means that, as far as possible, we look in a holistic way at her to determine the state of her tissues and how she is coping with the extra demand that pregnancy makes on them.

It has been this author's experience that patients tend to arrive by recommendation from their doctor, midwife, or health visitor, or through the personal recommendation of friends and relatives who know your practice. They also come after performing internet searches and reading articles in the local or national press, either about osteopathy in general or about your practice in particular.

Usually, the reason why first-time mothers come for treatment is pain, and the commonest place for that pain is the sacroiliac joint or symphysis pubis. Disc pain is not so common in pregnancy, and while other sources of musculoskeletal discomfort are frequently encountered, they are not as common as back pain. Visceral disturbances are not the main prompt for most expectant mothers, but if you address their pain problems first and then advise on other aspects of osteopathy related to the cardiovascular system or to digestive problems, they are usually very receptive. Then, later in the pregnancy, your help in getting them fit for labor through work to the breathing apparatus and pelvic joints means that, all being well, their labor will be easier and well controlled.

It is very common to see women again at second or subsequent pregnancies, and a frequent reason for presentation is prevention of the pain and discomfort they experienced last time.

When the osteopath evaluates the pregnant patient in front of him, he needs to understand not only if it is safe to treat her, but also the correct tools to apply for the best solutions to a problem.

Safety is paramount, regardless of who referred the patient or if they were self-referred. The osteopath must stand by his own decisions and not rely on the diagnosis of others. It would be unsafe to depend on the patient's idea of what is wrong with her, even if she has seen a family physician/GP or an obstetrician. She perhaps did not fully understand what she was being told. If in doubt, referring her back to her doctor can be the only premise under which to work.

Not all symptoms are clear-cut, and all too often pathology can present itself as what might seem at first to be a relatively simple problem. It is for this reason that, for their training to be effective, osteopathic students have to have a good working knowledge of the pathophysiological mechanisms of disease in every part of the body: firstly, to judge whether it is safe to treat the patient, and secondly, maybe to use myofascial or visceral techniques, as well as musculoskeletal maneuvers, to try to treat the patient and resolve the problem.

Then there is the issue of choosing a technique. A tight muscle can be addressed using a cross-fiber soft-tissue technique to stretch it; a longitudinal soft-tissue drainage technique; an exercise to stretch it; a functional technique to create a balance between the muscles contracting and relaxing around a joint; a high-velocity, low-amplitude thrust technique which will relax the tension around a joint capsule using the mechanisms of the neurological connections that go to and from the spine; and many other ways to restore physiological balance at the point of dysfunction. It goes without saying that this list of techniques is not complete; there are many more ways to encourage a muscle to release, if that is what the evaluation tells you needs to be done.

The choice of which technique to apply, in which order and when, is as old as manipulation itself. It will vary from patient to patient, and will change each time we see the patient, depending on the palpatory response, which in turn is part of the evaluation.

The subject of the human body is vast! Where to begin and what to do first are the most daunting questions facing a student. Of course, the answers lie in the word "experience." That is why, in many developed countries, all schools of osteopathy are associated with a school clinic where student osteopaths, under the training and guidance of more senior practitioners, have to undergo a minimum number of patient contact hours before they qualify. They gain the ability to take a case history and to make a pathophysiological evaluation. Then, combining this information with visual clues and a deep and thorough palpatory examination, they begin to understand "why this patient, why this problem, and why now" (that is, why did this patient present with this problem at this time?), and also to make a decision as to which tools to use, in which order, and for how long, to achieve maximum resolution of the patient's problem. The last part of this is fascinating. How long should a technique be applied for? The answer, again, is as old as osteopathy or manual medicine itself. Find it, fix it, and leave it alone!

The Case History Analysis

When treating a pregnant patient, the osteopath starts the consultation, as in general osteopathic practice, with a detailed case history analysis, based on the functions of the various tissues causing the presenting problem. This is not simply a structural analysis, but must include a detailed account of the problem, the woman's general physical and obstetric health, a full structural examination, and, if need be, a clinical examination of the various body systems, including the nervous system or visceral system as appropriate.

Boxes 2.1 to 2.6 present an example of the case history form used in the author's own practice. They are followed by an explanation of why the questions are deemed important.

The Case History Sheet

Evaluation of the obstetric patient begins with the case sheet. The case sheet is, in essence, the same as that used in regular practice for non-pregnant patients, but with some important differences.

Biographical details

As part of the biographical details, it is good practice to include weight gain, as well as current weight. Midwives use weight gain as an indicator of good obstetric health (Fig 2.1). It is common at the beginning of a pregnancy for the patient to lose weight, especially if she is vomiting a lot, but continued weight loss may be a sign that all is not well with the fetus. This might lead the midwife to request further tests and scans to assess the growth of the baby.

It is also sensible to include the names and ages of any previous children. Obstetrics is about treating families, as well as the pregnant patient. Lots of toys, games, and books in the osteopathic consulting room will encourage the mother to bring her child or children with her. This not only means that she does not have to find a babysitter each time she visits, but also, if children get to see and enjoy the atmosphere of the consulting room, it makes them less likely to be afraid to come in for treatment if they have a problem.

Obstetric details

Women often have a number of options when it comes to where they are going to give birth and the sort of care they would like.

BOX 2.1

Case history page 1

EXPECTANT MOTHER'S CASE HISTORY

Date:……………………………………

Patient's surname:……………………………………

Address ……………………………………

Osteopath:……………………………………

First name:……………………………………

Age: ……………………………………

Date of birth:……………………………………

Weight (kilos/pounds):……………………………………

Weight gain: ……………………………………

Height: ……………………………………

Telephone numbers and email: ……………………………………

Children, including names and ages:……………………………………

Occupation and interests:……………………………………

……………………………………

Family physician/GP or midwife's name and address:……………………………………

……………………………………

BOX 2.2

Case history page 2

OBSTETRIC DETAILS

Expected date of delivery:..........

Number of weeks pregnant:..........

Type of care (shared; family physician/GP, community midwives; consultant):..........

Where booked:..........

Scans (dates and results):..........

Blood tests (dates and results):..........

Miscarriages and terminations: (including dates and number of weeks):..........

Problems with previous pregnancies:..........

Length of previous labor:..........

Forceps, ventouse, or other interventions:..........

BOX 2.3

Case history page 3

TISSUE DIAGNOSIS

(based on questions)

Presenting symptoms: ....

History, onset, and treatment: ....

Aggravating factors: ....

Relieving factors: ....

Non-affecting factors: ....

BOX 2.4

Case history page 4

MEDICAL HISTORY

Illness and operations:...

Accidents:...

General health:...

1. Diet
2. Gastrointestinal
3. Renal and urinary
4. Cardiovascular and respiratory
5. Endocrine
6. Gynecological before pregnant...

Medications (to include proprietary medicines, vitamins, herbal preparations, and prescribed medications):

....

Smoking/alcohol:...

Remarks and impressions:...

Important social factors:...

BOX 2.5

Case history page 5. PSIS, posterior superior iliac spine; SIJ, sacroiliac joint, SLRT, straight leg raising test; VBI, vertebrobasilar insufficiency. See also Figure 2.13 for the circle system of notation.

POSTURAL EXAMINATION

From the side

ANTERIOR POSTERIOR VERTEBRAE

From the back

O
C1
C2
C3
C4
C5
C6
C7
T1
T2
T3
T4
T5
T6
T7
T8
T9
T10
T11
T12
L1
L2
L3
PSIS L4 PSIS
L5

COCCYX

SOFT TISSUES
REFLEXES ACTIVE/PASSIVE MOVEMENT
POWER
SENSORY
SLRT
SIJ TEST
VBI TEST

BOX 2.6

Case history page 6

EVALUATION

(To include tissues causing local and general pathology, etiology, predisposing and maintaining factors. Why did this patient present with this problem at this time?)

Aim of management in the short term: ....

Aim of management in the long term:...

Special precautions:...

Further examinations to be performed:...

First visit treatment given:...

Instructions to patient:...

Prognosis in both the long and the short term:...

Name:...

Date:...

Signature: ....

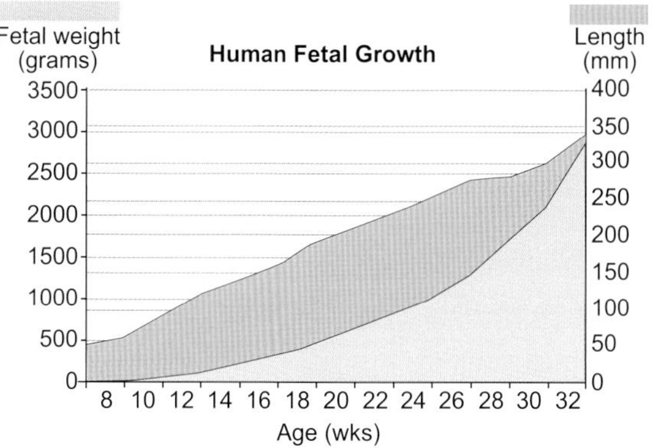

Fig 2.1

Fetal growth chart.

To convert millimeters to inches, multiply by 0.04. To convert grams to pounds, multiply by 0.002.

© Dr Mark Hill; https://embryology.med.unsw.edu.au/embryology.

Usually, as soon as they think they are pregnant because they have missed a period or had a positive pregnancy test, they will contact their family physician/GP. Home pregnancy tests are very accurate and work by detecting the presence of human chorionic gonadotrophin (HCG), a hormone produced by the very early fetal cells within the first 2 weeks after conception.

Antenatal care monitors the mother's health during pregnancy, as well as the health and development of her baby. It can help predict possible problems with the pregnancy or the birth, so that action can be taken to avoid or treat them. This is the essence of good modern obstetric care, and explains why maternal and perinatal mortality figures are as low as they are. Most women are healthy and will not need to see a doctor at all during their pregnancy. The midwifery service takes care of all of the antenatal appointments, which are designed routinely to check that all is well with the pregnant woman and her baby. Those cases that are high-risk are then booked into the local maternity unit for care under a consultant obstetrician.

What Happens at the Antenatal Visits?

The first antenatal appointment will probably be for booking in, and this usually happens at about 8 to 12 weeks. In some areas, it is carried out at home by a community midwife; in others, the patient may be asked to visit the hospital. If she plans to have her baby at home, the appointment will almost certainly take place at her home or at her local health center.

At the booking visit, she will be asked a number of questions about her health, family history, and any previous pregnancies. The aim is to build up a basic picture of her health and her pregnancy so far.

Routine checks at other appointments are likely to include blood pressure, weight, listening to her baby's heart, questions about the baby's movements, urine tests for protein and infections, and a check for any swelling in the legs, arms, or face. This swelling is referred to as edema, and high blood pressure, edema, and protein in the urine constitute the clinical triad called pre-eclampsia, a potentially serious condition which would require immediate referral by an osteopath to the labor ward.

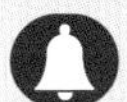

Warning

If you are treating a pregnant patient, it is highly likely that you will be seeing her more frequently than the midwife or doctor conducting routine antenatal visits. It might be that you are the first person to see this edema. If so, you should take the blood pressure and perform a dipstick urine test yourself, looking for proteinuria. This is very important. If in doubt, call the midwife or the labor ward while the patient is still with you. Depending on the advice given, she may even need to be taken to hospital by ambulance from your surgery.

BOX 2.7

Major antenatal complications

- Isoimmunization
- Bleeding
- Polyhydramnios
- Oligohydramnios
- Associated clinical conditions that pregnancy interferes with, e.g. cardiac or kidney problems

Follow-up tests at the clinic or the hospital will depend on how the pregnant patient is doing and how well the baby is growing. Not counting appointments for scans or other hospital-based tests, she can expect to attend appointments every 4 weeks after week 12, every 2 weeks from week 32, and every week during the last 3 or 4 weeks.

In the UK, the National Institute for Health and Care Excellence (NICE) guidelines recommend that healthy women have up to ten check-ups for a first pregnancy, including the booking visit. For second and subsequent pregnancies, seven visits is common.[1]

Major and minor antenatal complications are listed in Boxes 2.7 and 2.8.

Blood Tests During Pregnancy

Normally, a small sample of the pregnant patient's blood is taken at the first antenatal appointment. She may also be asked to give a sample in later pregnancy. The first test can:

- identify her blood group
- establish whether her blood is Rhesus-positive or negative
- look for conditions that could affect her own health or her baby's (this may or may not include HIV)

BOX 2.8

Minor antenatal complications

- Vomiting
- Gastric reflux
- Constipation
- Pruritus vulvae
- Vaginal discharge
- Cramps
- Varicose veins
- Hemorrhoids
- Back pain
- Fainting
- Paresthesia

- check for immunity to rubella (German measles)
- check for anemia.

Blood tests can also be used to estimate the risk of Down's syndrome. A blood sample is taken at about 16 weeks to measure three substances: alpha-fetoprotein (AFP), unconjugated estriol, and HCG. Together with the mother's age, these give an estimate of risk. The level of AFP can also indicate the risk of a neural tube defect, such as spina bifida.

Ultrasound Scans

Ultrasound scanning is used for different reasons at different times. It is safe, does not harm the baby as it does not involve ionizing radiation, and can be very reassuring for a mother who is concerned or worried that all is not well.

A scan at about 6–8 weeks is used to confirm or date the pregnancy, to establish whether it is ectopic (developing in the fallopian tubes, not the uterus), and to check that the fetus is alive by looking for a heartbeat.

A scan at about 10–14 weeks is used to confirm and date the pregnancy, to check for twins (especially if the pregnancy was achieved by in vitro fertilization, IVF), and, when offered alongside a nuchal scan (which looks at a pad of skin at the back of the baby's neck), to assess the risk of Down's syndrome or other chromosomal conditions.

A scan at about 20–23 weeks is used to look for spina bifida and other possible abnormalities, to examine the baby's major organs and skeleton in detail, to check the health of the placenta, and to monitor the baby's growth.

Later scans monitor the baby's growth and check the position of the placenta and the baby.

Different types of scan are available and some will reveal a wealth of detail about the baby. The normal ultrasound is a 2D scan in black and white, which shows all the information needed to assess growth, heartbeat, and so on (Fig 2.2). Then there are 3D scans, which provide greater detail and are usually obtainable privately (Fig 2.3). Lastly, there are 4D scans: mini video clips showing the child moving around and giving even greater depth of view.

Labor

At around 40 weeks, most women will go into labor. Regular contractions, the show or loss of the mucus plug, and the breaking of her waters are all accepted as signs that she has started to give birth.

During a first-time birth, labor lasts 16 hours on average; however, this can vary tremendously.

Labor can be divided into three stages. Stage one, when the cervix dilates, is subdivided into three phases: early, active, and transition.

Early labor is the longest part, lasting 8–10 hours. In this phase, the cervix opens from 0 to 3 cm (1.2 inches). Contractions are mild and occur between 5 and 20 minutes apart.

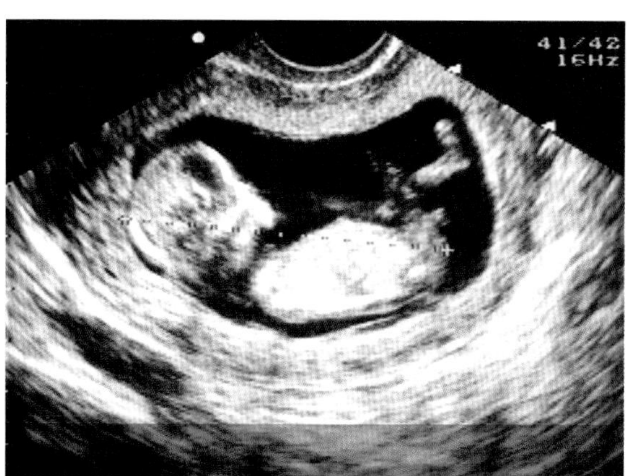

Fig 2.2
A classic early pregnancy scan.

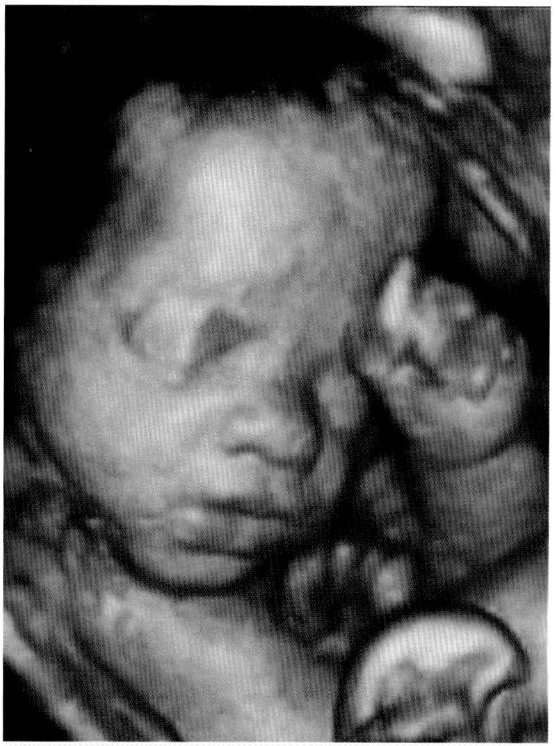

Fig 2.3
A 3D ultrasound image of the fetus at 30 weeks.

The patient may notice that it takes some effort to get through the contractions as she goes from early labor into active labor. In active labor, contractions last about 1 minute and occur about 2–5 minutes apart. Active labor lasts about 3–5 hours and the cervix dilates from 4 to 7 cm (1.6 to 2.8 inches).

The most intense phase of labor is transition. Contractions are only about a minute apart and may last up to 90 seconds as the cervix opens from 8 to 10 cm (3 to 4 inches). This is the shortest phase of labor and the patient will soon be ready to push.

Stage two is the part of labor where the baby is born. Some women have a little resting period after the cervix opens all the way and before they feel the urge to push. Contractions can be about 5 minutes apart during pushing and last for about 1 minute. During this phase, the baby descends through the pelvis, moves down through the birth canal, crowns on the perineum, and is then born. Pushing may last anywhere from 15 minutes to 2 hours on average.

The third stage of labor is delivery of the placenta. This may happen between 15 minutes and an hour after the baby is born.

Cesarean Section

There are two types of cesarean section: elective, where the decision is made a long while before the birth process starts; and emergency, where labor has started and the obstetrician decides for various reasons that there is a problem and operates to deliver the child surgically. Delivery by cesarean section has been the subject of intense debate in recent years. One thing that is for certain is that it is always better to deliver with a section that is planned rather than having an emergency operation.

The obstetrician might advise an elective cesarean if:

- the patient has serious pre-eclampsia (see earlier)
- she has a serious medical condition which means that she should avoid the stress of labor
- she is expecting a multiple birth
- the placenta is positioned across the neck of the womb, making it impossible for the baby to be born vaginally; this is known as placenta previa
- the baby is lying transverse across the uterus and cannot be turned to a head-down position
- the baby is too big to be able to get through the pelvis; this is called cephalopelvic disproportion (CPD)
- the baby is in the breech position.

Whether all breech babies should be delivered by cesarean is a matter of obstetric debate. Some obstetricians prefer to turn babies into a head-down position at the end of pregnancy (this is called external cephalic version, ECV), while others like to give the mother the chance to try for a vaginal delivery with her baby in the breech position.

An emergency cesarean might become necessary after labor has started because:

- the baby's heartbeat shows that it is not coping well with contractions (in medical terms, the baby is described as being "distressed")
- the cervix stops dilating or dilates very slowly, so that both mother and baby become exhausted
- the placenta starts to come away from the wall of the uterus and there is a risk of hemorrhage (bleeding); this called an abruption
- the baby does not move down into the pelvis, indicating that the pelvis is too small for the baby to get through (CPD).

It has traditionally been considered inappropriate for women to have an elective cesarean section on request in an uncomplicated pregnancy. In previous studies, female obstetricians and midwives were questioned on their preferred mode of delivery. One study asked 344 women attending a routine antenatal booking clinic what mode of delivery they would prefer in an uncomplicated pregnancy, and why. Of the women questioned, 14·5% opted for an elective cesarean section at 39 weeks' gestation, the main reasons being to avoid maternal trauma, to avoid a prolonged labor, and to promote fetal wellbeing. A cesarean section may have some potential benefits over a vaginal delivery, and it may be difficult for an obstetrician to refuse a well-informed woman an elective cesarean section on request, even if it results in a further rise in the rate of cesarean section.[2]

Diabetes and Pregnancy

It is estimated that between 2 and 3% of pregnant women are affected by diabetes occurring for the first time in pregnancy. This is called gestational diabetes. What causes a pregnant woman to contract gestational diabetes is still not known.[3] The hormones that are produced when pregnancy occurs may, in some ways, prevent the functioning of insulin. If the mother's body cannot produce sufficient insulin to overcome this, gestational diabetes may develop.

As with diabetes outside pregnancy, some women are more prone to developing gestational diabetes than others. Women at greater risk of gestational diabetes include those who are over 35 years of age, are obese, have previously had a still birth in the latter stages of pregnancy, and have already had a large baby. Also, any person is more at risk if they have a family history of type 2 diabetes.

One of the problems with gestational diabetes is that it does not manifest itself with clear symptoms. The symptoms common to high blood sugar (thirst, frequent urination, hunger) sometimes occur, but all of these are frequently encountered in the latter stages of pregnancy. The presence of high blood sugar levels during pregnancy may cause the fetus to grow larger than it usually would. This can make delivery more complicated and, in some instances, may provoke the need for a cesarean section.[4]

The Postpartum Period

Having had her baby, the patient may be allowed to go home on the same day if all has gone well. She will usually be visited at home within 24 hours by the family physician/GP or health visitor, who will assess her and the baby. Advice about breast feeding is commonly given at this point. Not every mother is able or wishes to feed the baby herself. It is important not to be judgmental and to be sympathetic to whichever choice she has made.

The osteopath may well be involved at this point, especially if he practices craniosacral techniques for the baby, as well as the mother. Otherwise, having taken care of your patient during her pregnancy, it is good practice to offer her a postnatal visit at 6 weeks to check her, to ensure that any problems you treated during the pregnancy have resolved, and to establish whether she can be discharged from your care. Of course, if she is still suffering from any pains that she consulted you about during the pregnancy or if issues have arisen during the course of the labor, she can and should be offered the earliest possible appointment for treatment, as long as she has been seen by the midwife and or the health visitor.

Osteopathy and Obstetrics: The Legal Issues in the UK

The law in the UK is very specific. Since 1902, only those people trained specifically as midwives or qualified as medical doctors are allowed by law to manage and treat a pregnant woman or a woman in labor. This was reinforced by midwifery legislation in 1958, 1956, and 1992. Therefore, we are quite clearly not allowed to be involved in the whole childbirth and labor process if the person who is managing that labor does not want us there, regardless of the feelings of the mother or father to be!

Classic osteopathy does give us some idea of what osteopathic physicians did in the past. Still writes in his lecture notes of the osteopathic physician and his role in labor, but remember that he was a Doctor of Medicine and therefore acting within the law in the USA. Today, osteopathic physicians in the USA are doctors, and are legally allowed to deliver children and take full responsibility for the mother's obstetric care. In this sense, they are in a unique position. In no other country in the world are osteopaths allowed or legally able to take part in childbirth.

A logical role for osteopathy would be to act as a supporting service to the midwifery profession, in particular in treating those minor problems in pregnancy that midwives are traditionally not well trained to deal with. Examples might include musculoskeletal pain: in particular, back pain, sacroiliac and pelvic pain, gastroesophageal reflux (GER, or GOR) and indigestion, uncomplicated headaches, and pubalgia (pain radiating from the pubis).

Once the initial presenting symptom has resolved, our role changes. By addressing issues that might arise from changes in maternal physiology and working to ensure that, during her pregnancy, those changes and adaptations take place with the minimum of discomfort and stress, we are acting to ensure that the optimum physiology leads to the best possible pregnancy, and thus a better outcome all round.

BOX 2.9

Questions that must be asked at every osteopathy visit

1. Expected date of delivery (EDD)?
2. Number of weeks?
3. Last antenatal visit?
4. Any further scans or blood tests?
5. Any obstetric abnormalities?
6. Is the patient fit and well?
7. Any abnormal vaginal discharge?
8. Any vaginal bleeding?
9. Any abdominal cramping?
10. Is the patient still fit to treat or should she be referred back to the doctor or midwife as a matter of urgency?

Questions to Ask at Every Osteopathy Visit

Certain enquiries should be made every time a patient visits you (Box 2.9).

1 and 2. A woman will sometimes have a scan that reveals that she is more, or sometimes less, advanced in her pregnancy than she thinks. The usual expected date of delivery (EDD) is based on her last menstrual period, but the ultrasound scan is more accurate and so the date can change. This can be important when she is near to her due date.

3. When did the patient last see the midwife? Does the midwife know about the problem you are discussing today or are you the first person to see it?

4, 5, and 6. These questions are self-explanatory.

7. Vaginal discharge is normal during pregnancy and is due to the effects of estrogens on the genital tract. The discharge should be clear or creamy, and will stain her underwear, but should not be foul-smelling or offensive. If it is yellowish, she may have a pelvic infection and should be referred to her family physician/GP or midwife immediately.
8. Vaginal bleeding must be referred for investigation or evaluation as a matter of extreme urgency.
9. Abdominal cramping might just be Braxton Hicks contractions, or if it occurs towards the end of her pregnancy may indicate that she is actually in labor. How many weeks pregnant is she? Are the pains regular or irregular? Are they rhythmic? How long has she been having them? Again, the midwife or family physician/GP should be notified.

The Tissue Diagnosis from a Structural Point of View

The questions and answers leading to a tissue diagnosis are no different from the ones that are asked of a patient who is not pregnant. They are based on a logical interpretation of structure and function. How the tissue or structure works is dependent on a clear understanding of normal physiology and biomechanics. A differential diagnosis leads logically to technique and treatment.

Low back pain in pregnancy is common. It has been estimated that up to 72% of pregnant women will develop back pain. Other studies put the figure around the 50% mark.[5,6,7] One researcher maintains that, during pregnancy, serious pain occurs in about 25% of patients studied, and severe disability in about 8%. After pregnancy, problems are serious in about 7%.[8]

Whichever figure is nearer to the truth, back pain and pelvic pain are common and orthodox medicine has problems dealing with them. Powerful analgesia and non-steroidal anti-inflammatory drugs (NSAIDs) can be harmful to the developing fetus during the first trimester of pregnancy, belts and corsets sometimes just do not work, and bed rest is contraindicated because it is better for a pregnant patient to be mobile, aiding the return of venous blood from the legs and pelvis to the heart. If a woman is suffering from low back or pelvic pain, her family physician/GP might well send her to a physiotherapist for care and treatment.

In the UK, physiotherapists undergo basic training and then go on to specialize by attending postgraduate courses. The availability of a physiotherapist who has also completed a course of postgraduate training in manipulation or back care and obstetrics and women's health care would not be common. For this reason, it would be fair to say that, because most schools of osteopathy include time spent in an expectant mother's clinic as part of the basic training, osteopaths have more techniques at their disposal and have had more specific training in treating pregnant women than physiotherapists. Back pain is something that we, as osteopaths, see on a daily basis, and so it is logical that we should be involved in the treatment of pregnant patients who are suffering in this way.

The commonest problems treated at the British School of Osteopathy Expectant Mother's Clinic in London (now the University College of Osteopathy) were found to be sacroiliac pain, facet pain, and disc pain.[9] Specific questions based on function can often be very helpful in making a differential diagnosis. The questions listed in the next section are not the only ones to be asked but are used as an example of the thought processes commonly employed to identify the structure that is causing the discomfort. Of course, if the patient has headaches, thoracic or extremity pain, or something else, questions appropriate to those problems are asked and the answers evaluated in each case.

Differential Diagnostic Questioning for the Three Commonest Structural Problems Causing Pain in Pregnancy

Sacroiliac joint pain

Sacroiliac joint (SIJ) pain has the following characteristics (Box 2.10):

Definite laterality. Sacroiliac pain alone does not cross the midline. If it does, it is more likely to be disc or facet pain. It can be referred pain to a myotome, sclerotome, or dermatome, or root pain due to entrapment syndrome. The piriformis muscle is usually pierced by the sciatic nerve, and an SIJ lesion, especially one involving the lower pole, can lead to sciatic nerve pain and clinical signs such as reflex and power changes in the area supplied.

BOX 2.10

Characteristics of sacroiliac joint pain

- Definite laterality to pain
- Pain does not cross the midline
- Can be referred or root pain
- Turning in bed provokes pain
- Getting in or out of the bath lifting the leg is painful
- Getting out of the car causes pain
- Going upstairs, i.e. taking the whole weight of the body against gravity, causes pain
- Pain referred to the groin or genitals
- Pain with opening legs during sex
- Pain related to menstruation prior to pregnancy

Turning in bed. This provokes pain. Sleep is disturbed by SIJ pain, especially if it is the pain of inflammation. Also, to turn in bed, you have to use the pelvic girdle to turn and swivel the hips to the new position.

Getting in or out of the bath. When getting in or out of the bath, lifting the leg is painful. This is all about unilateral weight-bearing. The act of stepping over the high sill of the bath involves separating the legs and standing on one leg. A person with SIJ pain will not be able to stand on the affected leg.

Getting out of the car. Again, this involves separating the legs and then unilateral weight-bearing. Depending on whether patients are driving or are passengers, and if the car is a left-hand or right-hand drive, this will be easier or harder. Certainly, they will not be able to get out of a low car seat without help or without grabbing hold of the door to pull themselves up.

Going upstairs. Moving the whole weight of the body against gravity causes pain on the affected side.

Pain referred to the groin or genitals. It goes over the hip, not to the hip. Patients use the back of the hand to show pain radiating from the posterior superior iliac spine, and then over the front of the hip and down to show the pain in the groin.

Walking on flat ground. This involves the weight-bearing phase on the affected side, not the swing phase of walking.

Pain with opening the legs during sex. Practitioners should not be coy about the subject of mechanical pain with sexual intercourse, especially with pregnant patients! Pregnancy is often a time of increased libido but if the patient has sacroiliac pain, sex may not be possible. If she is lying on her back with her knees abducted and hyperflexed, she will stretch the SIJ capsules to the maximum. If she is experiencing pain in this way, then suggest a side-lying position or a rear entry position, which involves separating the legs much less. If she is heavily pregnant, this may be more comfortable anyway.

Facet joint pain

Facet joint pain has the following characteristics (Box 2.11):

Weight-bearing not involved. Pain can occur when the patient is off weight-bearing, unless there is an anomaly and the facet joints become weight-bearing, leading to degeneration known as spondylarthrosis. Normal facet joints do not carry weight, and when they are called on to do so – for example, in the last weeks of pregnancy when she has a deep lordosis – they can start to hurt.

Pain related to movement, specifically rotation. There is only 1 degree of rotation per facet in the lumbar spine and so rotation in the neutral plane will

BOX 2.11

Characteristics of facet joint pain

- NOT related to weight-bearing
- Related to movement, specifically rotation
- Patient does not like lateral compression
- History of relatively small injury in relation to great pain
- Eased by rest
- Referred to an extremity
- Not affected by coughing or sneezing

engage the facet joints, quickly causing pain. If they flex and rotate, the pain will go away.

Lateral compression. The patient does not like lateral compression. This is for the reason described above. It is one of the principles behind the triangle test (see later).

History of relatively small injury in relation to great pain. There are thousands of nociceptive fibers around the facet joints,[10,11] and so a small injury can produce violent pain and muscle spasm, which can die down again very quickly.

Pain eased by rest. Pain is eased by rest in any position. Normally, lying on the side with the painful side up is most helpful.

Pain referred to an extremity. There is little evidence that facet pain will entrap a nerve root, but, as mentioned before, it will refer via a sclerotome, myotome, or dermatome.

Pain not affected by coughing or sneezing. This is because it does not cause a rise in intra-abdominal pressure, as disc pain does.

Disc pain

Disc pain has the following characteristics (Box 2.12):

Morning pain and stiffness. Care should be taken when asking about this because inflammatory back pain from rheumatoid disease or any of the seronegative arthritides will cause morning pain and stiffness; however, these are not common in pregnancy. If there is a structural fault or derangement of the internal architecture of the annulus fibrosus, it can lead to a disc bulge or herniation; if there is extrusion of material from the nucleus pulposus outside of the protective annulus fibrosus, this is a disc prolapse. The discs are like sponges and absorb water and nutrients from the bone end plates during the night when the patient is horizontal and not weight-bearing. When she rises, she puts all of her body weight onto the inflated disc, and this will encourage bulging and

BOX 2.12

Characteristics of disc pain

- Morning pain and stiffness
- Weight-bearing component
- Age of the patient
- Increased abdominal pressure
- Sleep not usually disturbed
- Daily pattern
- History of repeated micro-trauma
- Movement eases pain but not for long (patients tend to fidget)
- Pain on going uphill
- Pain on getting out of a chair

cause muscular hypertonia as a protective measure: hence the morning stiffness. Once she has been on her feet for a while, she literally squeezes the excess water out and has more freedom of movement as the hypertonia in the muscles dies down.

Weight-bearing component. There are only two tissues in the spine that support the body weight under physiological conditions: these are the intervertebral discs and the vertebral bodies (see facet joint pain in the previous section). The medical case history questioning should alert the osteopath to potential pathology involving the vertebral body, such that positive responses to weight-bearing activities suggest the involvement of the disc as a source of pain. Standing is possible but not for too long, such as when ironing, standing in the kitchen cooking, standing in line, or supermarket shopping at a slow pace involving frequent stops. These are the questions that elicit a positive response.

Age of the patient. The commonest age to develop a prolapsed disc is between 30 and 50 years. Twice as many men as women are affected.[12,13] In pregnancy, degenerative disc disease is not a common presenting symptom, despite the fact that the patient is working harder to carry both the extra weight of the baby and the extra weight that she has put on during the pregnancy. This is probably because the high levels of circulating estrogen have a strengthening effect on her skeletal muscles. Paradoxically, the levels of the hormone relaxin that are circulating will mean that the fibrous structures of the annulus can be weakened. This is why muscular back pain is so common in pregnancy: women have to work harder to protect a weak annulus and also, in the case of the postural muscles, to allow the postural changes of pregnancy.

Increased abdominal pressure. Patients with a weak annulus commonly report pain when sneezing or coughing, or on defecation, because the raised intra-abdominal pressure causes a disc to bulge, and also because these actions encourage an increase in lumbar flexion.

Sleep. Sleep is not normally disturbed, and patients with disc problems are able to sleep throughout the night if they can find a comfortable position. It is the SIJ patients who are disturbed by pain when they turn over in bed (see earlier). The further she progresses in the pregnancy, the more a woman's sleep is going to be disturbed by the need to empty her bladder, and that is when she may feel that her back is stiff and sore.

Daily pattern. Patients with disc disease commonly report that it is painful and stiff in the morning, easier at lunchtime, and then sore as the day progress into the afternoon and evening.

Repeated micro-trauma. It is not common for acute disc pain in pregnancy to indicate the first time that the patient has had an acute back pain incident. Much more common is a history of repeated small attacks, which culminate in a major disc prolapse.

Movement eases pain but not for long. People with disc pain tend to fidget because, as the small postural muscles contract to support the weak annulus, they fatigue and patients have to move so that they can relax. The new position repeats the action, such that they find it difficult to sit for long in the cinema or theater because of this constant need to change position.

Going uphill. When we walk uphill or up a slope, we lean forward into a flexed attitude. Likewise, when we walk down a hill, we adopt a position where the lumbar spine is held in extension. The flexed attitude will challenge the disc lesion.

Getting out of a chair. This usually involves spinal flexion, followed by extension, especially if it is a low sofa or easy chair. Pregnant patients should be encouraged to sit in a dining chair which is more upright because it means that they will not slump, challenging their lower esophageal sphincter, and thus helping with reflux, and also because an upright chair encourages them to sit supported, which is better for the lumbar discs.

The Medical History

Once again, the medical quiz is, in many respects, the same as in normal osteopathic practice, although more attention is perhaps given to the changes in normal function of each system since the patient has been pregnant. The physiological changes that occur during pregnancy can and do affect every system in the body. Her whole metabolism will change, and this can be reflected in her weight gain and factors such as dyspnea (breathlessness), constipation, or urinary frequency.

Questions regarding dyspnea are important in pregnancy. Dyspnea could be benign, relating to the fact that, in the last trimester, when the baby is sitting high under the diaphragm, there is less room for the patient to breathe, or the fact that she is undergoing the physiological anemia of pregnancy, which will make her breathless too. However, dyspnea might relate to hypertension and thus pre-eclampsia, which are important signs to look for; if found, they are reasons to refer (Box 2.13).

Likewise with her fluids: is she passing more urine for a simple benign reason, such as the pressure of the baby against the bladder, or could the polyuria (abnormally large amounts of urine) be associated with polydipsia (excessive thirst or drinking), and thus potentially gestational diabetes?

BOX 2.13

History-taking and pathological dyspnea

What to ask about	Pathology indicated
Dyspnea on exertion	Cardiac or pulmonary disease, deconditioning
Dyspnea during rest	Severe cardiopulmonary disease or non-cardiopulmonary disease (e.g. acidosis)
Orthopnea, paroxysmal nocturnal dyspnea, edema	Congestive heart failure, chronic obstructive pulmonary disease
Medications	Beta-blockers may exacerbate bronchospasm or limit exercise tolerance; pulmonary fibrosis is a rare side-effect of some medications
Smoking	Emphysema, chronic bronchitis, asthma
Allergies, wheezing, family history of asthma	Asthma
Coronary artery disease	Dyspnea with or without angina pectoris
High blood pressure	Left ventricular hypertrophy, congestive heart failure
Anxiety	Hyperventilation, panic attack
Dizziness, tingling in fingers and perioral area	Hyperventilation
Recent trauma	Pneumothorax, chest-wall pain limiting respiration

The answer to a simple question such as "When did you last visit your doctor for anything other than pregnancy?" is very revealing. It might reflect how a previous problem, such as thyroid underactivity, is being managed during the pregnancy.

Remarks and impressions, together with questions about social circumstances, are not intended to be intrusive. They are needed because a woman's social circumstances are important to how she is managing her pregnancy. Is she a single parent? Does she have other children or an elderly relative to look after, as well as herself? How is she coping with the pain that she is presenting with? If pain is a feature in the early months, especially if it is acute pain, then it will affect how she manages with the rest of the pregnancy. She cannot take extended powerful analgesics, cannot rest in bed if she has another toddler to look after, may not be able to get an appointment with the physiotherapy service, or may not have found their advice helpful. All these and other factors will affect her mental attitude and should be tactfully included in your case history questioning. Very few osteopaths are trained as psychotherapists and we should be very wary of any advice that we might offer with the best of intentions. However, if we promote ourselves as carers at this time, it is well within our remit to be aware of the social factors that might be playing a part in her managing the pregnancy or not; with her permission, we might even have a word with her family physician/GP or midwife, so that the whole team is involved and aware of what is going on.

Osteopathic Examination from a Structural Point of View

It would be usual to begin the osteopathic examination with a standing postural examination, just as in the majority of our patient assessments in regular practice. However, in pregnancy, a woman's posture is going to change over the three trimesters, if it is able to do so.

The Postural Changes of Pregnancy

During the different phases of pregnancy, a woman's posture in the antero-posterior plane will change radically three times over 40 weeks because of her weight gain and how this extra weight is carried.[14,15]

Many papers have investigated the relationship between low back pain and postural changes in pregnancy, but the results of the research have been inconclusive.[16] One paper published in 1987 suggested that, in the standing position, the lumbar lordosis and sagittal pelvic tilt increase and the head position becomes more posterior as women progress from the first trimester to the last trimester of pregnancy. It was found, however, that these postural changes were not related to back pain.[15]

Not every woman experiences back pain during pregnancy; rather, it is the body's inability to cope with the change that produces the problem. Osteopaths should be capable of analyzing the patient in front of them and assessing how her body is trying to change. Then, by treating the areas responsible for governing how she adapts, such as the cervicodorsal and the thoracolumbar junctions, to facilitate change as her baby grows, we have the power to reduce the amount of back pain significantly during pregnancy.

The first trimester

During the first 12 weeks, as the uterus grows, it starts to rise out of the pelvis. It pushes the abdominal contents in front of it, and an increased tension is noted in the rectus abdominis muscles as the uterus "leans" against them. These muscles are attached between the xiphoid process and the pubic symphysis. As they contract in response to the stretch imposed on them by the expanding uterus, there is a flattening of the lumbar lordosis and a posterior rotation of the pelvis (Fig 2.4).

The success of this change allows more room for the uterus and the fetus to develop. It relies on normal

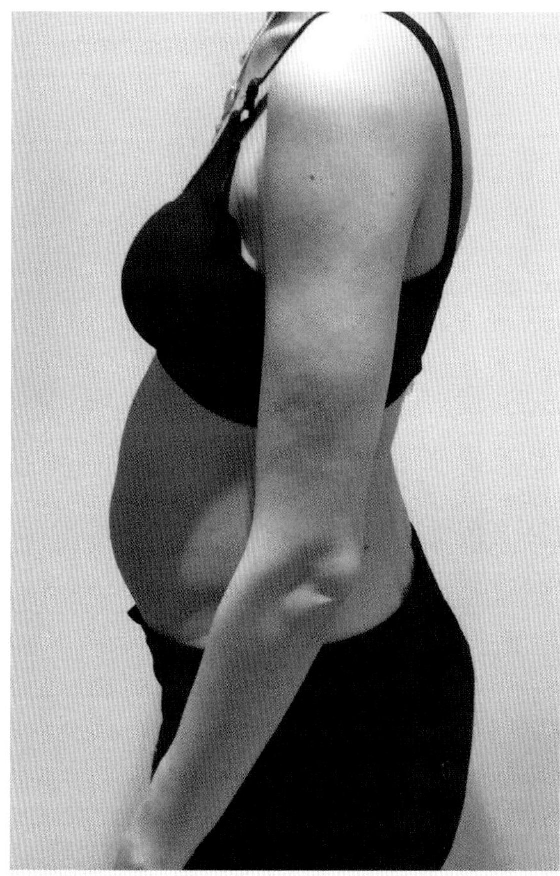

Fig 2.4
Posture at the end of the first trimester, showing posterior rotation of the pelvis.

mobility of the lumbar spinal segments, especially the L5/S1 segment. Unfortunately, anomalies of spinal segments are common; they can alter the relationship between the vertebrae, and thus their ability to adapt under conditions of changing demand.[17] The thoracolumbar junction too is an important area. The attachments of the ribs and the differing demands of muscles attached in this region, such as the diaphragm, quadratus lumborum, and the intercostal muscles, will again affect the ability of the thoracolumbar junction to allow normal change with advancing pregnancy.[18,19]

Scheuermann's disease (see Chapter 3) is a condition that commonly affects the growth plates of vertebrae in this region, producing a stiffening of segmental motion. During pregnancy, we can use the presence of the hormone relaxin, which unwinds the collagen in the patient's ligaments globally, to treat this area with short lever articulation and fascial unwinding techniques, again to facilitate the postural changes that are going to be necessary. Also, the weight of the baby falling posteriorly can cause pain on weight-bearing facet joints. Likewise, the increase in thoracic kyphosis can lead to rib muscle or diaphragm pain at this time.

The second trimester

By the end of the second trimester the growth of the abdomen is advanced, depending on the shape of the lumbar curves. If the patient has a deep lordosis (Fig 2.5), she will appear more pregnant than if she had a shallow curve (Fig 2.6).

It is at this time that the shape of the thoracic kyphosis is influenced. The breasts will change in shape and size at any time during pregnancy, but by the end of the second trimester they can cause an anterior rotation of the arms around the chest wall and a deepening of the cervical lordosis, bringing the eyes up to the horizontal plane. Thoracic spinal muscle pain is common at this time.

How the breasts change is as individual as a fingerprint. Some patients start to grow larger from the first trimester, others not until later. Some will enlarge by two or three cup sizes or strap sizes, while others will experience more modest changes. Advice about a correctly fitting bra is essential at this time. It is very common for women to wear a bra whose horizontal strap is too small and thus restricts their breathing. If they wear a bra that is not fitted correctly

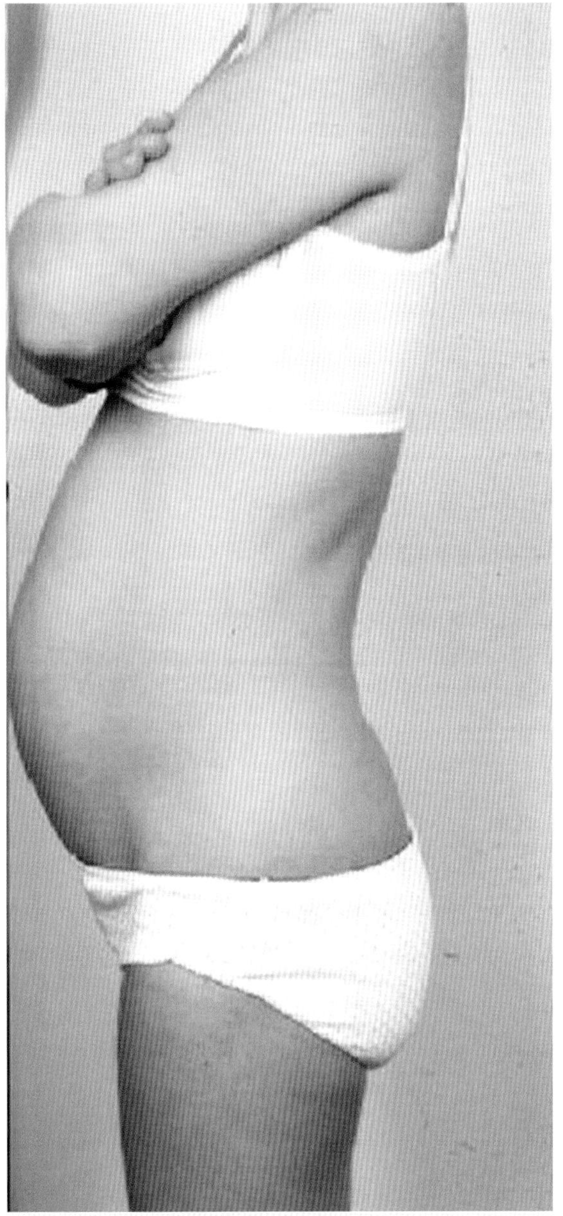

Fig 2.5
Posture at the end of the second trimester, showing a deep lordosis.

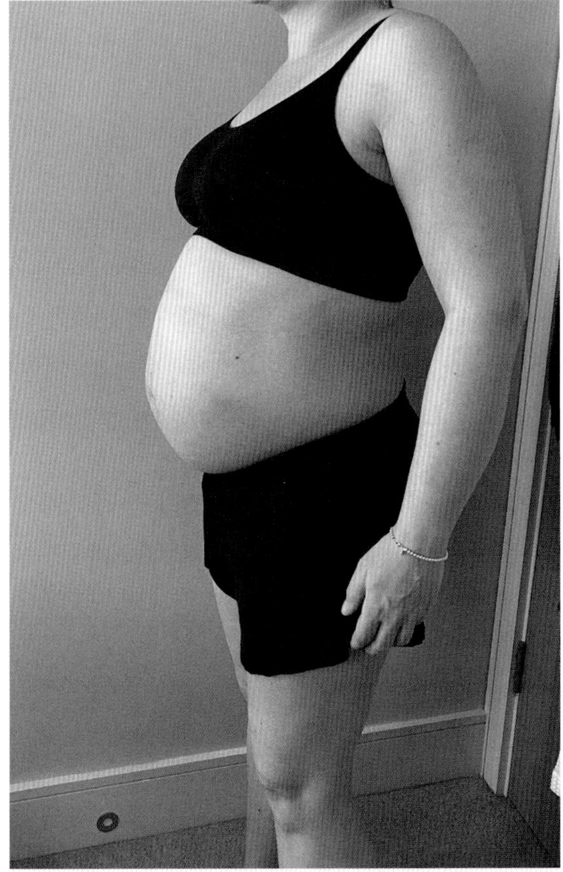

Fig 2.6
Posture at the end of the second trimester, showing a shallow lordosis.

or is simply too small, then their spinal muscles will fatigue, leading to thoracic muscle pain, costovertebral pain, or rib lesions. Intercostal pain can be mistaken for shingles, and anterior sternocostal pain for Tietze's syndrome (see Chapter 3). They should be advised to go for a bra fitting as soon as they feel that their bra is tight, and at night to wear a loose sports top so as to avoid stretch marks (although this is by no means a guarantee).

The third trimester

There are two distinct postures that can develop at the end of the third trimester. Both are dependent on pre-pregnancy posture. Approximately 75% of women will develop the typical deep lordosis of pregnancy (Fig 2.7). This is especially true if they are of Afro-Caribbean origin (Fig 2.8).

The increase in lumbar lordosis will put strain on the lumbar spinal facet joints and cause them to become symptomatic. The joints at L5/S1 are not usually weight-bearing, but if they are forced to carry weight they can produce symptoms. If the woman has a congenital defect at the pars interarticularis, she can develop back pain due to a spondylolisthesis at this time. Likewise, the extra weight on the SIJs can cause problems. If she carries the bulk of the developing abdomen on her pubic symphysis, this can cause pubalgia or symphysis pubis dysfunction. This

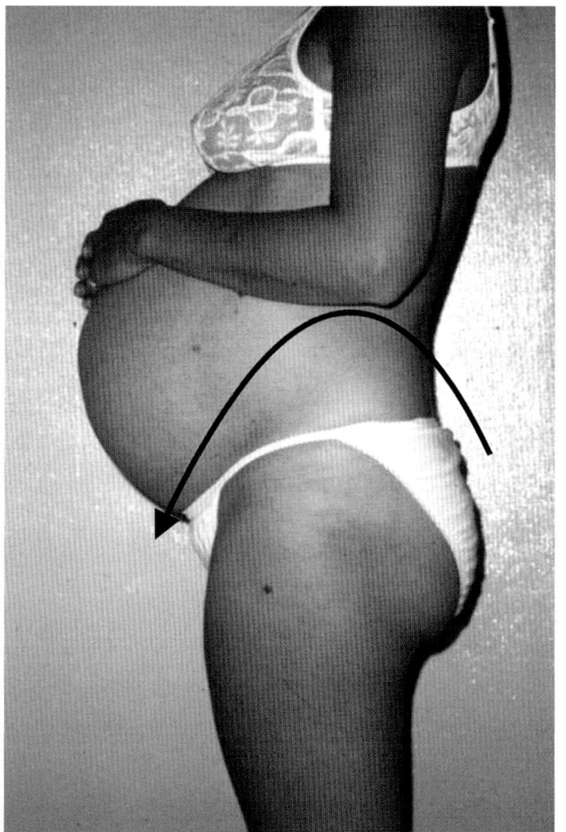

Fig 2.7
Posture at the end of the third trimester with a normal lordosis.

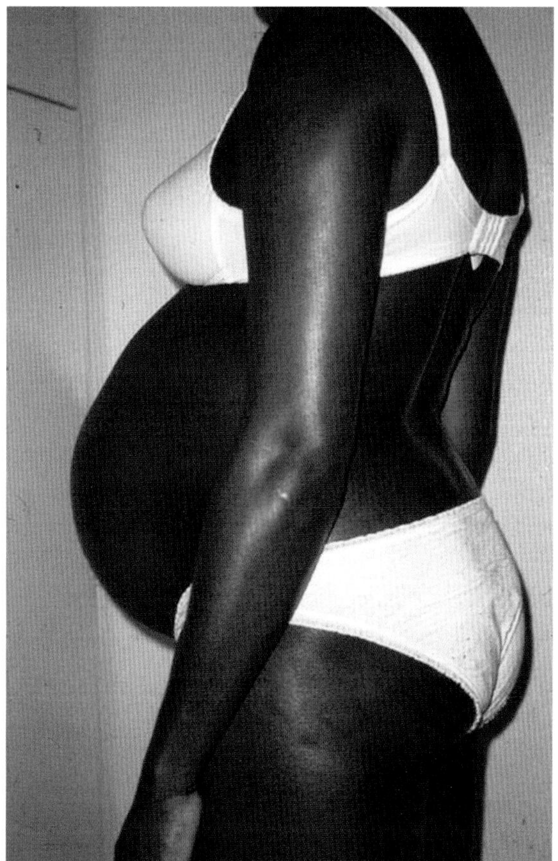

Fig 2.8
An Afro-Caribbean patient at the end of the third trimester with a very deep lordosis.

is a common problem and one which can vary from being very painful indeed (8–10 on a visual analog scale, VAS) to causing just minor discomfort when walking. Patients report not being able to turn over in bed, not being able to take weight on their feet for the first few steps, and needing elbow crutches or a walking frame in order to get about. The evaluation of the whole pelvic ring is of maximal importance at this time.

More pronounced lumbar lordosis will also cause increased pressure on the bladder and may lead to stress incontinence. It is important to quiz the patient about the sort of incontinence she is experiencing. Does she leak when she coughs, laughs, or sneezes, and how much does she leak? Is she losing a few drops that can be absorbed by a panty liner, or has she had episodes where she is neurologically incontinent, wetting herself without warning and losing control of the bladder completely? If the pressure on the last lumbar segments is such that she disturbs an otherwise stable spondylolisthesis, then it is possible that the loss of urinary control is a cauda equina symptom and the patient must be referred immediately to the local emergency room for assessment; this can be a neurosurgical emergency and you may be the first person to see it.

The other posture that may develop in the third trimester is the "sway back" posture (Fig 2.9). It is seen in approximately 25% of patients, and at the end of the pregnancy they appear to be hardly pregnant at all. Tall, thin women are more likely to be seen with this posture. There is nothing inherently wrong with it but these women do have a tendency towards hypermobility anyway, and so fatigue of the postural muscles as they protect the joints from overstrain is the main problem to be overcome in these cases.

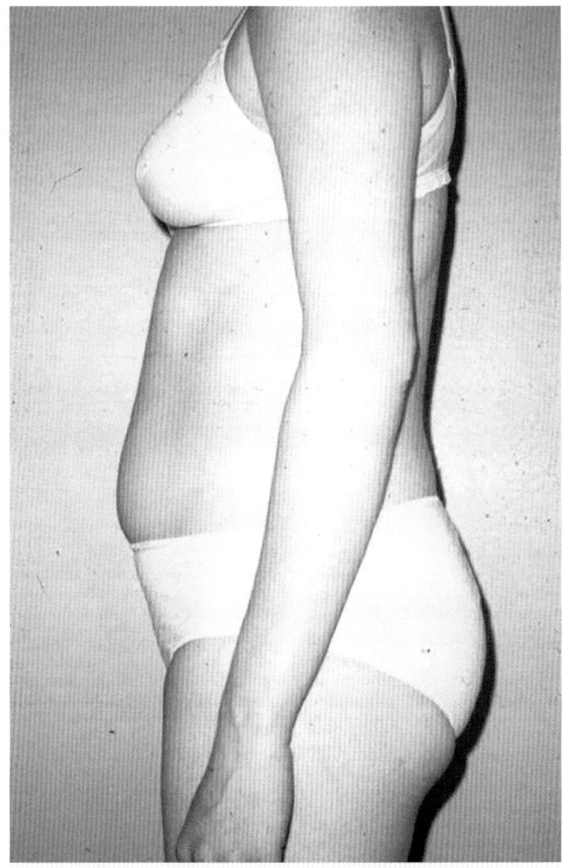

Fig 2.9
The "sway back" posture at the end of the third trimester.

Postural changes in the lateral plane

In pregnancy, because of the expanding abdomen and increasing weight, together with the actions of the pregnancy hormones on the muscles and supporting ligamentous tissues, changes to posture in the lateral plane are also exaggerated sometimes (Fig 2.10). The position of the placenta, and thus the room available for the baby to develop in the uterus, may themselves be dependent on the lateral plane curves, and vice versa. If there is a profound pelvic tilt, this will influence the way the child lies, and the space it enjoys for its normal growth and development.

The topic of how scoliosis develops in some individuals has been the subject of medical research for

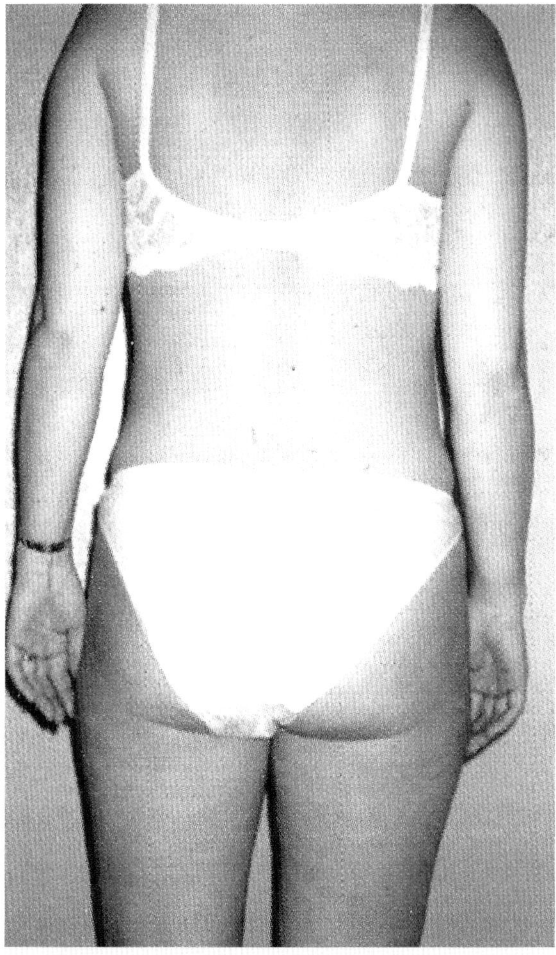

Fig 2.10
A lateral plane curve.

many years. In a recent paper, environmental factors, genetics, vitamin deficiency, chemicals, and drugs, singly or in combination, have all been implicated in the development of vertebral abnormalities. Whatever the cause, the physiological injury occurs early in the embryologic period, well before the development of cartilage and bone. The resulting defects can lead to full or partial fusion or lack of development of the vertebrae, which in turn causes a curvature which may be progressive during the growth of the child.[20]

This does seem to support the argument that the management of a scoliosis in the mother might have an important effect on the development of a scoliosis in the child.

If the tilt is such that a scoliosis is exaggerated, the effects on the descent of the diaphragm and the flaring of the rib cage may mean that a patient develops difficulty in breathing in the middle of the pregnancy, rather than at the end. The altered weight-bearing can cause extra weight to be delivered to the hips, knees, and feet on one side, again causing them to become symptomatic when they might otherwise have been compensating well for the scoliosis. Foot pain can develop if the longitudinal arches collapse under the increased weight and ligamentous laxity.

The Standing Examination

This starts with the observation skills taught on the basic courses in every reputable school of osteopathy. The patient is asked to undress down to her underwear (or bikini, if she prefers), and the antero-posterior and lateral curves are observed and noted. The horizontality – or not – of the occiput, shoulders, shoulder blades, and waist folds, and the height of the pelvis, together with any rotoscoliosis or leg length discrepancies, all form part of the routine assessment. Any changes in the antero-posterior curves compared to normal, and the development or not of the kypholordotic postures, should also be observed and noted at this time.

The integrity of the abdominal muscles is important to assess because if the patient has had previous abdominal operations, the scar tissue will be resistant to stretch, and this could prevent the lordosis from developing. Also, if the patient has had several children in a short space of time, her abdominal muscles are more likely to have lost tone and thus not support the weight of the growing fetus. This could lead to the lordosis being established too early, with all of the attendant problems.

Palpation of the static standing posture will reveal a lot about how a woman's body is coping with the postural shifts and weight gain of pregnancy.

With the patient standing comfortably upright, the osteopath stands at her side. Her bare feet should be around 20 cm (8 inches) apart and her weight should be resting comfortably over her hips and pelvis. Her arms rest by her sides.

The osteopath places one of his flat hands on her sternum and the other on her thoracic spine (Fig 2.11). His center of gravity is back towards his heels, so that he has the minimum of weight in his hands. Ideally, his hands are passive palpatory tools.

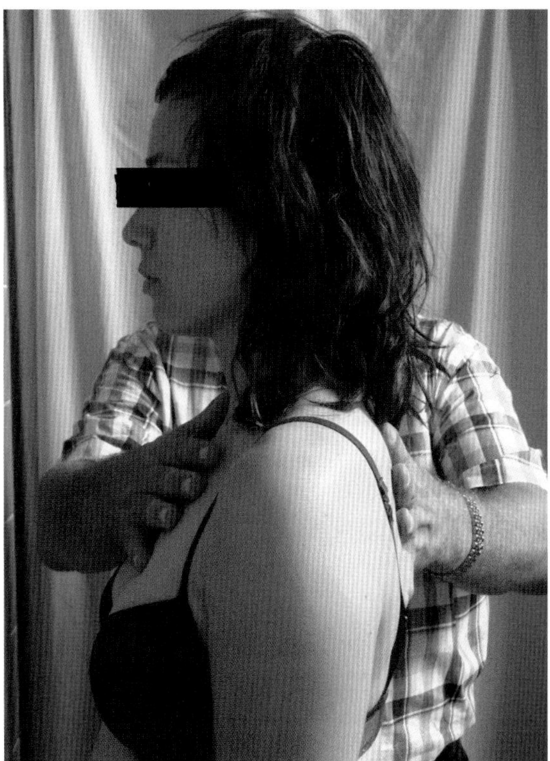

Fig 2.11
Standing examination to assess postural strains reflected in the chest region.

He should wait for 20 or 30 seconds for his hands to become quiet and unobtrusive. Now he very gently induces a motion from his center of gravity through his hands to the patient in the antero-posterior plane. This is not a push or a pull force; instead, it is a "belt buckle" technique because he transfers his weight through his belt buckle and via his hands, noting the response in the patient to this diagnostic movement.

It should be possible to assess where her center of gravity lies, either anterior or posterior to the normal point of balance, or if there is a tendency for the osteopath's hands to be pulled one way or the other, according to the drag of the fascial chains. If her breasts are large and the shoulders rotated around the chest wall, this will cause an anterior pull. If there is a deep lordosis, this might cause a posterior pull.

Now the osteopath moves his hands below the diaphragm, with one hand on her belly and the other at the thoracolumbar junction. The postural muscle and fascial pulls are assessed as before.

He now places one hand under her swollen abdomen and the other over the spinal muscles (Fig 2.12). The abdominal hand lifts the bump, taking the weight, and the spinal hand palpates the response to this movement in the spinal muscles. The muscles usually relax immediately as the task of holding the weight of the gravid uterus is temporarily taken by the osteopath's abdominal hand.

Moving behind the patient, he places the palms of his hands on her shoulders and hips, again very lightly, to assess any postural drag pulling the body to one side or the other.

In pregnancy, because of the weight changes and because of the importance of the fascial chains supporting the organs above and below the diaphragm, these assessments form an integral part of understanding how a woman's body is coping with the various physiological changes.

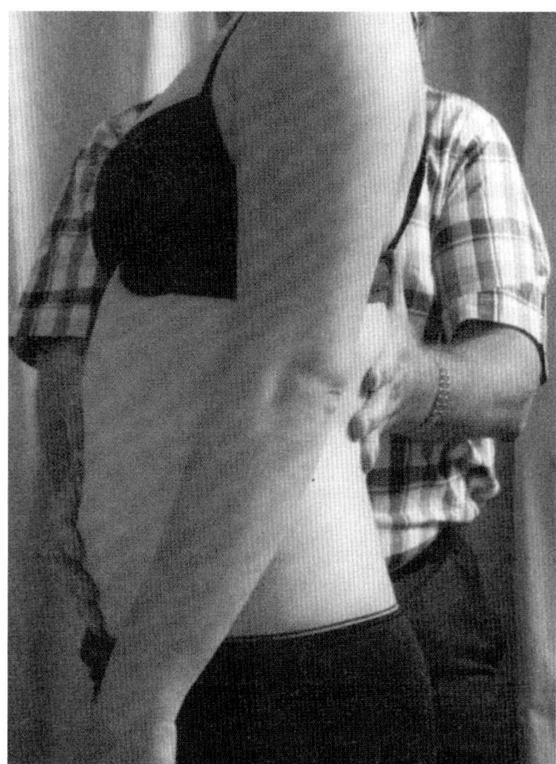

Fig 2.12
Standing examination to assess postural strains reflected in the abdominal region.

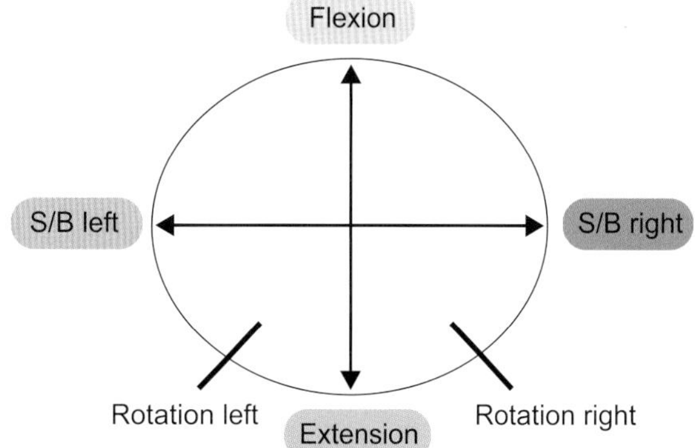

Fig 2.13
The circle system of notation. S/B, side-bending (lateral) flexion.

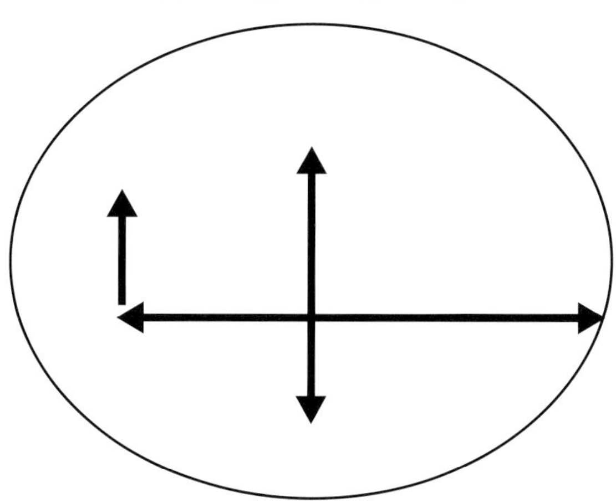

Fig 2.14
Diagram depicting the quantity of motion restricted.

Active Movement Examinations

The patient is asked to undergo active movements in both planes. Range of motion and quality of motion are observed and palpated – both globally and regionally, and at each individual segment – for flexion and extension, lateral flexion or side-bending, and rotation to each side. The results are noted.

Notation of these active movements is a subject of personal choice and training. At the Expectant Mother's Clinic of the British School of Osteopathy, a circle system of notation is taught and used (Fig 2.13). Here an aerial view of the patient is represented by a circle. The edges of the circle represent the ends of the normal ranges of motion for the patient under examination. These will depend on her age, morphology, and any associated previous history.

If motion is limited, then both the quality and quantity of that motion limitation can be noted on the chart with a smaller arrow pointing in the relevant direction (Fig 2.14). The edge of the circle represents

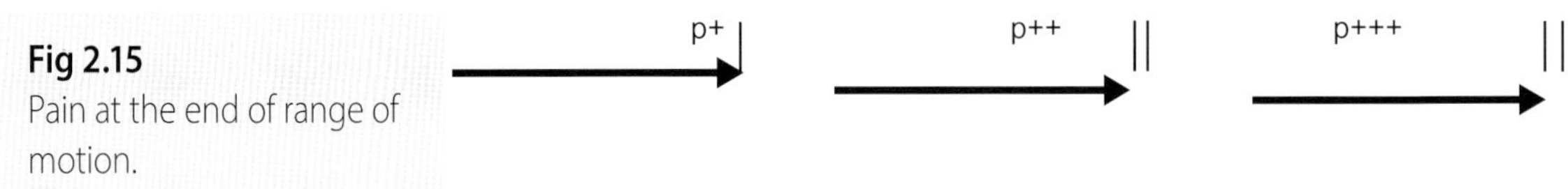

Fig 2.15
Pain at the end of range of motion.

the normal range. Likewise, if the patient were found to be hypermobile, the arrow would extend beyond the edge of the circle. Rotation is noted by lines around the edge of the circle.

The quality of motion can be depicted by the use of bars at the end of the arrows (Fig 2.15). One bar represents mild pain, two indicate moderate pain, and three severe pain. If the circle has grid lines, this can provide an accurate representation of the patient's pain if she is asked to fill in the circle chart at each visit. It is a variation on the VAS scale.

The triangle test

This test is used for the differential diagnosis of pain arising in a facet joint, SIJ, hip joint capsule, and/or the iliopsoas muscle.

Looking at the patient from the back, visualize a triangle, with the apex passing through the body of L4 and the base horizontally level with the hips. From the side, this triangle is at approximately 30 degrees, as shown in Figure 2.16.

The patient stands as before, with the weight evenly distributed between the feet, which are placed approximately 20 cm (8 inches) apart.

Firstly, she is asked to bend to the right and then the left in a pure side-bending movement with no flexion and extension (Fig 2.17). Because of the way that the facets are arranged at this level, she will compress the L5/S1 facets; if they are the main pain generator, she will be reluctant to perform the movement because it will cause pain as the facet joints are compressed.

If the test is negative for facet joint pain, to test the left SIJ, she is asked to take a step forward on her right foot and side-bend left, extending her spine as if passing down the side of the triangle (Fig 2.18). The weight transfers from the non-symptomatic facet joint and is transmitted to the SIJ. If this is the source of the problem, there will be some reluctance to perform the movement, as it will be painful.

If the second part of the test is pain-free, she continues the side-bending and extension movement until the movement is halted by the stretch on the anterior capsule of the hip joint and the tension in the iliopsoas muscle (Figs 2.19 and 2.20). If this is the source of the pain, then the test is positive at this point.

This is not intended as a definitive and accurate stand-alone test, but instead, if performed with the passive supine and side-lying tests, it allows the osteopath to infer the correct source of pain.

Standard orthopedic and neurological tests are used if there is an indication in the case history to do so.

The Sitting, Side-lying, and Supine Examinations

The main problem with the passive motion examinations is the position of the patient. We usually examine and treat our patients prone or supine, and both of these positions have their problems in pregnancy.

If she lies on her back, especially in late pregnancy, the weight of the gravid uterus on the great vessels in the abdomen is going to restrict blood flow from the lower extremities back into the chest, and thus to the heart (Fig 2.21). Your patient can become breathless very easily, which can be quite frightening for her.

Laying her face down can also be problematic. In early pregnancy you do not want to put any pressure

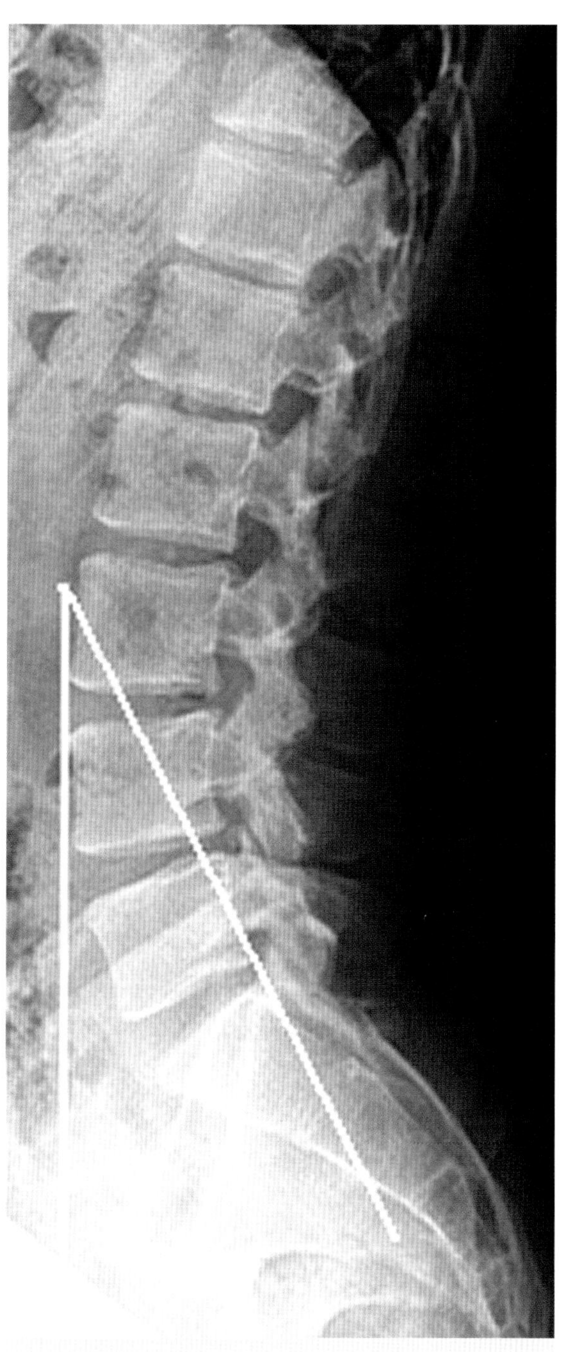

Fig 2.16
X-ray showing the triangle test.

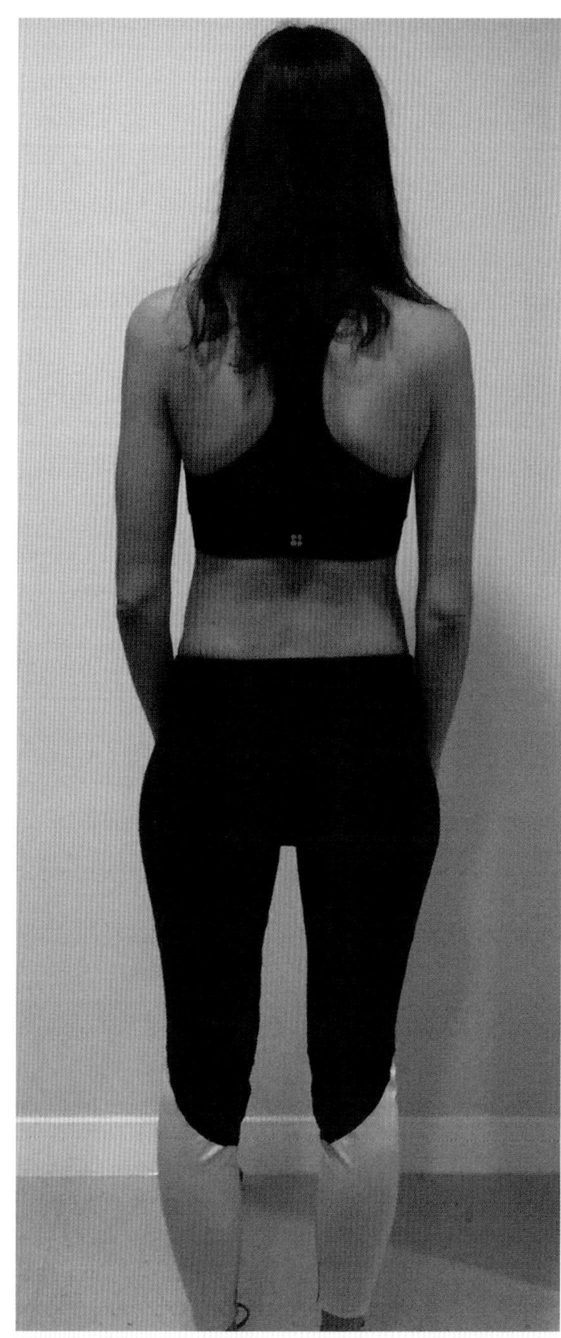

Fig 2.17
Triangle test 1.

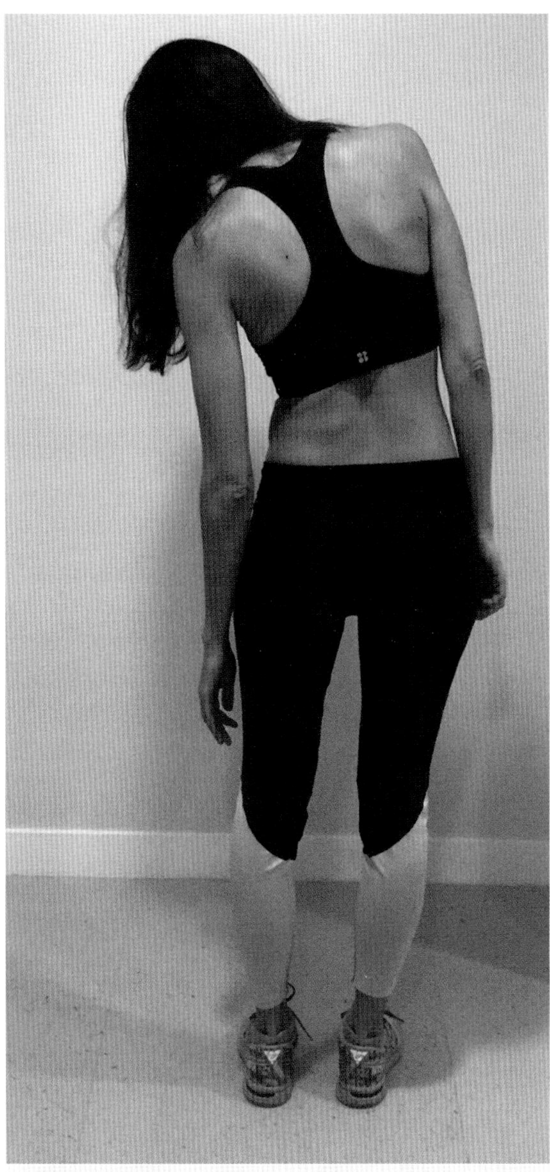

Fig 2.18
Triangle test 2.

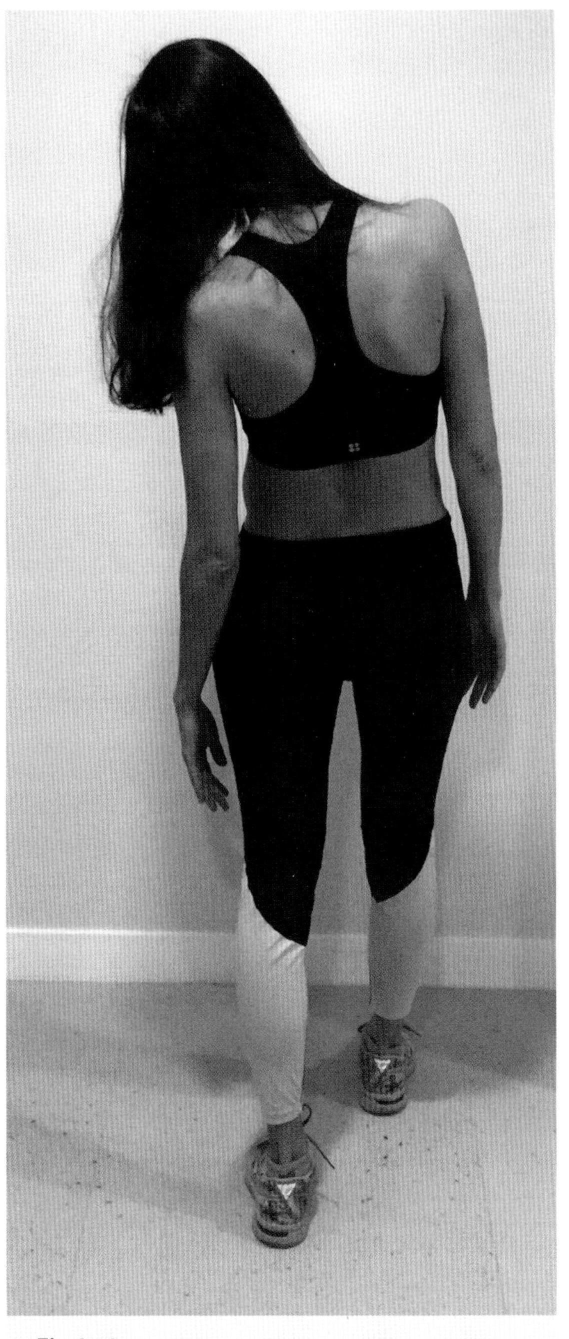

Fig 2.19
Triangle test 3.

straight down onto the sacrum or abdomen, for obvious reasons. As the bump gets bigger, lying face down becomes impossible. Sometimes, women sleep in a "semi Sims position," half prone, half side-lying,

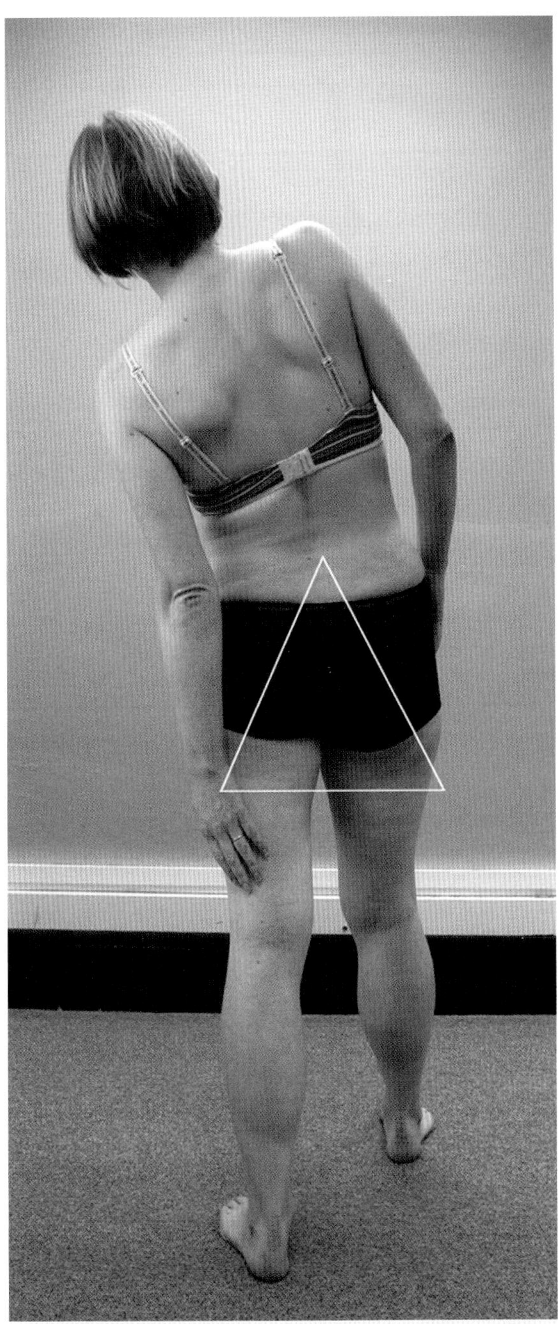

Fig 2.20
Triangle test 4, showing the triangle.

with a pillow between the knees to separate them and to support the pelvis, which you can try (Fig 2.22).

Laying her on her side is the obvious solution but, again, is not without its problems. Firstly, do not have your patient too near to the side of the treatment table, where she can see the floor, as this might cause her to be anxious. Secondly, you cannot use both legs to flex the spine, as this compresses the abdomen and causes discomfort. The solution is simply to use just one leg, the top one, which allows you to access the interspinal spaces and to diagnose problems in the joints and underlying muscles in the usual way (Fig 2.23). This is also an ideal position to assess the SIJs with gentle compression techniques through the femur, while palpating the superior and inferior SIJs, respectively.

If you position the patient supine to examine the SIJs, then prop her up at about 40 degrees, as this will be better tolerated than lying flat.

With the patient in this position, be careful when assessing the SIJs not to lift her foot off the treatment table as you flex the hip joint. Posterior rotation of the innominate bone will cause tension at the level of the iliolumbar ligament, which is attached between the iliac crest and the transverse process of L5. By itself, it is a pain-sensitive structure. Therefore, if the foot is lifted off the treatment table, it is no longer a differential diagnostic test. It is better to leave the foot flat on the table and to simply palpate at the posterior superior iliac spine as you direct your force through the femur via the hip to the SIJs directly (Fig 2.24).

If it is symptomatic, the test is positive, and the diagnosis is a lesion of the SIJ on the side tested. Both the superior and inferior poles of the SIJ can be tested in this way, depending on where the palpating fingers are located, either at the posterior superior or posterior inferior iliac spine, respectively. Common findings might include a superior lesion on one side and an inferior lesion on the other.

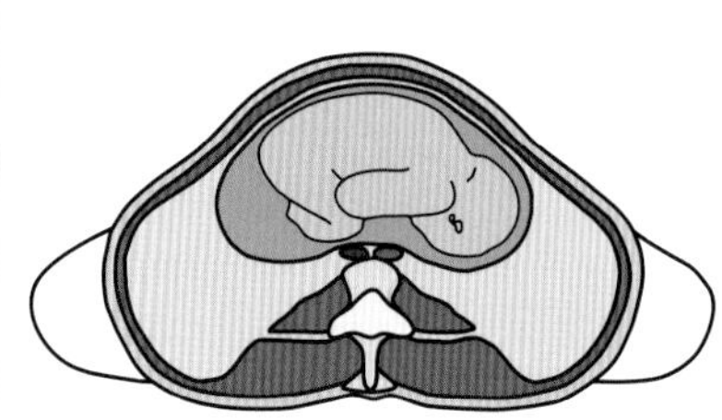

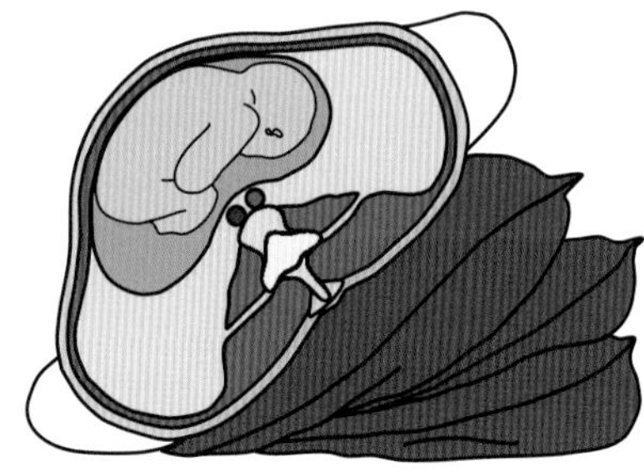

Fig 2.21
Patient lying on her side to avoid vena cava compression.

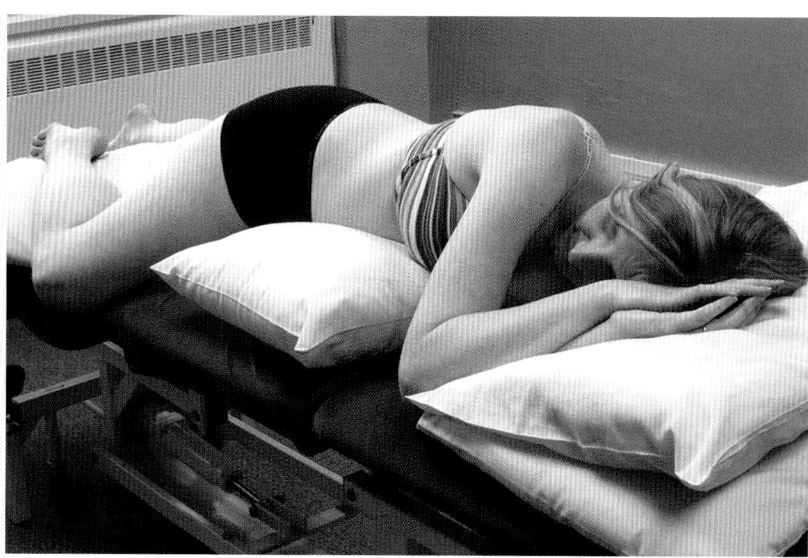

Fig 2.22
Patient semi-side-lying, with a pillow supporting the bump.

The test is then repeated with the foot off the treatment table and the hip in half-flexion. If there is pain, it suggests that the iliolumbar ligaments are the pain generators (Fig 2.25).

The abduction test

If testing the right SIJ, the operator stands on her right side and turns to face the feet of the patient, who is still supine with one knee flexed. It is important for the internal malleolus of the leg to be tested to be in line with the opposite knee joint (Fig 2.26). In this way, when the test is repeated on the other side, you will be comparing like with like. Holding her left iliac crest down with his left hand, the osteopath allows the leg to fall open into full abduction. The adductor magnus muscle is inserted onto the ramus of the pubic bone, and if the SIJ is in lesion there will be a restriction in full opening.

Warning

There is an ethical issue here that involves the patient's modesty. It is better to face her feet when doing this test, rather than her groin. It can be difficult for her to relax if she feels immodest at this time. Also, during a normal pregnancy, a vaginal discharge is a common finding. If her underwear is stained in this way, she will again feel uncomfortable, and so by facing her feet you avoid this potential source of embarrassment.

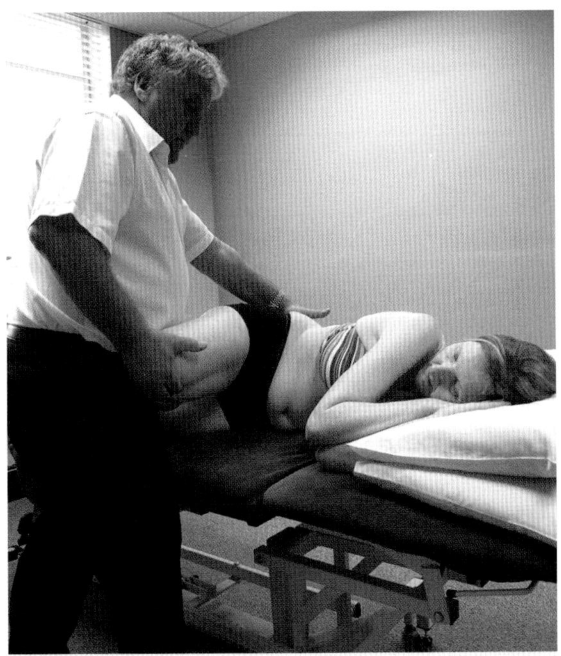

Fig 2.23
Single leg flexion.

Side-lying Examination of the Sacroiliac Joints

The patient is lying on her side, with the painful side uppermost. The osteopath places the patient in the form of a three-sided square, as shown in Figure 2.23.

The fingers of both hands palpate the joint line. Using his chest, he gently compresses the ilium, rocking his weight forwards and backwards, and assessing how the joint opens and closes. In this way, hyper- and hypomobility of the anterior, posterior, and interosseous ligaments can be assessed (Fig 2.27). Likewise, locking at the superior and inferior poles can be evaluated.

The joints of the spine can be tested from occiput to sacrum, including the SIJs, and an assessment made of how they have changed from normal and how they have adapted their function. The evaluation of individual joints – not only against the background of the morphology of the patient, as in routine practice, but also against the changes caused by the pregnancy to the muscles and ligaments, as well as to the viscera and fascial supports – will influence

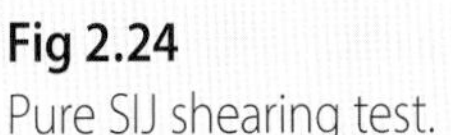

Fig 2.24
Pure SIJ shearing test.

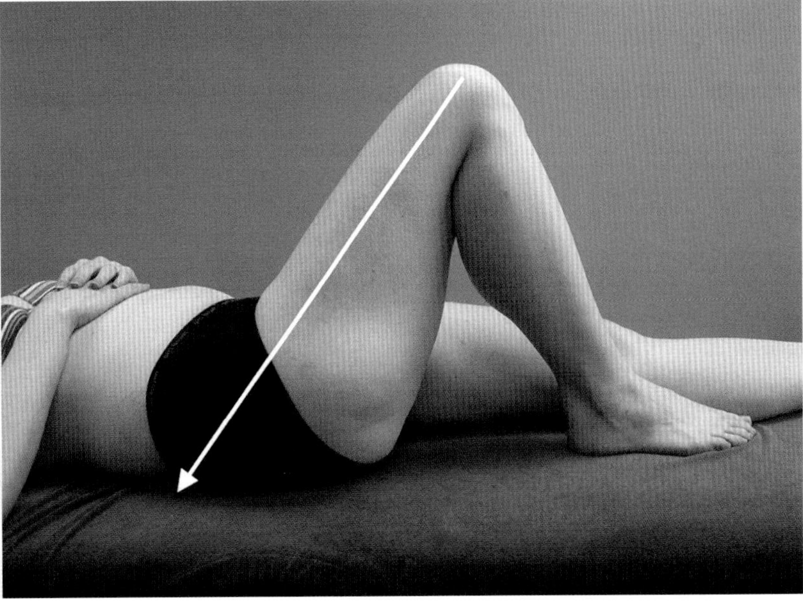

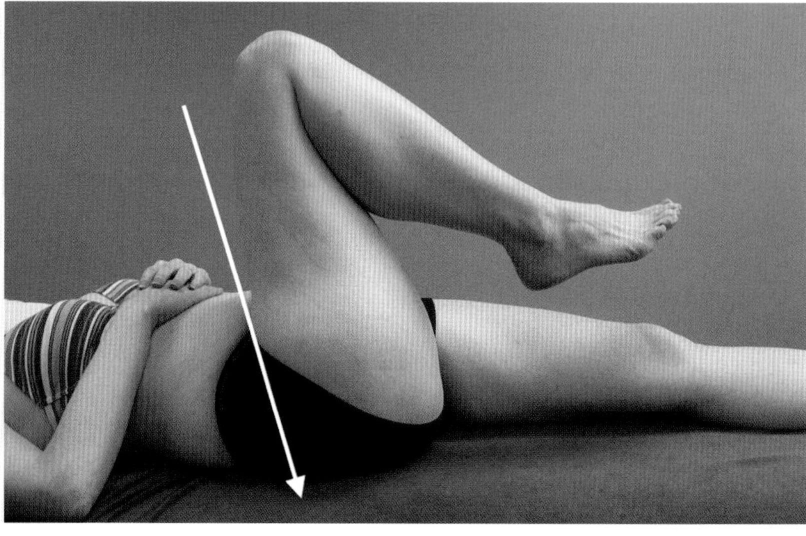

Fig 2.25
Test involving the iliolumbar ligament.

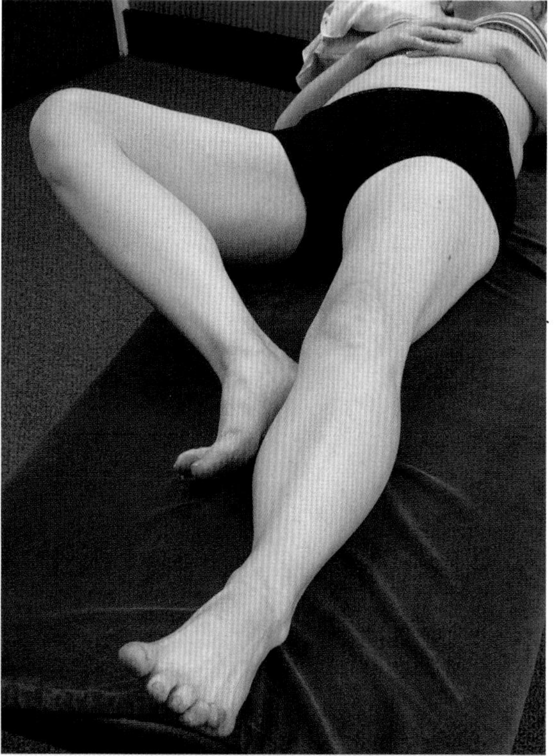

Fig 2.26
The position of the feet for the adduction test.

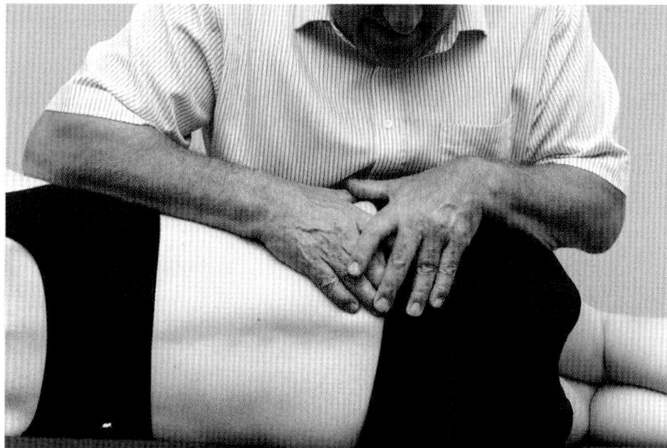

Fig 2.27
Palpation of the superior pole of the SIJ with the patient side-lying.

amplifier for the palpatory response. This, together with the laxity effects of the hormones on ligaments and muscles, means that palpation of the craniosacral system can be easier during pregnancy than at any other time, except as an infant.

Once again, it is not a good idea to have the patient lying supine for too long, and so the side-lying position is best for actual treatment (Fig 2.28). The usual position for evaluation begins supine; however, the

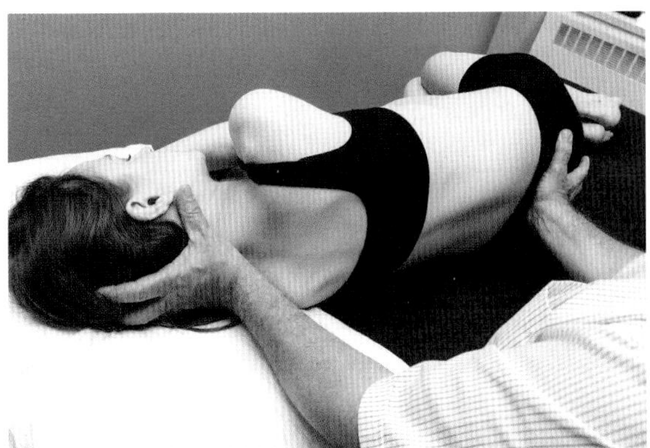

Fig 2.28
Palpation of the craniosacral system with the patient side-lying.

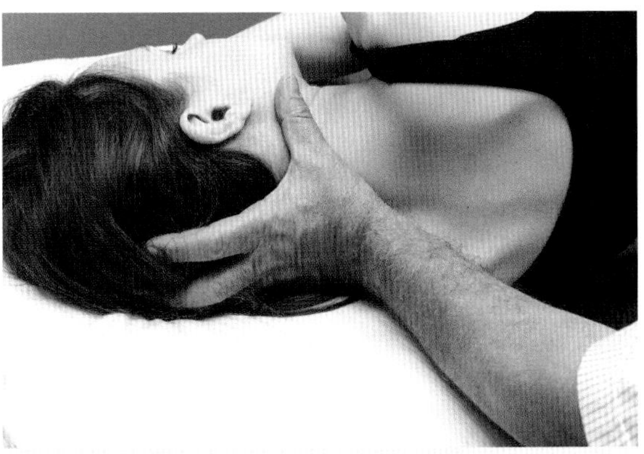

Fig 2.29
The cranial hold, cradling the occiput.

head should be comfortably propped up by a pillow, with another pillow or bolster supporting the knees.

It is easier to begin with the classical holds used in regular palpatory assessment of the cranial bones and sutures (Figs 2.29 and 2.30). Any area of dysfunction can be looked at both locally and in relation to neighboring structures. The basiocciput is very important because of the change in the attitude of the skull on the cervical spine, caused by an alteration in

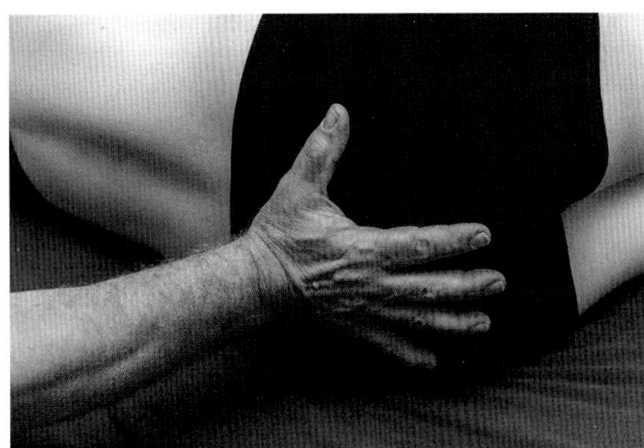

Fig 2.30
The sacral hold.

the patient's posture, as mentioned earlier. Muscular attachments on the bones of the skull from the long strap muscles in the neck and beyond can become unbalanced and tense, resulting in a distortion of cranial bone motion. Suboccipital tension headaches are not uncommon in pregnancy.

Once the bony motion has been assessed, palpation at a deeper level of the ligamentous tensions reveals the relationship between the skull and the sacrum. The long connections between the occiput and sacrum can soften during pregnancy, and again, patterns of normal motion will be distorted due to weight changes and postural changes at different phases of pregnancy.

Lastly, fluid dynamics are assessed and the health and vitality of the primary respiratory mechanism are noted (Fig 2.31). Changes to the cardiovascular and respiratory systems, and alterations in the kidneys and their fascial supports, have an important effect on the fluid volumes in the body during pregnancy. These include the fluid volumes within the skull and the spinal cord. Vitality and essential energy can be depleted during the last trimester simply due to exhaustion. Osteopathic treatment using cranial techniques at the level of the primary respiratory mechanism can give the patient the energy she is

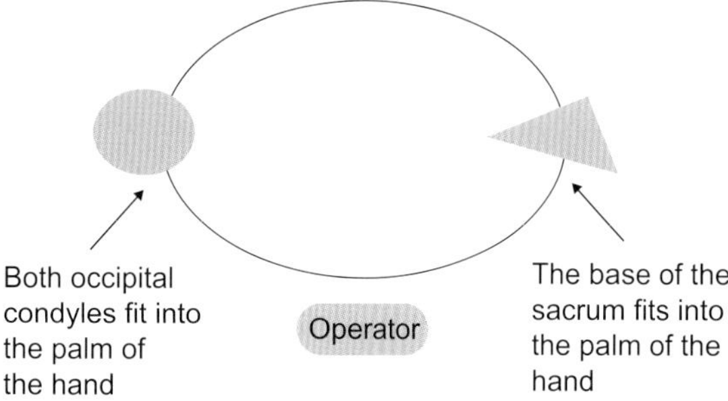
Both you and the patient form parts of a greater circle
Both occipital condyles fit into the palm of the hand
Operator
The base of the sacrum fits into the palm of the hand

Fig 2.31
Volumetric assessment of the primary respiratory mechanism with the patient side-lying.

going to need for labor and the puerperium, the time immediately after childbirth. Many osteopaths treat their patients within 48 hours of delivery, or even earlier if it is practical. This gentle and subtle approach to the recovering tissues can help the recovery process, and provide support through the following months and through all the physical changes that are to be expected.

Summary

The evaluation of the pregnant patient is not just an assessment of the structural mechanical system. This will form a major part of what can be done with pregnant women, but it is by no means the only thing that we assess. An evaluation of the fascial chains, both above and below the diaphragm and into the pelvis, is essential if we are to comprehend the effects they are having on our patient during the pregnancy. Just how much change is taking place and how successfully? Are the tissues supporting the viscera and organs being overstretched because of the growing fetus? The organs themselves have to be assessed where possible, given that their position is going to change because of the rising bulk of the gravid uterus. Changes in the cardiovascular and respiratory systems, and in the position of the abdominal organs and the uterus and bladder, which should take place physiologically as she progresses through the pregnancy, will all have a part to play in how comfortable she is and how able she is to cope with the incredible demands that pregnancy places on her. The osteopath is ideally placed to evaluate these changes, and to see if his techniques can improve and facilitate that change and play their part in the structure–function equation.

References

1. National Institute for Health and Care Excellence. Intrapartum Care for Healthy Women and Babies. Clinical guideline [CG190], December 2014; https://www.NICE.org.uk.
2. Edwards GJ, Davies NJ. Elective caesarean section - the patient's choice? J Obstet Gynaecol. 2001 Mar;21(2):128–9.
3. Damm P. Gestational diabetes mellitus and subsequent development of overt diabetes mellitus. Dan Med Bull. 1998 Nov;45(5):495–509.
4. Pregnancy and Diabetes, January 2019; www.diabetes.co.uk/diabetes-and-pregnancy.html.
5. Orvieto R, Achiron A, Ben-Rafael Z, Gelernter I, Achiron R. Low back pain of pregnancy. Acta Obstet Gynaecol Scand. 1994;73(3):209–14.
6. Sturesson B, Uden G, Uden A. Pain patterns in pregnancy and “catching” of the leg in pregnant women with posterior pelvic pain. 1977. Spine. 22(16):1880–3.
7. Mogren IM, Pohjanen AL. Low back pain and pelvic pain during pregnancy: prevalence and risk factors. Spine 2005;30(8):983–91.
8. Wu WH, Meijer OG, Uegaki K, Mens JMA, van Dieën JH, Wuisman PIJM, et al. Pregnancy-related pelvic girdle pain (PPP), I: Terminology, clinical presentation, and prevalence. Eur Spine J. 2004 Nov;13(7):575–89.
9. Sandler SE. Unpublished survey information, 1988. British School of Osteopathy, Expectant Mother's Clinic.
10. Giles LG, Taylor JR. Human zygapophyseal joint capsule and synovial fold innervation. Br J Rheumatol. 1987 Apr;26(2):93–8.
11. Giles LG, Taylor JR. Innervation of lumbar zygapophyseal joint synovial folds. Acta Orthop Scand. 1987 Feb;58(1):43–6.

12. Tidy C. Prolapsed Disc, October 2020; https://patient.info/bones-joints-muscles/back-and-spine-pain/slipped-disc-prolapsed-disc.
13. Prasad R, Hoda MF, Dhakai M, Singh K, Srivastava V. Epidemiological characteristics of lumbar disc prolapse in a tertiary care hospital. Internet J Neurosurg. 2006;3(1).
14. Dumas GA, Reid JG, Wolfe LA, Griffin MP, McGrath MJ. Exercise, posture, and back pain during pregnancy: Part 1. Exercise and posture. Clin Biomech (Bristol, Avon). 1995 Mar;10(2):98–103.
15. Bullock JE, Jull GA, Bullock MI. The relationship of low back pain to postural changes during pregnancy. Aust J Physiother. 1987;33(1):10–17.
16. Franklin ME, Conner-Kerr TJ. An analysis of posture and back pain in the first and third trimesters of pregnancy. Orthop Sports Phys Ther. 1998 Sep;28(3):133–8.
17. Paściak M, Besler K, Doniec J, Smigiel M. The effect of joint facet asymmetry on the pathogenesis of lower segments of the lumbar spine. Chir Narzadow Ruchu Ortop Pol. 1997;62(3):219–23.
18. Lowe TG, Line BG. Evidence based medicine: analysis of Scheuermann kyphosis. Spine (Phila Pa 1976). 2007 Sep 1;32(19 Suppl):S115–19.
19. Zaina F, Atanasio S, Ferraro C, Fusco C, Negrini A, Romano M, et al. Review of rehabilitation and orthopedic conservative approach to sagittal plane diseases during growth: hyperkyphosis, junctional kyphosis, and Scheuermann disease. Eur J Phys Rehabil Med. 2009 Dec;45(4):595–603.
20. Zheng L, Yu X, Shen J. Environmental aspects of congenital scoliosis. Environ Sci Pollut Res Int. 2015 Apr;22(8):5751–5.

Above the Diaphragm: Changes in Anatomy and Physiology During Pregnancy

3

Many common problems that are not in themselves life-threatening occur in pregnancy. Very often, our patients are given advice or told to live with the problem, as it will resolve itself once they deliver. Sometimes, these problems in pregnancy are the result of a compromise to the structure–function relationship.

There are also profound physiological changes that accompany pregnancy and these can present as symptoms in your practice (Box 3.1).

Physiological Changes in the Cardiopulmonary System During Pregnancy

Physiological changes during pregnancy affect nearly every organ system. In the thorax, the diaphragm elevates by as much as 4 cm (1.6 inches) because of displacement of the abdominal organs by the gravid uterus, resulting in lower lung volumes. Maternal blood volume and cardiac output are increased by approximately 45% by mid-pregnancy. Cardiac output can rise by as much as 80% during vaginal delivery and by up to 50% with cesarean section. These changes result in pulmonary vascular engorgement, progressive left ventricular dilatation, and mild hypertrophy.

BOX 3.1

Common symptoms presenting to osteopathic practice in pregnancy

- Respiratory distress (dyspnea)
- General tiredness and fatigue
- Nausea and vomiting in early pregnancy
- Musculoskeletal pains in the thoracic spinal structures and ribs
- Costochondral pain
- Headaches, especially suboccipital headaches
- Thoracic outlet syndromes, including carpal tunnel syndromes
- Changes to breast tissues

Patients with pre-existing cardiovascular disease – for example, rheumatic heart disease – will need consultant care during pregnancy if they are to avoid cardiac complications.

During pregnancy, great changes occur to the maternal physiology to give the fetus nutrition for growth and to provide the mother with the energy she needs to sustain this growth, both for labor and for lactation. Looking first at the changes in the physiology of the cardiothoracic system, we can start with the gases.

Oxygen Supplies and Carbon Dioxide Disposal

The supply of oxygen to the growing fetus is protected by changes occurring in the mother in terms of ventilation, number of red cells, and circulation.

The need for oxygen increases progressively during pregnancy with the growth of the mother and the fetus. By term, resting oxygen consumption has increased by 15% over non-pregnant levels.[1]

More oxygen is also needed for the extra energy expended in daily activities because of the mother's weight gain. The total weight gain on average will be 12.5 kilos (22 pounds), amounting to 20% of her body weight.

> **BOX 3.2**
>
> **NICE guidelines on weight control in pregnancy**
>
> - Base meals on starchy foods such as potatoes, bread, rice, and pasta, choosing wholegrain where possible
> - Eat fiber-rich foods such as oats, beans, peas, lentils, grains, seeds, fruit, and vegetables, as well as wholegrain bread and brown rice and pasta
> - Eat at least five portions of a variety of fruit and vegetables each day, in place of foods higher in fat and calories
> - Eat a low-fat diet and avoid increasing fat and/or calorie intake
> - Eat as little as possible of fried food; drinks and confectionery high in added sugars (such as cakes, pastries, and fizzy drinks); and other food high in fat and sugar (such as some take-away and fast foods)
> - Eat breakfast
> - Watch the portion size of meals and snacks, and keep an eye on how often you are eating
> - Make activities such as walking, cycling, swimming, aerobics, and gardening part of everyday life and build activity into daily living – for example, by taking the stairs instead of the elevator or going out for a walk at lunchtime
> - Minimize sedentary activities, such as sitting for long periods watching television, at a computer or playing video games
> - Walk, cycle, or use another mode of transport involving physical activity

Women will be more likely to achieve and maintain a healthy weight before, during, and after pregnancy if they follow the guidelines of the UK's National Institute for Health and Care Excellence (NICE) on weight gain in pregnancy (Box 3.2).[2]

Progesterone increases the sensitivity of the respiratory control centers in the hypothalamus to carbon dioxide (CO_2), so that ventilation is greater at any specific level of arterial CO_2 than in the non-pregnant state. The depth of breathing increases but the number of breaths per minute does not change.

As a result of this increased ventilation, the partial pressure of oxygen (PO_2) in alveolar air increases, so that the maternal arterial PO_2 increases and the partial pressure of carbon dioxide (PCO_2 falls by about 10 mmHg). This increases the rate of diffusion of gases across the placenta, improving fetal oxygen uptake and carbon dioxide excretion (Fig 3.1).[3]

Changes in Red Cell Numbers

Red cell production by bone marrow is stimulated by the hormone erythropoietin, leading to a 20% increase in the total number of red cells in the circulation.

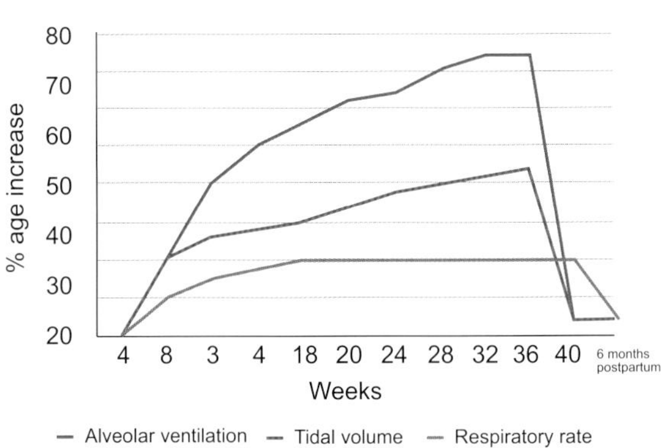

Fig 3.1
Respiratory factors in a normal pregnancy.

However, as the plasma volume increases by an even larger amount, the red cell count actually falls due to hemodilution. This is the physiological anemia of pregnancy.[3]

Changes in the Circulation

Pregnancy has a profound effect on the circulatory system. Most of these hemodynamic changes start in the first trimester, peak during the second trimester, and plateau during the third trimester.

The growth of maternal tissues causes an increase in the number of blood vessels in the circulation, notably in the placenta. Progesterone levels increase, causing a relaxation of vascular smooth muscle and leading to a fall in peripheral resistance. There is also a decreased response to the hormone angiotensin II.[4]

Circulatory pressure is maintained by an expansion of blood volume and an increase in cardiac output.

Changes in Blood Values

The expansion of blood volume is made up by an increase in plasma volume of about 2 liters (more than a 40% increase). Most of this change occurs in the mid trimester and there is a progressive increase in the number of red cells throughout the pregnancy (Fig 3.2).

Heart rate and stroke volume increase by 15% and 20%, respectively.[5]

As a result of these changes in volume and cardiac output, arterial blood pressure is normally fairly constant. Towards the end of the pregnancy, there is a small decrease in diastolic pressure of about 10 mmHg.

The main symptom that your pregnant patient will present with in relation to these changes will be dyspnea; this is physiological and not pathological, and your differential diagnosis should reflect this. Pathological dyspnea is described in Chapter 2 (see Box 2.13).

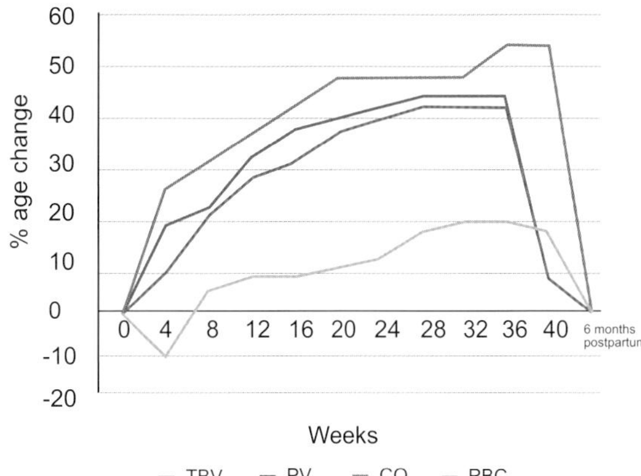

Fig 3.2
Blood values in a normal pregnancy. CO, Cardiac output; PV, Plasma volume; RBC, Red blood cells; TBV, Total blood volume.

Pregnancy is associated with vasodilatation of the systemic vasculature and the maternal kidneys. The systemic vasodilatation of pregnancy occurs as early as at 5 weeks and therefore precedes full placentation and the complete development of the uteroplacental circulation.

In the first trimester, there is a substantial decrease in peripheral vascular resistance, which decreases to its lowest level during the middle of the second trimester, with a subsequent plateau or slight increase for the remainder of the pregnancy (Fig 3.3). The decrease is approximately 35–40% of baseline. Systemic vascular resistance increases almost to pre-pregnancy levels postpartum, and by 2 weeks after delivery, maternal hemodynamics have largely returned to non-pregnant levels.

The effect of the rising uterus under the diaphragm will mean that, as the pregnancy progresses, the pregnant patient feels less able to take a deep breath (Fig. 3.4). Deep inspiration relies on good diaphragmatic excursion and good "pump handle" and "bucket handle" mechanics of the rib cage. The attention you pay to maintaining good rib and diaphragmatic excursion (see later) will be greatly appreciated by your pregnant patients.

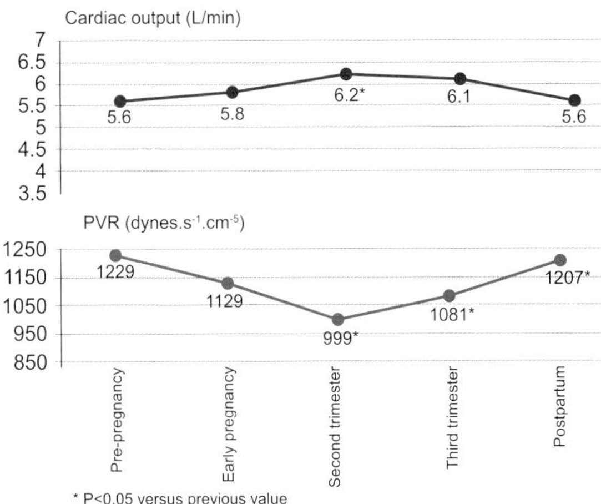

Fig 3.3

Cardiac output and peripheral vascular resistance (PVR) in pregnancy.

From Sangavi M, Rutherford JD. Cardiovascular Physiology of Pregnancy. Circulation. 2014 Sep;130(12):1003–8. Reproduced by kind permission of the publishers.

During the third trimester, cardiac output is further influenced by body position, where lying supine causes caval compression by the gravid uterus. This leads to a decrease in venous return, which can cause supine hypotension of pregnancy. As we have seen, stroke volume normally increases in the first and second trimesters, and decreases in the third trimester. This decrease is due to partial vena cava obstruction.

The delivery and immediate postpartum period is associated with further profound and rapid changes in the circulatory system. During delivery, cardiac output, heart rate, blood pressure, and systemic vascular resistance increase with each uterine contraction. Delivery-related pain and anxiety aggravate the increase in heart rate and blood pressure.

Immediately postpartum, delivery of the placenta increases afterload by removing the low-resistance circulation, and increases preload by returning placental blood to the maternal circulation. This increase in preload is accentuated by elimination of the mechanical compression of the inferior vena cava. Blood loss is typically 300–400 mL (0.07–0.09 gallons) during vaginal delivery and 500–800 mL (0.1–0.2 gallons) during cesarean delivery. These changes

Fig 3.4

Compression of the abdominal organs in pregnancy.

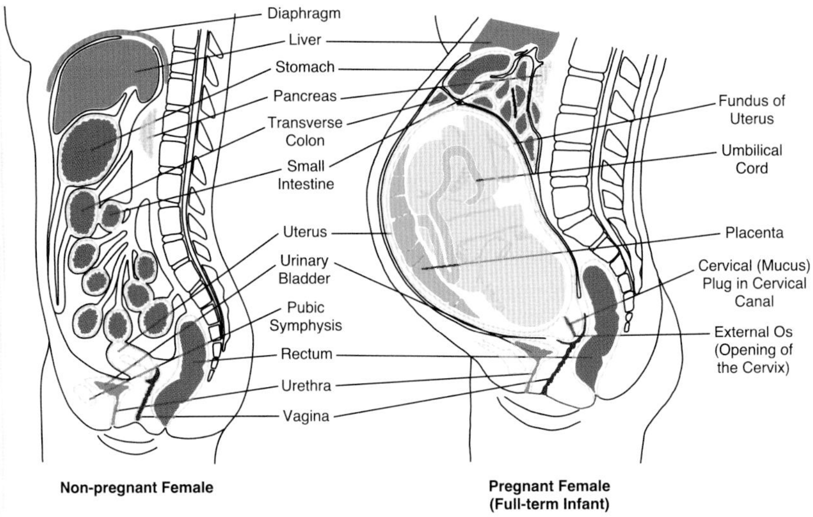

can place an intolerable strain on an abnormal heart, necessitating invasive hemodynamic monitoring and aggressive medical management.[5] Postpartum, the cardiac output is typically reduced for 2–6 weeks.

As we have seen, the changes in blood cells and blood gases described above are all physiological, not pathological; as the pregnancy progresses, the changes and compensations will take place with time in most cases. Where there are mechanical restrictions in the thoracic spine or intercostal joints and muscles, your work to the muscles joints and fascias is essential to meet the compensatory changes that pregnancy demands.[5]

Common Symptoms due to Changes in the Physiology of the Heart and Lungs During Pregnancy

Tiredness and Fatigue

Tiredness, or fatigue, is very common in early pregnancy and reaches a peak at the end of the first trimester. Advising rest, suggesting that the patient tries to do a little less, and reassuring her that all is well can help a great deal. Speaking to the midwife or health visitor about diet and iron levels is important because there might be a physiological anemia of pregnancy that relates to a lower than normal iron level due to expansion of the blood volume (see earlier). A multivitamin and iron tablets might be all that is needed. Consulting the internet for changes to the diet to alleviate fatigue can often provide a wealth of information. Fatigue also occurs in late pregnancy, when it is important to make sure that the patient does not have anemia.

Insomnia

Pregnant patients may lose sleep during pregnancy for a variety of reasons. Whatever the cause may be, it is important to understand that insomnia is not harmful to the baby. Insomnia during pregnancy is normal and affects approximately 78% of pregnant women.

Insomnia is the perception of inadequate or poor-quality sleep. Inadequate sleep may be the result of difficulty falling asleep, waking up frequently during the night, difficulty returning to sleep, or unrefreshing sleep.

There are a variety of causes, some of which are treatable and some of which are not. They include discomfort due to the increased size of the abdomen, back pain, heartburn, frequent urination during the night, frequent and vivid dreams, and the hormonal changes of pregnancy.

Heartburn and back pain will be dealt with in Chapter 6. It is not advisable to sleep on the back during pregnancy, as the weight on the gravid uterus might compress the inferior vena cava and thus compromise venous return from the legs, abdominal organs, and pelvis back to the heart. People change position all the time during sleep and it would be very unusual to wake in the same position you fell to sleep in. Turning in bed can be very difficult and if the sacroiliac joints are painful and sore, turning over will wake you up, again contributing to disturbed sleep, fatigue, and insomnia.

Good osteopathic management of pregnancy will always look at the sacroiliac joints and ensure good physiological mobility, so that problems such as turning in bed and thus disturbed sleep are alleviated. Patients often ask for advice about using pillows in pregnancy. One folded pillow placed at the neck will help to ensure that the neck and head are lined up with the spine, and a large pillow between the thighs will keep the thighs level and avoid sacroiliac joint strains as the patient grows bigger. Gentle exercise, such as yoga or Pilates, half an hour before bed will relax the body and help prepare for sleep. Probably the best advice for those who have difficulty sleeping is to try to nap during the day if they can, especially at the end of the pregnancy or at weekends when at home. When the child is born, it is also sensible to try to take a nap when the baby does, as this will help with the fatigue that comes with the disturbed sleep at night that is so common in newborn babies.

Headaches

Headaches can be a common problem in pregnancy, especially early on when the body is trying to adapt to the many changes in hormones. They are also often due to muscular tensions caused by spasm of the suboccipital muscle insertions and occipitofrontalis, the muscle that goes over the head. These tension headaches are often caused by the demand placed on the muscles with the changing posture of pregnancy.

Although most headaches seen in women are primary headache disorders (migraine, tension-type headache), complications or conditions associated with pregnancy can present with a secondary headache. Headaches are common symptoms in idiopathic intracranial hypertension, eclampsia, and reversible cerebral vascular syndrome. Migraines may begin or worsen during pregnancy, but pregnancy tends to reduce migraine frequency and severity. Approximately two-thirds of women with migraines experience headache improvement during pregnancy.[5]

Your case history needs to be very specific. Did the patient suffer from migraines before she became pregnant and was it associated with a particular phase of her menstrual cycle? Some migraine headaches can be much better with the change in hormone profiles in pregnancy.[6] Is this, in fact, a migraine headache or a pseudo-migraine? Migraine is usually a unilateral condition, and headache that crosses the midline or just sits under the skull is unlikely to be pure migraine. Likewise, did she suffer from tension headaches before the pregnancy and are these headaches similar to those headaches?

Your patient might consult you between her routine antenatal appointments. She may have seen her midwife before the headache started and not have another appointment for 2 or 3 weeks. The osteopath who treats pregnant patients must be aware of potentially serious obstetric complications and, if need be, refer as a matter of urgency.

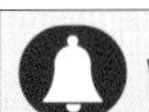

Warning

One such complication is pre-eclampsia, which presents with the triad of hypertension, protein in the urine, and edema. Patients who present with headache should always have their blood pressure taken and be examined for peripheral edema. If the blood pressure is high (140/90 mmHg is considered to be gestational hypertension),[7] they should be referred to the midwife for further monitoring.

Manipulation is safe in pregnancy. It has been this author's experience, over more than 40 years, that there is no evidence to suggest that, in the correct hands, a manipulation that is specific and gentle has any detrimental effect on the mother or her baby. Gentle craniosacral and unwinding techniques, such as functional or myofascial release techniques, can quickly ease a headache caused by the muscular spasms which can occur at any stage of the pregnancy.

Changes in Normal Cardiac and Respiratory Anatomy During Pregnancy

The heart lies in the center of the thoracic cavity, above the diaphragm and behind the sternum (Fig 3.5). The posterior mediastinum contains the esophagus and the descending aorta, which separate the heart from the 5th to 8th thoracic vertebrae. Above are the aorta and the pulmonary arteries, along with the two main bronchi into which the trachea divides.

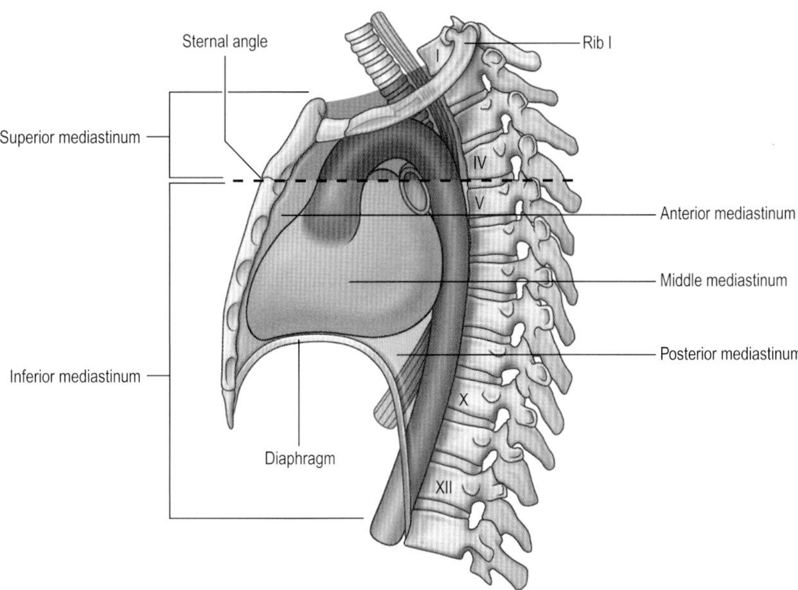

Fig 3.5
The heart in the mediastinum.
From Gray's Anatomy for Students, 4th edn, Richard Drake, A. Wayne Vogl, Adam Mitchell. Copyright Elsevier, 2019. Reproduced by kind permission of the publishers.

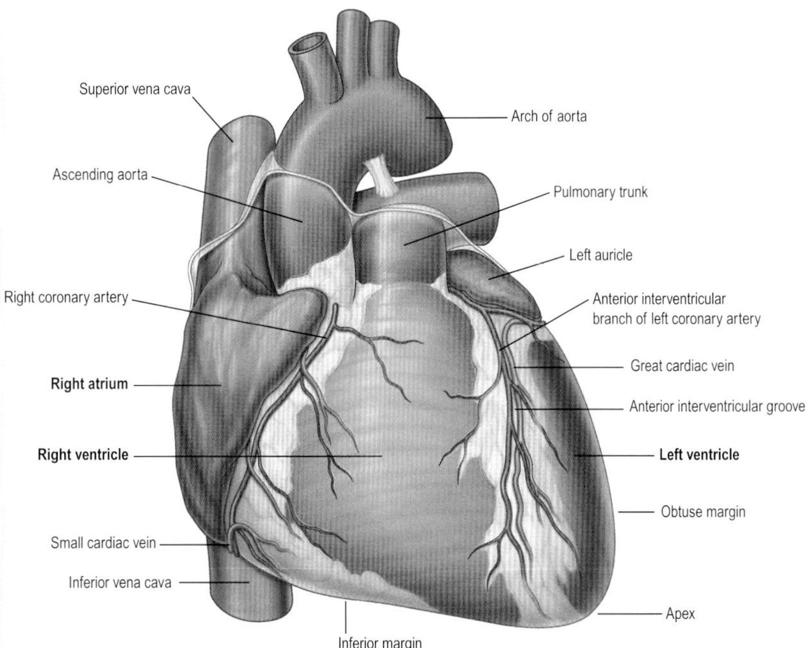

Fig 3.6
The heart: gross anatomy.
From Gray's Anatomy for Students, 4th edn, Richard Drake, A. Wayne Vogl, Adam Mitchell. Copyright Elsevier, 2019. Reproduced by kind permission of the publishers.

The two venae cavae enter the right atrium from above and below, and form most of its upper and lower walls (Fig 3.6). The coronary sinus is the main vein draining the heart muscle and it also enters the right atrium. Because of the oblique position of the heart in the chest, when the atria enlarge during pregnancy they do so into the right side of the thorax. When the left ventricle enlarges, it does so in the antero-posterior plane.

The Fascia, Heart, and Pericardium

The surface of the heart muscle is continually moving relative to the other contents of the thorax. Like the lungs, the heart is contained within a serous cavity, the pericardium, which allows free movement. According to Paoletti, the pericardium is part of a global fascial chain extending from the base of the cranium to the pelvis (Fig 3.7).[8] In the adult, the pericardium has an outer fibrous layer which encloses the whole heart, and deeper parietal and visceral layers. The fibrous layer is continuous with the serous layer covering the great vessels of the heart. It is the continuation of the fascial chain containing the pharyngeal fascia.

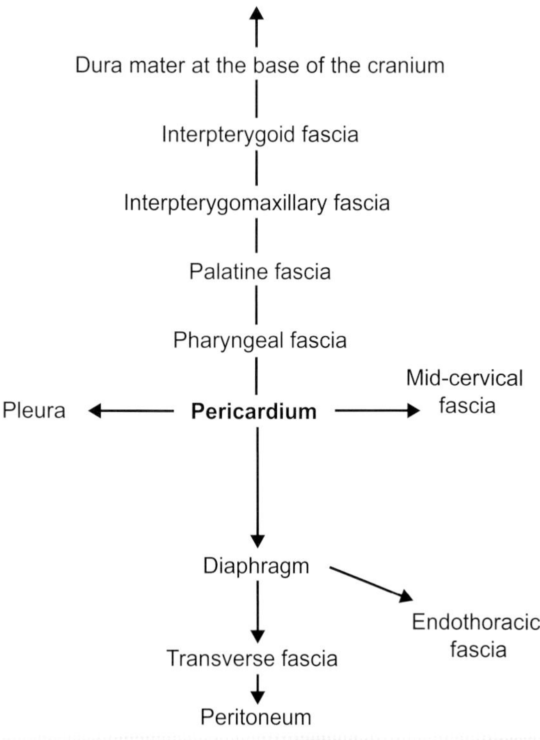

Fig 3.7
The fascial chain.
(After Paoletti.) ©Sully Editions.

There are some thick ligaments connecting the pericardium to the structures of the neck, thoracic spine, and diaphragm: for example, the central tendon of the diaphragm, which is fused to the inferior surface of the fibrous pericardium as the phrenicopericardial ligament. The fibrous pericardium forms a cone shape, which is flat at the base and encloses the heart; it is separated from it by a thin layer of fatty tissue that is continuous with the endothoracic fascia.

The endothoracic fascia is the extrapleural fascia that lines the wall of the chest, extending over the cupola of the pleura as the suprapleural membrane and forming a thin layer between the diaphragm and the pleura. The anterior surface corresponds to the anterior surface of the lungs and the sternum, and the posterior surface corresponds to the organs of the mediastinum, particularly the thoracic part of the esophagus. In the superior part, the endothoracic fascia covers the dome of the diaphragm on its pleural surface, attaching to the periostium of the 1st rib. It is also attached to the vascular sheath of the subclavian artery. On the inferior part, after the diaphragm, it becomes continuous with the transverse abdominal fascia. On the internal surface, it is attached to the parietal pleura and thus to the thoracic wall. In the mediastinum, it is thick and soft. However, it forms a fibrous lamina on the surface of the pericardium where it is united to the pericardium immediately underlying the pleura.

There are two sternopericardial ligaments, one superior and one inferior (Fig 3.8). The superior one attaches to the manubrium sternum. It is a continuation of a deep slip of the middle cervical aponeurosis, and according to Paoletti, is continuous with the anterior wall of the visceral sheath of the

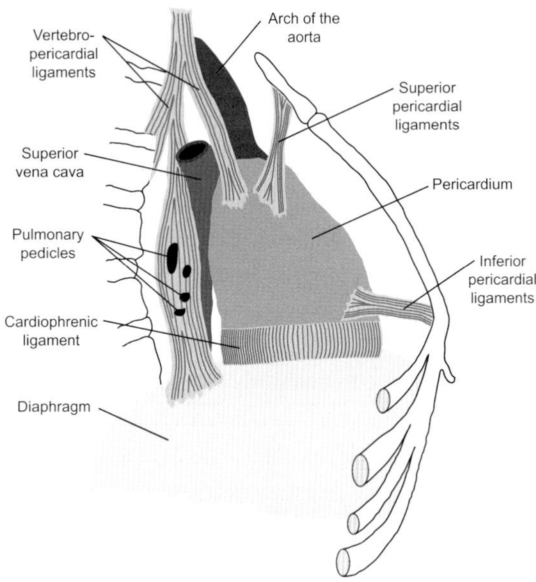

Fig 3.8

The ligaments of the pericardium.
(After Paoletti.) ©Sully Editions.

fascia of the neck. The inferior sternopericardial ligament attaches the base of the xiphoid process to the pericardium. The vertebropericardial ligaments are thin bands of fibrous tissue running from the 6th cervical vertebra to the 3rd thoracic, terminating below at the superior part of the pericardium.

The significance of these fascial chains and connections is of paramount importance to the osteopath. In order for there to be physiological changes in the mother during her pregnancy, anatomical changes have to take place in the supporting mechanisms of the heart and respiratory systems, mediated by the ovarian hormones.

Fascial relaxation techniques, such as functional and myofascial release techniques, are important technical tools used by the osteopath to facilitate changes in the cardiovascular and respiratory systems.

The treatment of structures that often lie far from the sites of palpable tensions may be necessary because of the fascial chains and their remote connections. From the base of the cranium to the pelvis, their influences on the fluid pumping systems in the chest have to be factored into a global treatment plan when addressing the treatment of pregnant patients.

Position and Size of the Heart

As the uterus enlarges and the diaphragm becomes elevated, the heart is displaced upwards and somewhat to the left with rotation on its long axis, so that the apex beat is moved laterally.[5] Cardiac capacity increases by 70–80 mL; this may be due to increased volume or hypertrophy of cardiac muscle. The size of the heart appears to increase by about 12%. The heart is enlarged by both chamber dilatation and hypertrophy. Normally, there is an increase in cardiac output in early pregnancy, reaching 40% above the non-pregnant state by 12 weeks' gestation.

The heart rate and stroke volume increase by 15% and 20%, respectively.[5]

The obstruction of the inferior vena cava posed by the uterus and the pressure of the fetal presenting part on the common iliac vein can result in decreased blood return to the heart. This lowers cardiac output, leads to a fall in blood pressure, and can cause edema in the lower extremities. This is why it is important not to have the pregnant patient lying supine for too long during treatment. Sitting or side-lying positions are much better.

One cause of back pain in pregnancy has been attributed to congestion in the veins of the vertebrovenous (Batson's) plexus in the lumbar spine. Side-lying lumbar flexion techniques will increase the pumping mobility of the spine during pregnancy treatment.

Structural Changes Above the Diaphragm During Pregnancy

Review of the Biomechanics of the Thoracic Spine

The heart, lungs, and mediastinum are contained within the rib cage. The rib cage, costal cartilages, and vertebrae, together with the sternum and the clavicles, are the local attachment points for the fascia that encloses and supports the heart.[5]

The thoracic spine is less mobile than other parts of the vertebral column because of the attachments of the ribs and the costal cartilages.[9] It is nevertheless capable of movements into flexion, extension, lateral flexion or side-bending, and axial rotation. According to *Grieve's Modern Manual Therapy*, one of the factors affecting the amount and direction of intervertebral movement is the elasticity of the musculoskeletal elements. He maintains, in general terms, that the most restricting element in the case of the thoracic spine is the behavior of the intervertebral discs.[10] During pregnancy, due to the action of hormones on connective tissues, this can change dramatically.

During flexion of the spine, the interspace between the vertebrae opens out posteriorly and the nucleus pulposus of the intervertebral disc moves posteriorly. The articular surfaces of the articular processes slide upwards. Flexion is limited by the tension developed in the interspinous ligament, joint capsules, ligamentum flavum, and posterior longitudinal ligament. The anterior longitudinal ligament is relaxed.

During extension of the spine, the vertebrae are approximated posteriorly and so crush the disc posteriorly. As a result, the nucleus pulposus of the intervertebral disc moves and expands anteriorly. Extension is limited by compression of the articular processes and the fact that the spinous processes almost touch. The ligaments anteriorly are stretched while the posterior ligaments and capsules are relaxed (Fig 3.9).

During lateral flexion, the articular facets slide on each other. On one side they move into flexion, while on the opposite side they move into extension relative to each other (Fig 3.10). This is a function of the angles of the facet joints in the thoracic spine. The motion is limited, once again, by joint apposition and by the tension of the ligaments on the opposite side.

Movements of the thoracic column are not just governed by the movements of the individual joints, however, as it is connected to the whole thoracic cage by multiple joints. All of the bony, cartilaginous, and articular components of the cage play a part in controlling and limiting the movements of the thoracic spine.

During lateral flexion of the thoracic column on the convexity, the thorax is elevated, the intercostal

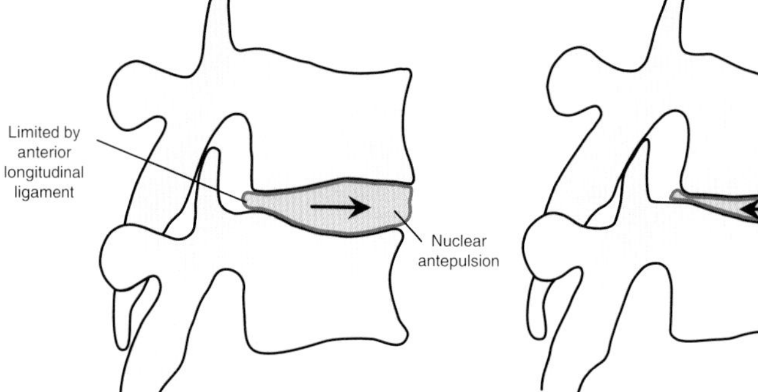

Fig 3.9
Flexion and extension of the spine to show movement of the nucleus of the disc.

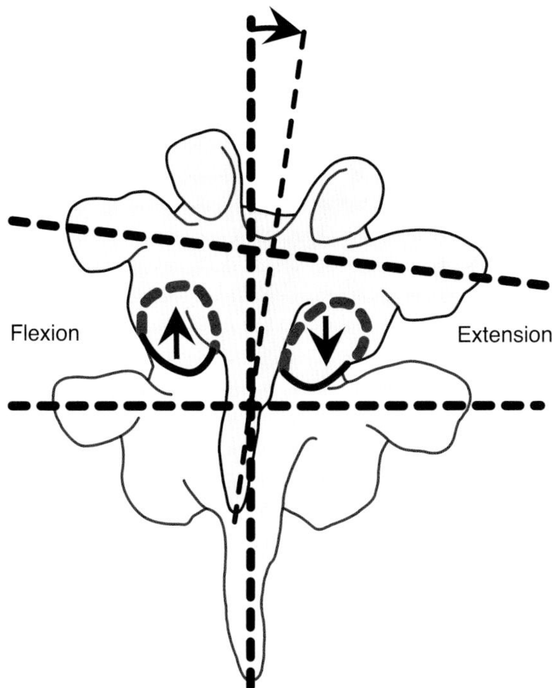

Fig 3.10
Lateral flexion of the spine to show one facet moving into flexion and the other moving into extension.

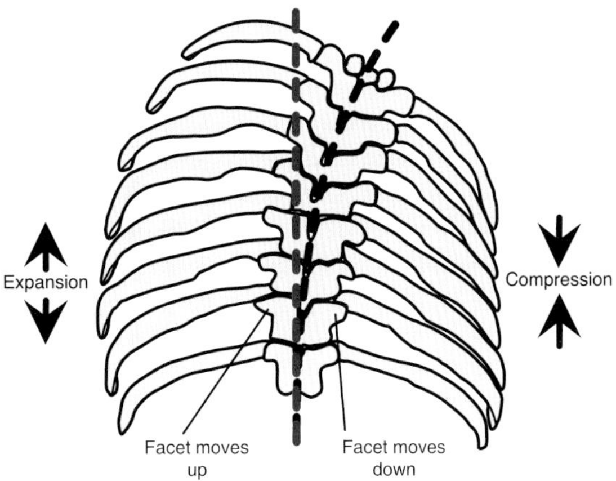

Fig 3.11
Lateral flexion of the thoracic cage to show compression on one side and expansion on the other.

spaces widen, the thoracic cage is enlarged, and the costosternal angle of the 10th rib opens up. On the concavity, the opposite happens: the intercostal spaces are compressed, the thoracic cage is reduced, and the costosternal angle becomes smaller (Fig 3.11). During flexion, all the angles between the various segments of the thorax open out, and during extension they are reduced.

Ranges of Spinal Movement

The possible ranges of movement depend on the angles of the facets and on the fact that, in the thoracic spine, the ribs and costal cartilages restrict the overall movement potential. A comparison of the ranges of motion reveals that the cervical column is mainly a rotation column; the thoracic has the same potential for lateral flexion as the cervical spine but less than the lumbar spine; and the lumbar spine has very poor axial rotation compared to the rest of the spine because of the angulations of the facet joints. These factors assume maximum importance when building leverages in osteopathic techniques.

All of the above presupposes normal motion of the thoracic spine; however, life is rarely normal and there can be many pathological changes in the thoracic spine which will compromise its ability to adapt and change in pregnancy. They range from serious disease processes, such as rheumatoid disease and the seronegative arthropathies, to muscular aches and strains of the ribs and spinal facet joints.

One condition to be aware of is Scheuermann's disease (also called Scheuermann's kyphosis or spinal osteochondrosis). Figures vary as to its incidence but one study showed that evidence of Scheuermann's

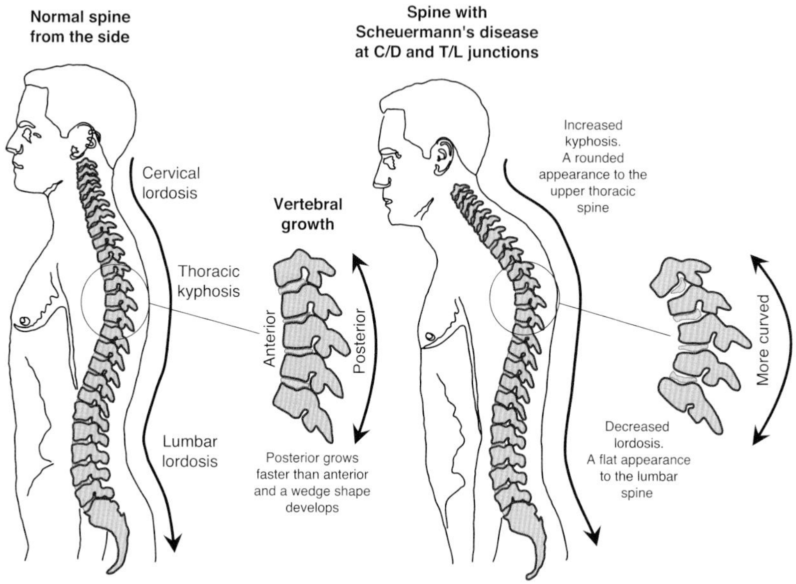

Fig 3.12
The development of Scheuermann's disease.

disease was detected in 60% of males and 23% of females.[11] However, another study put the figure much lower at 0.4–0.8% of the population.[12] This benign condition results in a restriction of segmental motion and a change in shape of the vertebral bodies, probably due to abnormal growth. During pregnancy, your patient will undergo changes in posture, segmental vertebral motion, and rib mechanics, and the presence and extent of Scheuermann's disease will materially affect her ability to change. It is usually quite difficult to find techniques to treat these fixed areas, but due to the actions of the various hormones of pregnancy, which soften the ligaments globally, this is one time when the condition is amenable to a degree of limited change.

Scheuermann's disease occurs when the front of the upper spine does not grow as fast as the back of the spine, causing the vertebrae to become wedge-shaped, with the narrow part of the wedge in front. The wedge shape of the vertebra creates an increase in the amount of normal kyphosis (front angulation of the thoracic spine; Fig 3.12). The wedging of vertebrae is most common in the thoracic spine, with the apex of the curve typically between the T7 and T9 levels of the spine. It can also occur at the junctions between the cervical and thoracic spines, and the thoracic and lumbar spines.

Patients who have this condition have greatly restricted motion between the vertebrae in those areas of the thoracic spine that are affected. This will interfere with the ability of the pregnant patient to change her posture as the pregnancy progresses (see later). The changing function of the thoracic spine and ribs during pregnancy is due in part to the need for mechanical adaptation as her posture alters. It is also caused by changes in the mediastinal contents, the heart and the lungs, during pregnancy in response to the alterations in physiological demands that the pregnancy places upon them.

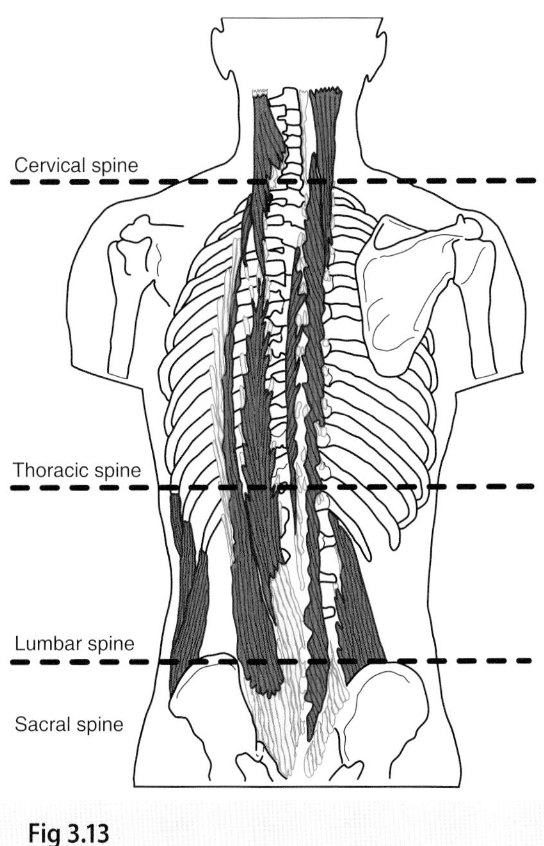

Fig 3.13
The erector spinae muscles.

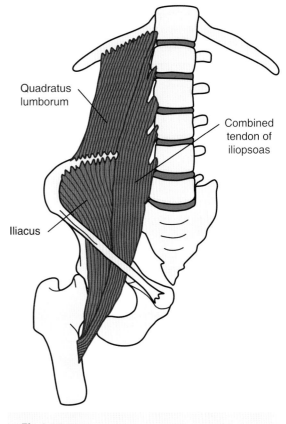

Fig 3.14
The iliopsoas muscle.

Muscles Involved in Spinal Movements

The erector spinae muscles arise from the sacrum, the spines of all the lumbar and last two thoracic vertebrae, the supraspinous ligaments, the sacrotuberous and sacrospinous ligaments, and the fibers of the gluteus maximus muscle (Fig 3.13).

Thoracolumbar extension is produced by contraction of the superficial fibers of the erector spinae muscles, such as the iliocostalis and longissimus muscles. Rotation is produced by contraction of the deep fibers of the erector spinae, such as the multifidus, the intertransverse muscles, and the rotatores muscles. Flexion is produced by contraction of the rectus abdominis muscle and by contraction of the iliopsoas muscle (Fig 3.14). Lateral flexion is caused by contraction of all of the muscles of one side of the trunk, particularly quadratus lumborum and the oblique and transverse abdominal muscles.

These actions should be considered in relation to the effects of gravity on movement and posture.

In standing, because of the lumbar lordosis and thoracic kyphosis, the force of gravity naturally leads to thoracic spine flexion and lumbar spine extension. This is again of major importance in pregnancy because the patient changes her posture radically three times during the pregnancy to accommodate growth of the uterus and fetus.

Postural Changes to the Thoracic Spine and Ribs During Pregnancy

During the first trimester, as the uterus expands and grows, it will rise out of the pelvis and into the abdominal cavity. Pressure on the rectus abdominis muscle, which runs from the xiphoid process on the sternum to the pubis, causes it to contract. This will lead to a posterior rotation of the pelvis and a gentle flattening of the spine (Fig 3.15). At this stage, the thoracic spine does not need to change. However, if your patient undergoes early growth and change of her breast tissue during the first trimester, she might start to develop an increased thoracic kyphosis at this stage. As she progresses through the first trimester to the second trimester, there will be a flaring of the lower ribs, especially the 11th and 12th, to accommodate growth. Dyspnea is not an uncommon symptom around 12–16 weeks. It is during the second trimester that the patient starts to develop the normal kypholordosis of pregnancy.

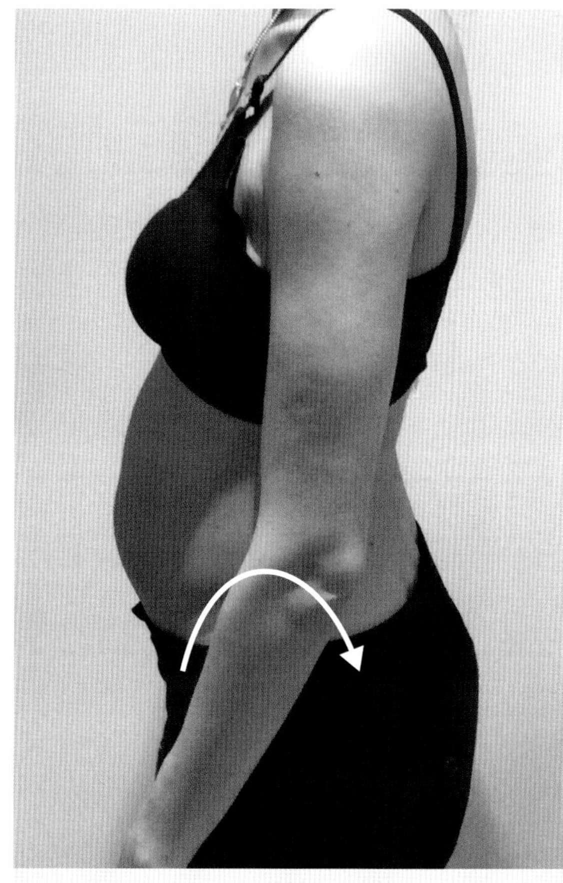

Fig 3.15
Posterior pelvic rotation at the end of the first trimester causing a flattening of the thoracolumbar junction.

The transition of the spinal curves at the thoracolumbar junction is very important, in both the antero-posterior and the lateral planes. If stiffness or Scheuermann's disease is present, it may well prevent good antero-posterior transition and thus contribute towards back pain. Also, the weight of the baby falling posteriorly can cause pain on weight-bearing facet joints. Likewise, the increase in thoracic kyphosis can lead to rib muscle or diaphragm pain at this time. The weight of the growing breasts, if they are heavy, will cause a round-shouldered posture as both upper extremities rotate around the chest wall. This can provoke thoracic spinal muscle pain, as well as shoulder pain, and it may well compromise the structures in the thoracic outlet, causing arm pain (brachalgia) and nerve root pains, or disturbances in the fluid mechanics of the upper extremity.

During the last trimester, there is not a lot of change in the thoracic spine and ribs compared to the middle trimester. If the patient continues to undergo breast development at this time, thoracic outlet syndromes may again cause arm and hand syndromes.

More information on the postural changes of pregnancy is provided in Chapter 5.

Common Symptoms due to Structural Changes Above the Diaphragm During Pregnancy

Costochondral Pain

As the fundus of the uterus rises out of the pelvis and into the abdomen, it occupies space normally taken up by the abdominal organs. The lower ribs and associated costal cartilages spread laterally, and if there is a pre-existing stiffness of the cartilages or a spinal stiffness involving the thoracolumbar junction (see Scheuermann's disease above), then this will become symptomatic – sometimes as early as the start of the second trimester. This is governed by the pre-pregnancy posture and the amount of fat in the mesentery.

Costochondritis describes an inflammation of the costochondral junctions of ribs or the chondrosternal joints of the anterior chest wall. It is sometimes called Tietze's syndrome, but this is not, in fact, synonymous with costochondritis, as it is distinguished by the presence of swelling over the affected joints. Tietze's syndrome is more localized, whereas costochondritis tends to be more diffuse. The cause of costochondritis and Tietze's syndrome is unknown; however, preceding upper respiratory infections and excessive coughing have been described in some patients. It is more common in pregnancy for the reasons described above.

In primary care, costochondritis has been found to account for 13% of presentations with chest pain. The figure may, in fact, be higher, as chest wall pain accounts for 20% of presentations and much of this may be costochondritis. Costochondritis is more common than Tietze's syndrome, which can present at any age but is most frequently found in those under the age of 40 years. Costochondritis is more common over the age of 40 years. Both conditions occur in men and women, and in adults and children. In 70% of those with Tietze's syndrome, it is unilateral and only one joint is affected. More than one rib is likely to be affected by costochondritis.[13]

Onset may be acute or gradual. The patient complains of pain that is often localized to the costal cartilage (that is, anteriorly on the chest wall). It may be described as aching or sharp, or as a pressure. Tietze's syndrome usually affects the upper ribs, especially the 2nd or 3rd. Costochondritis can affect any of the costochondral joints, but most commonly the 2nd to the 5th ribs are involved. The pain is aggravated by physical activity, movement, deep inspiration, coughing, or sneezing. There is commonly a history of recent illness with coughing, or recent strenuous exercise. There is localized tenderness; in Tietze's syndrome, this takes the form of a tender, fusiform swelling of the costal cartilage at the costochondral junction, which is tender to palpation. Although the pain usually disappears spontaneously, the swelling of Tietze's syndrome may persist long after the tenderness has disappeared. In the pregnant patient, the presence of the hormone relaxin, secreted by the corpus luteum of pregnancy, can weaken or soften the costochondral articulations and their capsules and ligaments. In the upper chest, the weight of the developing breast tissue can be very heavy and drag the ribs down. From the third trimester onwards, pregnant patients should be encouraged to wear a loose crop top or a sports bra at night, again to support and protect the developing breast tissues.

There are many causes of chest pain in both pregnant and non-pregnant patients, and these should be included in your diagnostic thought process; they are listed in Box 3.3. However, it is important to note that, in pregnancy, musculoskeletal pain is the commonest reason for rib and chest pain presenting to osteopathic practice.

BOX 3.3

Common pathological causes of chest pain in the non-pregnant patient

- Acute coronary syndrome
- Pericarditis
- Heart failure
- Pneumonia
- Pulmonary embolism (PE)
- Thoracic aortic aneurysm dissection
- Rib fracture
- Chest wall pain
- Gastrointestinal causes

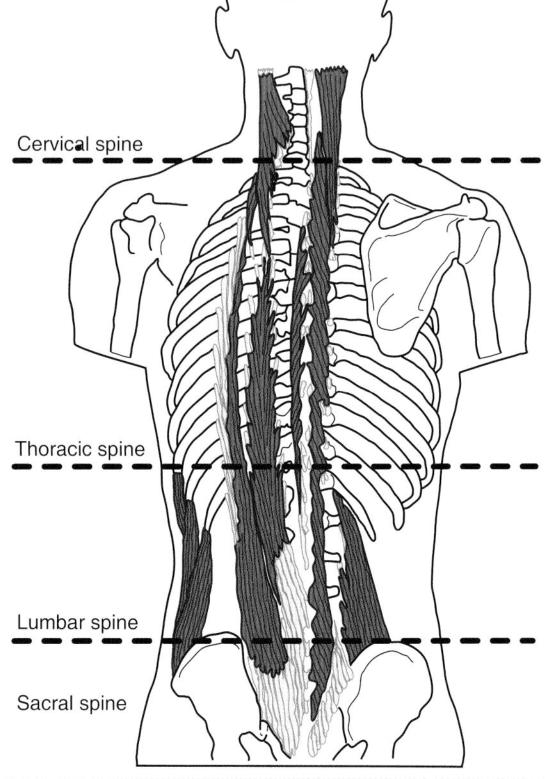

Fig 3.16
The erector spinae muscles.

Thoracic Spinal Pain

The changes in posture in both the antero-posterior and the lateral planes that should take place during the 40 weeks of pregnancy are often accompanied by pain and tension in the spinal muscles and joints of the thoracic spine (Fig 3.16).

These muscles run from the sacrum to the occiput and are responsible for holding us in an upright posture. Like any muscles, if they are made to contract for an extended period of time, they will fatigue and cause back pain. This can be ischemic pain due to poor oxygenation, or chronic congestive pain because the venous blood in the capillary beds does not adequately drain away.

Chapter 4, on treatment techniques, contains many examples of soft tissue and ligamentous stretch techniques that have been found to be useful when treating thoracic spinal pain in pregnancy.

Review of the Respiratory Movements of the Thoracic Skeleton

As a normal pregnancy progresses, expansion of the uterus and fetus up towards the diaphragm means that breathlessness is a common symptom from 20 weeks' gestation onwards. The severity of this symptom and its global consequences with regard to oxygenation of the tissues are really a function of the efficiency of the whole respiratory mechanism.

Inspiration depends on a rise in volume of the thoracic cavity by increase of one or more of its three diameters: vertical, antero-posterior, and transverse. As a result, air is sucked into the lungs and venous blood and lymph are drawn into the thoracic cavity from the surrounding parts. Incidentally, venous stasis syndromes, such as varicose veins in the lower extremities and hemorrhoids or even vaginal varices, are directly related to the ability of the thoracic mechanisms to move this venous blood.

The vertical diameter is increased by a straightening of the normal thoracic kyphosis, and by a contraction of the diaphragm down towards the abdominal cavity. The efficiency of the diaphragm contraction is dependent both on the stability of the ribs from which it arises, and on the compressibility of the abdominal contents. If the woman is in late pregnancy or is carrying a very big baby, this can be seriously compromised.

The origin of the diaphragm is stabilized by fixation of the 11th and 12th ribs by the posterior abdominal muscles. Accommodation of the displaced abdominal contents occurs because of relaxation of the anterior abdominal walls, and because of an increase in the transverse diameter of the upper part of the abdominal cavity, resulting from passive lateral displacement of ribs 8–10 by pressure from the displaced abdominal viscera. This passive lateral movement of the lower ribs increases the transverse diameter of the lower thorax, as well as the upper part of the abdomen. When the dome of the diaphragm is brought to a halt by the pressure on the abdominal contents, the costal fibers of the diaphragm act from a fixed central tendon and elevate the lower ribs.

The transverse and antero-posterior diameters of the rest of the thorax are increased by an elevation of the upper seven ribs by the muscles of the thoracic wall and the neck. Each rib is moved simultaneously about its transverse and antero-posterior axes, and the resulting forward displacement of the costal cartilages and sternum, and the lateral displacement of the shafts of the ribs, increase the antero-posterior and transverse diameters, respectively.

Expiration in quiet respiration is a function largely of the elastic recoil of the lung tissue. Any additional force required in forced expiration will result from contraction of the anterior abdominal muscles, such as in labor.

During forced respiration, as in violent exercise with forced inspiration, or in the forced expiration seen in coughing, sneezing, defecation, or labor, the body uses secondary muscles of respiration to aid and reinforce the respiratory movements (Box 3.4).

Once again, the relationship between the thoracic cage and the muscles of the neck, the chest, and the upper extremities is very important for the correct functioning of the breathing mechanisms, even more so in pregnancy when respiratory demand is so high. Attention to these accessory muscles during the pregnancy will mean that the patient will suffer less dyspnea and that her ability to exchange respiratory gases will be enhanced.

BOX 3.4

The muscles of respiration

Secondary muscles of inspiration	Secondary muscles of expiration
Sternocleidomastoid	External oblique
Scalenes	Internal oblique
Pectoralis major	Rectus abdominis
Pectoralis minor	Lower iliocostalis
Serratus anterior	Lower longissimus
Serratus posterior superior	Serratus posterior inferior
Upper iliocostalis	

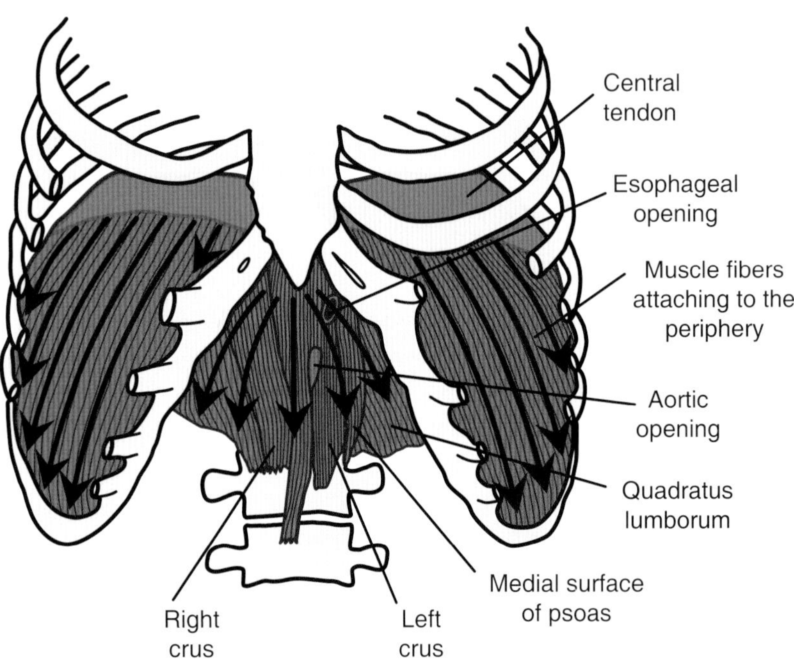

Fig 3.17
The diaphragm.

The relationship between the abdominal muscles and the muscles of the lower spine is essential for efficient expiration. During pregnancy, the abdominal muscles undergo extreme stretch, and the expansion of the gravid uterus can be accompanied by muscular pain and rib pain. Attention to these structures, especially in the last trimester, will mean not only that the final few months of pregnancy are more comfortable for the patient, but that when she needs to use these muscles to push during the expulsive phase of her labor, she can work from a position of optimal efficiency. A muscle that has been stretched and trained for hard effort is less likely to be damaged during extreme performance.[14,15]

The Diaphragm and its Mode of Action (after Kapandji)

The musculotendinous dome of the diaphragm separates the thoracic and abdominal cavities (Fig 3.17). Seen from the side, it reaches down farther posteriorly than anteriorly, and its apex is the central tendon (Fig 3.18). From this center, bands of muscle fibers radiate out to the periphery of the floor of the thorax and gain attachments to the deep surfaces of the costal cartilages, the tips of the 11th and 12th ribs, the costal arch, the vertebral bodies by means of the two crura, the medial surface of the psoas muscle, and the quadratus lumborum muscle.

When the diaphragm contracts, the central tendon is pulled down, thus increasing the vertical diameter of the thorax. The depression of the central tendon is checked by the contents of the mediastinum as they are stretched and by the contents of the abdomen as they are compressed. From this moment, the central tendon is fixed and the muscle fibers, now acting from the periphery of the central tendon, elevate the lower ribs.

The diaphragm is the principal muscle of respiration because it increases the vertical diameter

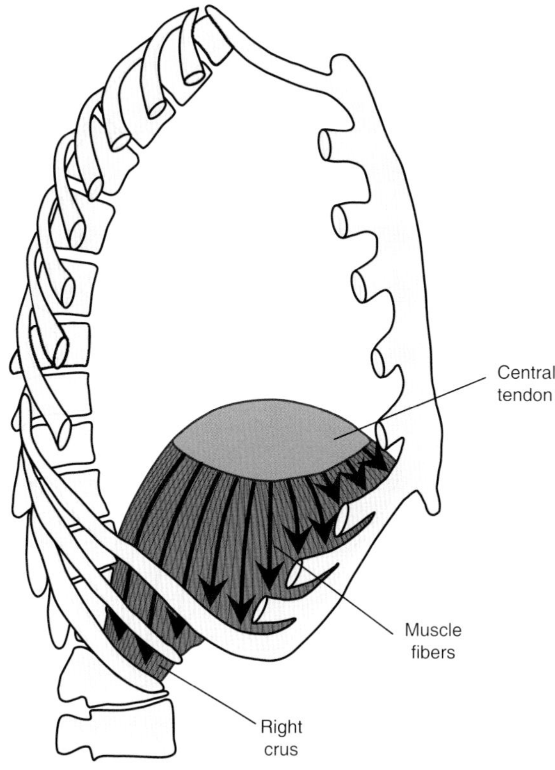

Fig 3.18
The ribs and diaphragm.

by pulling down the central tendon, increases the transverse diameter by elevating the lower ribs, and finally, increases the antero-posterior diameter by elevating the upper ribs with the help of the sternum.

Downward displacement of the diaphragm is dependent on fixation of ribs 11 and 12 by the quadratus lumborum muscle. As the diaphragm descends, there is passive lateral displacement of ribs 8, 9, and 10.

The antero-posterior and transverse diameters of the thorax are increased by elevation of the upper seven ribs. In quiet respiration, this is achieved mainly by the external intercostal muscles. In deep inspiration, these muscles are aided by the scalene and sternocleidomastoid muscles in the neck, and also by muscles that act on the ribs from the fixed upper extremity, such as pectoralis minor.

Increase in the vertical diameter of the thorax is due to extension of the thoracic column by contraction of the erector spinae muscles.

Quiet respiration is a passive process caused by elastic recoil of the lung tissues. In forced expiration in defecation and childbirth, contraction of the oblique and transverse abdominal muscles increases the intra-abdominal pressure and thereby passively raises the diaphragm. Contraction of the intercostal muscles prevents bulging of the intercostal spaces.

During defecation and childbirth, in order to stop the breath leaving the body and retaining the expulsive pressure on the pelvic floor, the glottis is closed by adduction of the vocal cords, as in a Valsalva maneuver.

Review of the Functions of the Trunk Muscles

Excluding the muscles of the pelvis and the perineum, the muscles of the trunk have two main functions. Firstly, they create pressure changes in the thoracic and abdominal cavities, including those involved in respiration. Secondly, they are concerned with displacement of one part of the trunk in relation to another through movements of the vertebral column.

Autonomic Circulatory Control During Pregnancy

From the earliest days, the history of osteopathy is peppered with references to the effects of manipulations of various sorts on the autonomic nervous system. Louisa Burns, in 1910, experimented with dogs and discovered the effects of peripheral lesions on the autonomic circulation. The work of Korr,

Denslow, and others led the way for practitioners to build a practice based on sound scientific principles.[16,17] In 2001, Patterson published some special reprints from the archives of the *Journal of the American Osteopathic Association*,[18] and again we see praise for workers who published more than 60 years ago and who must have contributed greatly to the understanding of osteopathic medicine at its outset.

It cannot be denied that, since then, many thousands of osteopaths all over the world have based their practices on these fundamental researchers and their patients have felt the benefit. Let us not forget that osteopathy, as it was set out by our founders, was propounded as a system of medicine, not a manual therapy for musculoskeletal pain.

However, recent evidence shows that the exact role of the autonomic nervous system in pregnancy is still unclear. Fu and Levine reviewed what is known about the hemodynamic adaptation, changes in vascular endothelial function, sympathetic neural control, and vascular responsiveness in pregnancy, and baroreflex function during pregnancy, too.[19] They maintain that whether and how the sympathetic nervous system (Fig 3.19) plays a role in hemodynamic homeostasis during *early* human pregnancy remains completely unknown.

Another paper by a Finnish research group[20] suggests that, in late pregnancy, parasympathetic deactivation towards term is likely to contribute to increased heart rate and cardiac output at rest, whereas restored sympathetic modulation with modest responses may contribute stable peripheral resistance and sufficient placental blood supply under stimulated conditions. Both papers seem to suggest that the sympathetic nervous system is of paramount importance to the control of blood pressure and circulation during pregnancy, even if the exact mechanisms behind that control are unknown. For osteopaths treating pregnant patients in practice, the effects of somatic dysfunctions in the upper thoracic spine might give us an input into this area of changing physiology because of the relation of the position of the sympathetic ganglia to the spine and the first rib (Fig 3.20).

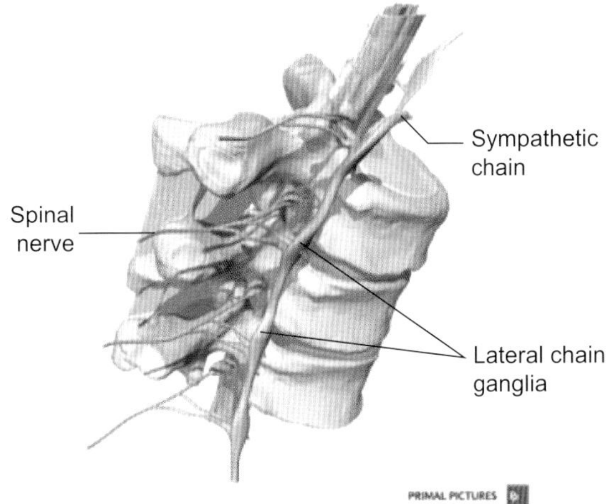

Fig 3.19
The sympathetic nervous system.

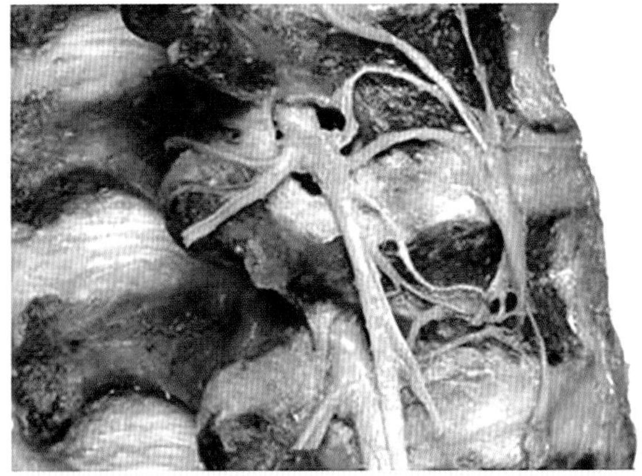

Fig 3.20
The spinal nerves and the lateral chain and sympathetic ganglia.

References

1. LoMauro A, Aliverti A. Physiology masterclass: respiratory physiology of pregnancy. Breathe (Sheff). 2015 Dec;11(4):297–301.
2. National Institute for Health and Care Excellence. Weight Management Before, During and After Pregnancy. Public health guideline [PH27], July 2010; https://www.NICE.org.uk.
3. Chandra S, Kumar Tripathi A, Mishra S, Amzarul M, Kumar Vaish A. Physiological changes in haematological parameters during pregnancy. Indian J Hematol Blood Transfus. 2012 Sep;28(3):144–6.
4. Stennett AK, Qiao X, Falone AE, Koledova VV, Khalil RA. Increased vascular angiotensin type 2 receptor expression and NOS-mediated mechanisms of vascular relaxation in pregnant rats. Am J Physiol Heart Circ Physiol. 2009 Mar;296(3):H745–55.
5. Soma-Pillay P, Nelson-Piercy C, Tolppanen H, Mebazaa A. Physiological changes in pregnancy. Cardiovasc J Afr. 2016 Mar–Apr;27(2):89–94.
6. NHS. Headaches in Pregnancy; Feb 2018, https://www.nhs.uk/pregnancy/related-conditions/common-symptoms/headaches/.
7. Children's Hospital of Philadelphia. Gestational Hypertension, https://www.chop.edu/conditions-diseases/gestational-hypertension.
8. Paoletti S. *Les Fascias.* Sully, 1998.
9. Oda I, Abumi K, Lü D, Shono Y, Kaneda K. Biomechanical role of the posterior elements, costovertebral joints, and rib cage in the stability of the thoracic spine. Spine. 1996;21(12):1423–9.
10. Boyling J, Palastanga N. *Grieve's Modern Manual Therapy.* Churchill Livingstone, 1994.
11. Fisk JW, Baigent ML, Hill PD. Incidence of Scheuermann's disease: preliminary report. Am J Phys Med. 1982 Feb;61(1):32–5.
12. Nowak JE. Scheuermann Disease: Practice Essentials, Pathophysiology; Sep 2020, https://emedicine.medscape.com/article/311959.
13. WebMD. Costochondritis, https://www.webmd.com/pain-management/costochondritis.
14. Small K, McNaughton L, Matthews M. A systematic review into the efficacy of static stretching as part of a warm-up for the prevention of exercise-related injury. Res Sports Med. 2008;16(3):213–31.
15. Woods K, Bishop P, Jones E. Warm-up and stretching in the prevention of muscular injury. Sports Med. 2007;37(12):1089-99.
16. Denslow J, Korr I, Krems A. Quantitative studies of chronic facilitation in human motoneuron pools. Am J Physiol. 1947;150;229–38.
17. Korr IM. The neural basis of the osteopathic lesion. J Am Osteopath Assoc. 1947;48:191–8.
18. Patterson MM. A research program for the osteopathic profession, our great and only hope. JAOA 2001 Sep;101(9):534.
19. Fu Q, Levine BD. Autonomic circulatory control during pregnancy in humans. Semin Reprod Med. 2009 Jul;27(4):330–7.
20. Heiskanen N, Saarelainen H, Valtonen P, Lyyra-Laitinen T, Laitinen T, Vanninen E, et al. Blood pressure and heart rate variability analysis of orthostatic challenge in normal human pregnancies. Clin Physiol Funct Imaging. 2008 Nov;28(6):384–90.

Treatment Techniques for Above the Diaphragm During Pregnancy 4

If she were not pregnant, your patient could be treated in any position that was comfortable for her, be it supine, prone, side-lying, or sitting. Due to the circumstances outlined in Chapter 1, she cannot lie flat on her back for any prolonged amount of time, but it is perfectly safe for her to be treated supine for a short period. As a general rule, however, sitting or semi-side-lying techniques are best.

Soft Tissue Techniques

What is the ambition of the technique? Are you aiming to stretch tight tissue and make it more comfortable, increase fluid flow through congested tissue, or reduce tone in painful hypertonic tissue? The answer to these questions is important, as it will dictate which technique is chosen by the osteopath. The difference between a massage and a soft tissue technique relates to diagnosis and to evaluation of why the tissue needs to be treated in the first place. It was Dr A. Clark Kennedy in 1945 who asked, "Why this patient? Why this problem? And why now?"[1] These questions cause us to ask how the patient became sick or decompensated, and lead us to address these points to correct the problem. Simply relaxing a tight muscle without asking why it was tight in the first place may well provoke an unwanted painful reaction if that muscle is guarding another sensitive structure. It should be evident, then, that the choice of technique will be dictated by evaluation of the pregnant patient, which tells you not only which tissue is causing symptoms, but also what predisposing and maintaining factors are present in this individual.

This book is not going to describe every technique for every region. I refer readers to books by Professor Laurie Hartman and Professor Phillip Greenman for a clear analysis of modern manual techniques for use in most circumstances.[2,3] Instead, it will show how techniques can be changed for the pregnant patient for her safety and comfort.

Soft Tissue Technique for the Neck and Suboccipital Tissues with the Patient Sitting

Techniques are not generally taught with the patient sitting down. In pregnancy, however, and especially in the third trimester, this is the most comfortable position for her. These techniques should be practiced so that you are familiar with them and feel comfortable with their use. Of course, they are also available for non-pregnant people who do not like to lie too flat, such as your elderly patients.

Position of the patient

The patient sits at the side of the treatment table, propped up with pillows and arms folded (Fig 4.1).

If the treatment table is too wide, the patient can sit across the corner of it, so that the osteopath can reach down to her upper thoracic spine.

Position of the osteopath

He stands facing the patient. His weight is spread, with 75% of it on his back foot.

As seen in Figure 4.2, the two hands come together over the patient's occipital protuberance, with as much of the palms of the hands in contact with the skull as possible. The pressure is no more than a few grams; certainly, there is no force compressing the skull.

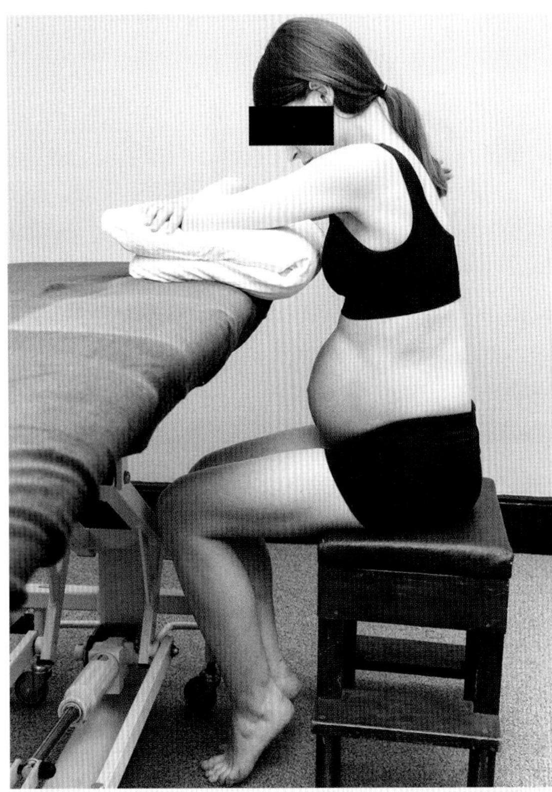

Fig 4.1
Patient sitting for cervical techniques.

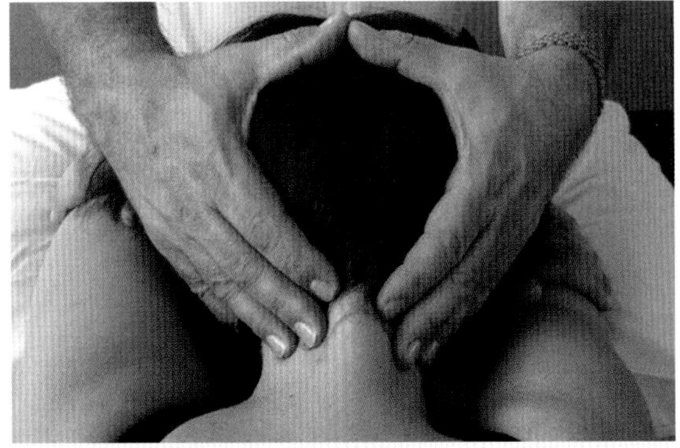

Fig 4.2
The position of the osteopath's hands for suboccipital work.

Ambition of the technique

This is a kneading, relaxing technique for the suboccipital muscles.

Application of the technique

Applying gentle pressure, with the right hand moving in a clockwise direction and the left counterclockwise, the osteopath gently kneads the suboccipital and upper cervical muscles with the tips of his fingers, and the scalp tissues with the palms of his hands, aiming to release any hypertonia and increase blood flow. At the same time, he rocks from the front foot to the back foot to introduce rhythm into the technique, which is slow and works synchronously with the patient's breathing. This can be particularly effective in patients who are suffering from tension or postural muscle headaches during their pregnancy. The action is continued until the muscles release.

Soft Tissue Technique for the Neck and Shoulders with the Patient Sitting

Position of the patient

She sits at the side of the treatment table, propped up with pillows and arms folded. Alternatively, she may sit across the corner of the treatment table, again with the head resting on pillows.

Position of the osteopath

He stands facing her, with his hands placed on her shoulders and looking down her spine as before. The technique starts with the hands together at the base of the skull. If she has long hair, this should be tied up. He stands with one foot in front of the other, 75% of his weight on the back foot to reduce the body weight that is going to be transmitted through the hands.

Ambition of the technique

This is a cross-fiber soft tissue release technique.

Application of the technique

The osteopath gently moves his hands down the patient's neck and onto her shoulders, with a gentle pressure on the soft tissues as they run under his fingers. When his hands reach the base of the neck, they run laterally across the fibers of trapezius bilaterally as it runs up to the skull (Figs 4.3 and 4.4). They then pass down and into the base of this muscle in the thoracolumbar junction. The overall shape of the technique is a diamond or trapezius as it crosses the fibers of the trapezius muscle, performing a cross-fiber soft tissue release.

The technique is performed in rhythmic and gentle fashion, in time with the patient's breathing, and the osteopath assesses the tissue response as he works. As the operator moves his hands down the spine, he gradually transfers his body weight from the back foot to the front foot in a rocking motion, to aid delivery of the downward movement of the hands and to induce a fluid pumping motion. He stops when the tissue has relaxed and changed sufficiently.

This technique can also be performed with the osteopath standing behind the patient, working upwards from the thoracolumbar junction across the muscles.

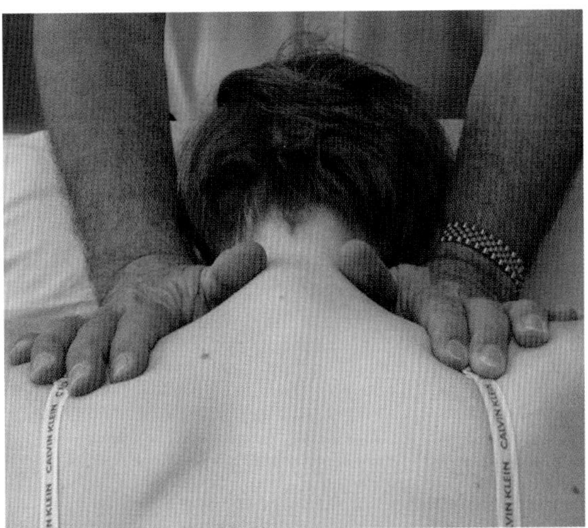

Fig 4.3
Cross-fiber technique for the upper fibers of trapezius.

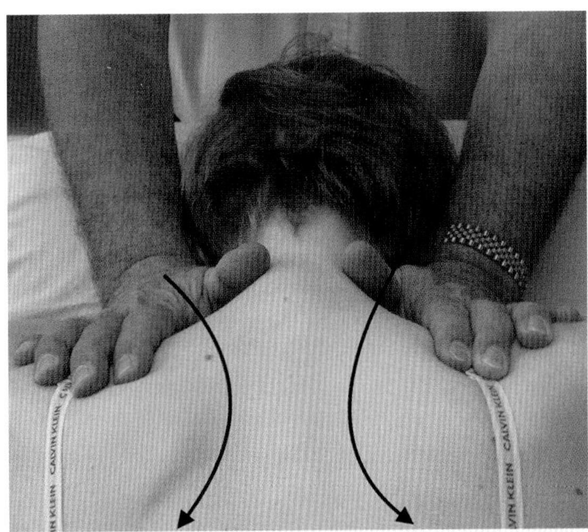

Fig 4.4
The thumbs pass out and lateral to cross the upper fibers of trapezius.

Modification of the Periscapular Soft Tissue Technique

Position of the patient

The patient lies on her side in the position of a three-sided square (Fig 4.5). Her head, neck, and abdomen are supported by pillows, and her cervical spine is held in a neutral position: "Mabel is stable on the table"! This position is fundamental. It allows for maximum stability of the patient, so that she

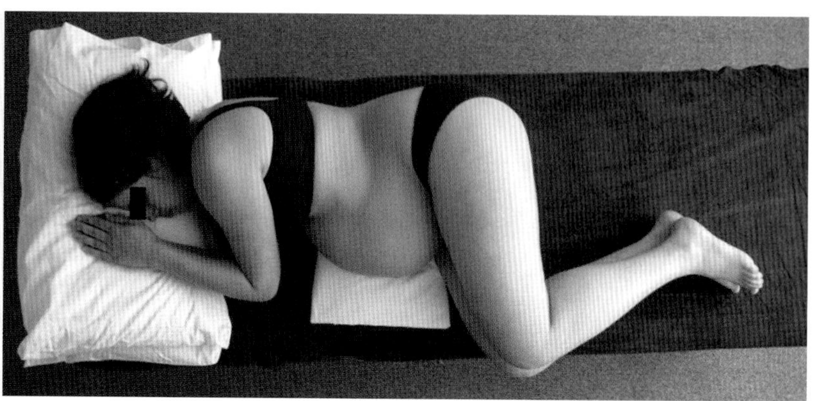

Fig 4.5
"Mabel stable on the table."

can relax, and permits the osteopath to do his job while allowing him to access all the areas he needs to without changing her position more than is necessary. The hips and shoulders are at 90 degrees to the table. She should be far enough back to allow for access, and not too near to the edge of the table so that she can see the floor.

Position of the osteopath

He stands in front of the patient and faces her. She lies on her side, facing him.

Ambition of the technique

The technique aims to release tension in the periscapular muscles and accessory muscles of respiration. It is helpful in cases of shoulder tension in women whose breast tissue is heavy, and so it is used during the mid and final trimesters of pregnancy. It is useful for treating cases of dyspnea, and for encouraging circulation and drainage back to the heart and lungs in pregnancy.

Application of the technique

The patient is treated side-lying in a similar way to the classic technique, but here the arm is not bent at the elbow; instead, it is used as a lever to assist the stretching motion of the upper limb muscles where they are attached to the spine. If she is lying on her left side, he takes her right arm at the elbow and loops it over his left arm at the elbow. His left hand grasps his right forearm below his elbow to form a brace or strut. This is a very important feature of this modified technique, as it means that all his movements, from his hips, knees, thorax, and shoulders, and not just the movements of his hands or arms, are transmitted to the patient.

Using her right arm as a brace and holding his own forearm as in Figure 4.6, he uses his right hand to contact the interscapular muscles and the muscles connecting the upper limb to the spine. During pregnancy, the breast tissues can become quite sensitive and sore, so any undue compression to the chest is best avoided if possible. However, there is a very small movement of the osteopath's body towards the table through the patient's arm, which has the effect of releasing the scapular muscles.

He moves his whole body in a clockwise direction from his feet, fixing the scapula but allowing the periscapular soft tissues to release and stretch. A small element of traction to the upper limb takes place too. Depending on the patient and her

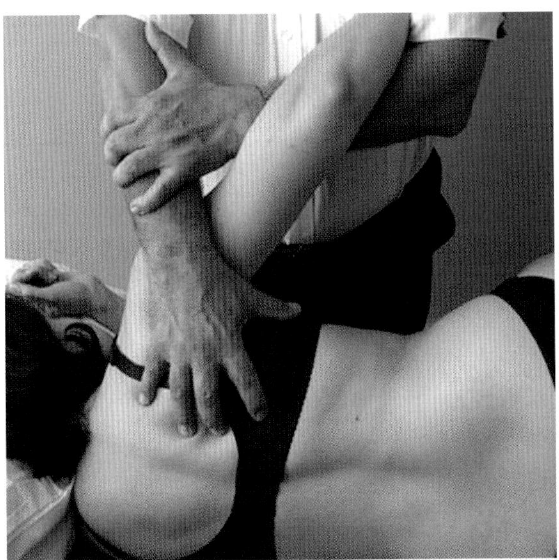

Fig 4.6
Periscapular muscle technique.

response, his movements are smaller or larger, and the desired effect is achieved either locally or more globally.

Cranial Techniques

Compression of the Fourth Ventricle: Technique CV4

This technique is a foundation of craniosacral approaches in osteopathy. It can be used alone or in a combination or protocol of other osteopathic cranial techniques when treating pregnant patients.

According to Greenman, "The CV4 technique seems to enhance the movement of fluid, changes the rhythm of the diaphragms, and increases the temperature of the suboccipital region."[3] Upledger and Vredevoogd go further and believe that the technique affects diaphragm activity and autonomic control of respiration, and seems to relax the sympathetic nervous system to a significant degree.[4] Other researchers disagree.[5]

What is not in dispute is the effect it has on the patient, enabling her to relax and release general body tension. It is excellent in the first and second trimesters when she can lie supine, with her knees supported by pillows. In the last trimester, it is performed in the side-lying position to avoid undue pressure on the inferior vena cava.

Position of the patient

She lies on her back at an angle of approximately 45 degrees, but certainly not flat on her back for the reasons mentioned in Chapter 1. Her head and neck are supported by a pillow, and her knees by a pillow or bolster.

Position of the osteopath

He sits at the head of the treatment table, the arms resting on the table and the fingers interlaced in a bowl.

Ambition of the technique

It can be used at the start of the treatment process as an evaluative technique, during the treatment as a fluidic technique, or at the end of the treatment to relax the patient as a finishing technique.

It has been postulated that compression of the fourth ventricle and use of the still point techniques (see later) have an effect on the release of specific brain hormones such as serotonin, dopamine, and even endorphins.

Application of the technique

The patient lies down so that the osteopath's thenar eminences are lateral to the external occipital

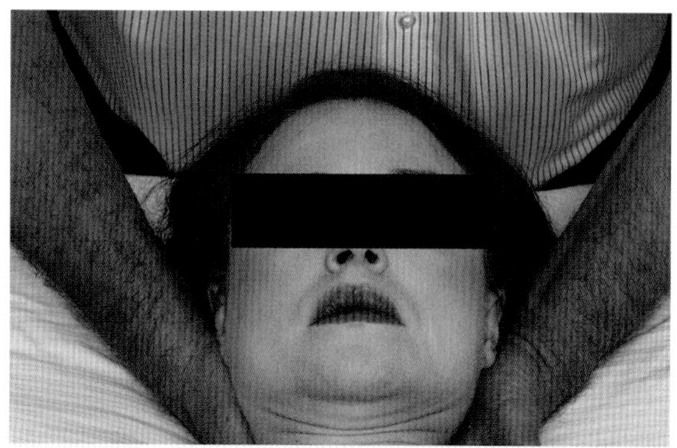

Fig 4.7
The CV4 technique.

masses but medial to the lower angles of the occiput (Fig 4.7).

The osteopath relaxes his own breathing and tunes in to the very gentle but subtle rhythm of the patient's cranial motion, otherwise known as the primary respiratory mechanism (PRM) or cranial rhythm. If the osteopath is inexperienced in the use of cranial techniques, pregnancy is an ideal time to try to palpate the PRM, as the amount of fluid in the body acts as an amplifier of the cranial rhythm. For many practitioners, pregnancy is the first time that they palpate an easily interpreted expansion and contraction of the membranes inside the skull.

There is a flexion and an extension phase. During the extension phase, or the rotation or exhalation phase, the osteopath begins to apply very slight but persistent pressure medially through his thenar eminences, exaggerating the normal cranial motion of the phase.

This pressure should not be generated by hand action but by contraction of the deep flexor muscles of the forearm. The slight "compressive" pressure is maintained and the cranial rhythm slows with each successive cycle, until no motion is perceived at all. This is what is known as a still point, and it can be accompanied by an alteration in the patient's breathing pattern. The still point can be held until a feeling of expansion occurs within the tissues. This might be after 20 or 30 seconds or may take a few minutes; the osteopath must learn to be patient and listen to the tissue dialog. At this point, the "compressive" force is allowed to release and a feeling of warmth occurs under the hands.

A variation of the above might be to hold the end of extension between the hands with absolute minimum pressure, until the cranial rhythm is felt to slow and stop. The hands are now gently removed, as the technique has achieved its aim of relaxing the patient.

The osteopath waits until he feels a gentle expansion again; then, following the expansion to its maximum amplitude, he follows the cycle to release once more. The maneuver is repeated a number of times, and with each cycle the relaxation of the tissues becomes deeper and breathing calmer and more regular.

If the patient is in her third trimester, putting her supine is probably not a good idea because of the weight of the gravid uterus on the inferior vena cava. Craniosacral techniques performed in the side-lying position are better at this time. The aim of the technique is the same. For details, see Chapter 6 on techniques below the diaphragm.

Techniques for the Ribs and Diaphragm

During all the stages of pregnancy, the ribs and diaphragm are much easier to treat if the patient is in the sitting position. This is especially the case in the third trimester, when having her supine for any length of time is contraindicated, as we have seen. During the first trimester, if she experiences nausea and vomiting, the intercostal muscles and the diaphragm can be very tense and uncomfortable (see Chapter 6 for treatment

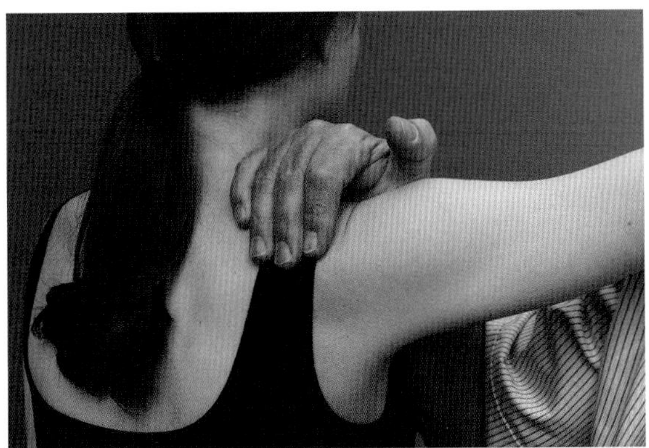

Fig 4.11
The position of the osteopath's upper hand, seen from behind the patient.

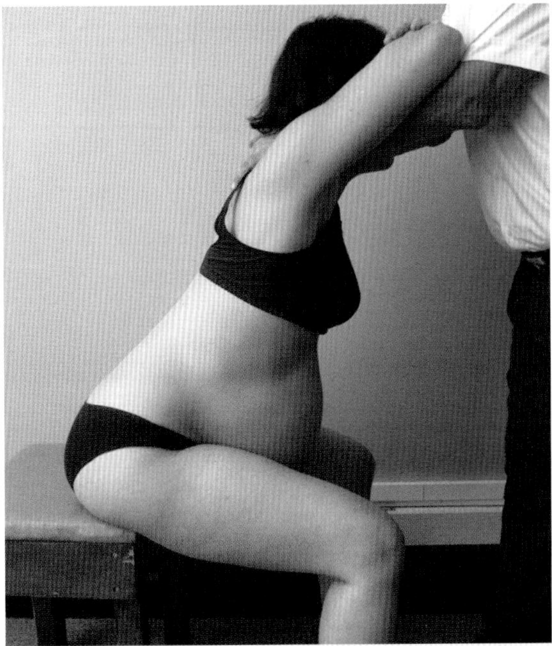

Fig 4.12
Patient sitting for flexion and extension of the thoracic spine.

Sitting Stretch Technique for the Thoracic Spine into Flexion and Extension

This is a particularly good technique for the upper ribs and thoracic spine, and the "pump handle" movements.

Position of the patient

She sits on the treatment table or on a chair. She needs to sit in the middle of the chair for this technique, and not too near the front or back (Fig 4.12). She folds her arms and firmly holds each biceps. She rests her head on her arms.

Position of the osteopath

The osteopath is in front of the patient. He stands with one foot either side of hers.

Ambition of the technique

This technique is similar to the previous one, except that this is used to mobilize, articulate, and stretch the ligaments and capsules of the upper thoracic vertebrae and ribs in an antero-posterior direction. The techniques are designed to stretch the intercostal muscles and to stretch the diaphragm at the costal margin. This can also be used as a longitudinal stretch technique for the long spinal muscles and as a semi-traction technique for the whole spine.

Application of the technique

The osteopath threads his hands under her arms and rests them on the upper thoracic spine in a wedge shape, with the fingers forming an arrowhead.

If one specific segment in the upper thoracic spine is found to be stiff and lesioned, the osteopath can use this position for an articulation or short lever ligament stretch technique. The transverse processes are fixed by the osteopath's index and

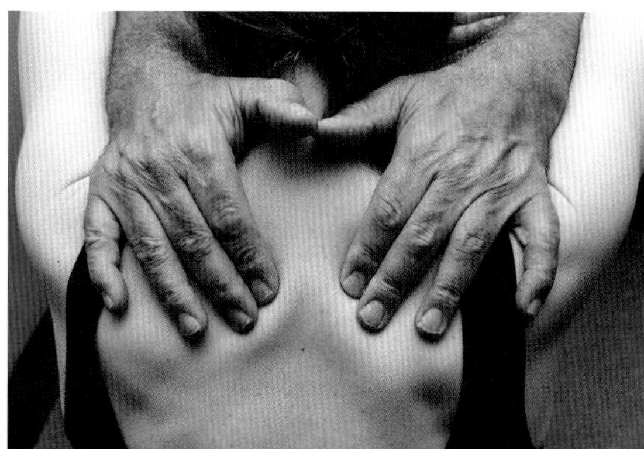

Fig 4.13
The index and middle fingers fix the transverse processes.

middle fingers (Fig 4.13), and the segment is taken into a gentle figure of eight movement, the center of the figure eight being the spinous process of the vertebra concerned.

If the technique is being performed with the ambition of stretching the upper ribs and their interspaces, or as a whole-spine stretch, the osteopath stands in the same position as before, but now he performs a forward–backward movement as he transfers his body weight from the front to the back foot. As he reaches the end of the movement, he lifts his arms, creating an arc of motion as the upper thoracic spine falls into extension (Fig 4.14). The 1st to 3rd ribs are mobilized in the same way but the focus is at the costal transverse junction.

Technique to Stretch the Periphery of the Diaphragm, Performed from Behind

Position of the patient

The patient sits on the treatment table, with her feet over the edge and with her hands on her hips, keeping them there at all times.

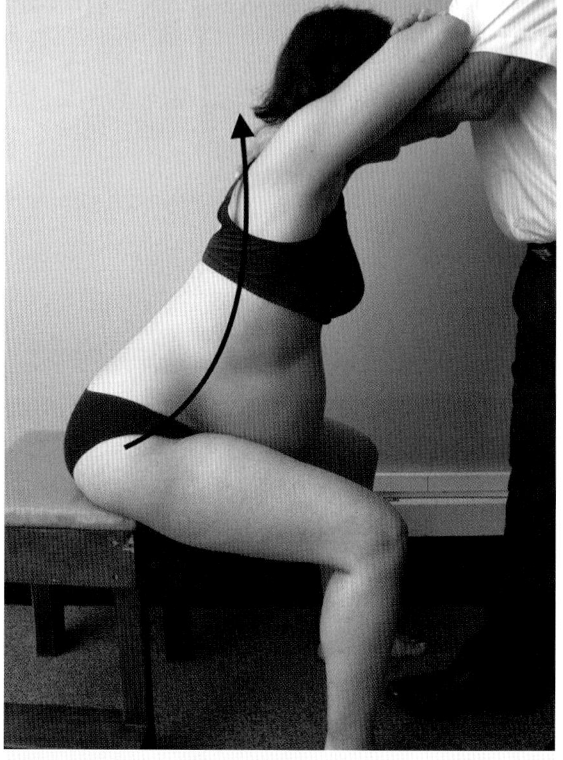

Fig 4.14
The osteopath lifts his arms to create an arc of movement in the antero-posterior plane.

Position of the osteopath

The osteopath stands behind the patient, with one foot in front of the other as before.

Ambition of the technique

The technique is used to stretch the diaphragm laterally to enhance breathing, and towards the end of pregnancy when she is particularly dyspneic due to the height of the fundus under the dome of the diaphragm, to allow it to drop back down into the abdominal cavity.

Application of the technique

The osteopath threads his hands though her arms and they come to rest around the costal margin laterally, with the ulnar borders under the breasts (Fig 4.15).

Warning

A word of caution is important here. The osteopath's hands are very near to the breast tissue. Quite apart from being tender, this a sensitive area as far as ethics and patients' comfort are concerned. The osteopath must explain very clearly to the patient what he intends to do and why, in order to ensure that she is clearly informed as to the ambition of the technique and is in a position to give her informed oral consent. If English is not her native language, then use of a suitable adult interpreter must be considered. Once the explanation has been given and accepted, then the technique can proceed.

The patient is instructed to take a deep breath. As she does so, the osteopath uses his hands to contact the patient's costal margin, gently reaching under it and leaning backwards in an extension movement of his own spine. His hands and elbows move in a lateral direction, pulling the costal margins in a lateral direction (Fig 4.16).

As she reaches the maximum of inspiration, she is asked to hold her breath for 3 or 4 seconds; then, as she breathes out, the osteopath uses the thenar eminences of his hands to push down gently but firmly on the sides of her ribs, until she reaches the point of maximum exhalation (Fig 4.17).

It is the movement into extension which is important in this technique, as it literally pulls the diaphragm open at the costal margins and the intercostal interdigitations where the diaphragm is inserted.

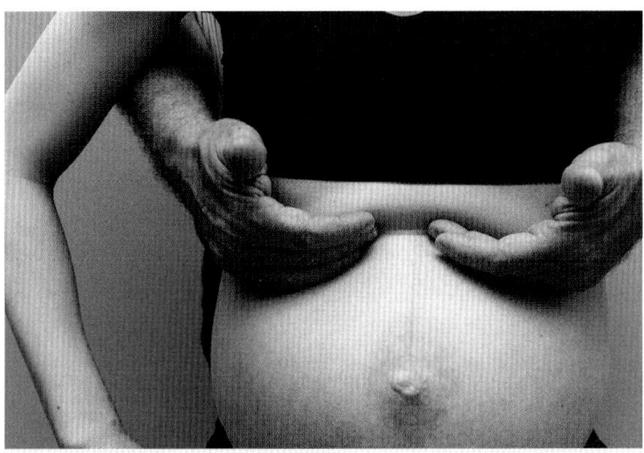

Fig 4.15
The osteopath's hands on the costal margin under the breasts.

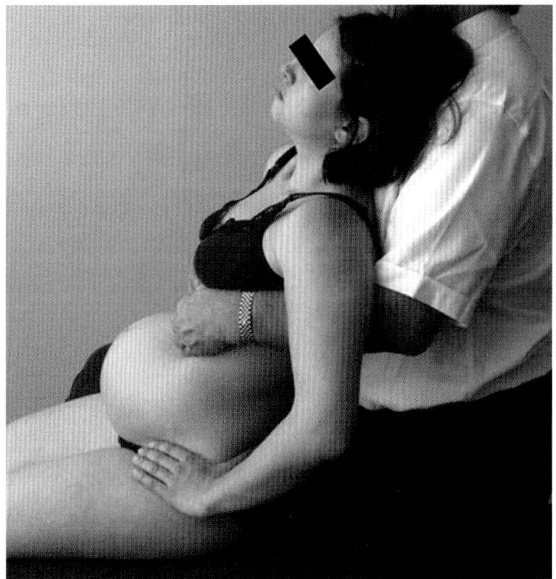

Fig 4.16
The movement into extension opens the ribs and allows the diaphragm to descend.

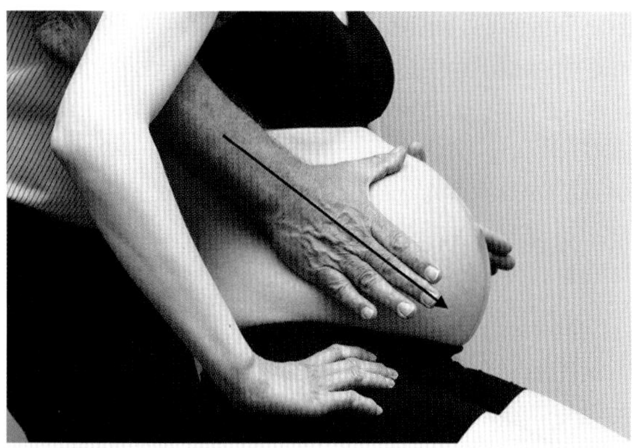

Fig 4.17
As the patient breathes out, the osteopath exerts gentle pressure with the palms of the hands in a downward direction, towards the pelvis but not compressing the abdomen. N.B. The pressure here is on the lower ribs, not the abdomen.

The effects of this technique on the position of the gravid uterus in late pregnancy are dramatic, with the patient feeling immediate relief and regaining the ability to take a deep breath.

Myofascial Release for the Thorax and the Mediastinum

As mentioned in the previous chapter, the mediastinum contains fascia and ligamentous tissues, and, in the thorax, is part of a continuous chain of tissue that extends from the top of the head down to the feet. There are many techniques to release the fascia in this region. In pregnancy, however, it is better to have the patient sitting, in order, once again, to reduce the pressure of the gravid uterus on the inferior vena cava. Also, because the ambition of this technique is to release tension within the mediastinum that might be impeding venous return from the lower extremities, it is better to perform it with the patient sitting than supine. Lastly, sitting techniques give her a chance to breathe as, under the effects of gravity, the weight of the gravid uterus naturally gravitates towards the pelvis.

Position of the patient

The patient sits at the end of the treatment table, with her feet over the edge. She is upright, with the spine in a neutral position and her hands in her lap (Fig 4.18).

Position of the osteopath

The osteopath stands at her right side, one hand on her sternum and the other on her upper thoracic spine.

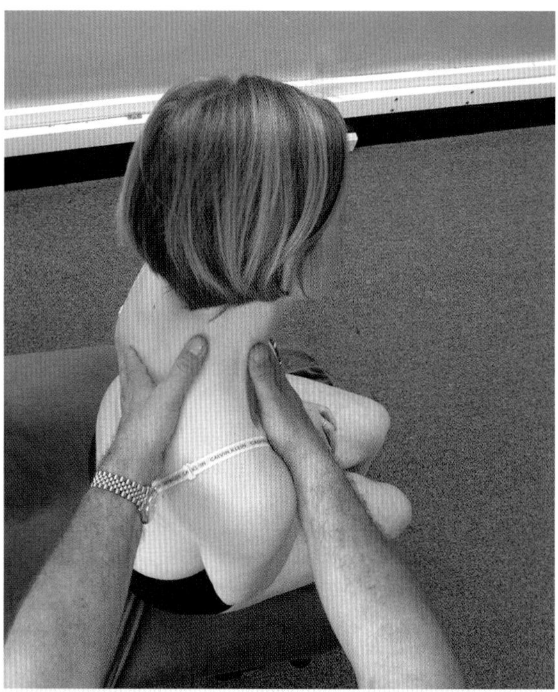

Fig 4.18
A myofascial release for the thorax and the mediastinum.

 **Warning**

The same note of caution regarding ethics and the breast tissues (mentioned earlier) will apply here too.

Ambition of the technique

The ambition of the technique is to normalize tension within the mediastinum by balancing the fascial tensions and creating a point of minimal tension (also known as the still point). The heart, pericardium, lungs, and great vessels will also reach their point of minimal tension and ease as the technique is performed.

Application of the technique

The normal axis of the heart runs from the right shoulder to the left hip, and the osteopath's hands must reflect this by being angled in the same axis. If need be, the treatment table must be very low to allow this to happen, or the patient can sit on a chair.

This technique is used for patients who suffer from dyspnea in pregnancy, where the gravid uterus is pushing up under the diaphragm and compressing the mediastinum and its contents. The mediastinum is released using a myofascial technique in this instance.

The osteopath is going to use the usual vectors of flexion/extension/rotation left and right, and side-bending left and right. In addition, he will add the vectors of translation of anterior–posterior motion and lateral motion, and a final vector of cephalad motion (towards her head) and caudad motion (towards her sacrum).

The osteopath balances his weight on his heels, so as not to transfer the weight to his hands. He should think of his belt buckle as being the center point of motion with this approach. Very gently allowing the flexion/extension parameter to enter his consciousness, he tries to perceive which vector is dominant: that is, which of the two vectors of motion the tissue between his hands prefers to move in. He holds that vector and adds the next vector of rotation to it, then side-bending, and so on. He stacks each vector of ease onto the next, and when he has each of the ease directions or vectors in place, he holds the point of minimal tension for around 90 seconds. At this time, he should perceive warmth or softening in the tissues under his fingers as the tension within the myofascial chain in the thorax releases. For more information on these techniques and an explanation of how they are thought to work, the reader is referred to Leon Chaitow's excellent books on the subject.[6,7]

The technique described here is one part of the mechanism whereby tensions and torsions within the mediastinum are addressed. Figure 4.19 shows the whole of the fascial chain that involves the pericardium. If your history and evaluation reveal tension within the pericardial space as the focus of your attention, then you should use cranial techniques at the base of the skull and then other myofascial techniques along the chain before addressing the pericardium directly. Structural techniques on the upper ribs, the clavicles and sternum, and the diaphragm where the pericardium is attached also form an important part of the rationale behind treatment in this region. Tension within the mediastinum will increase the pressure on the heart and the great vessels within the thorax, and thus have a negative effect on venous return.[8,9]

By working not just on the fascia of the mediastinum but also on the fascia within the neck and the base of the skull, and down into the abdomen and beyond, the osteopath uses a global appreciation of the effects of the technique in treating the whole patient

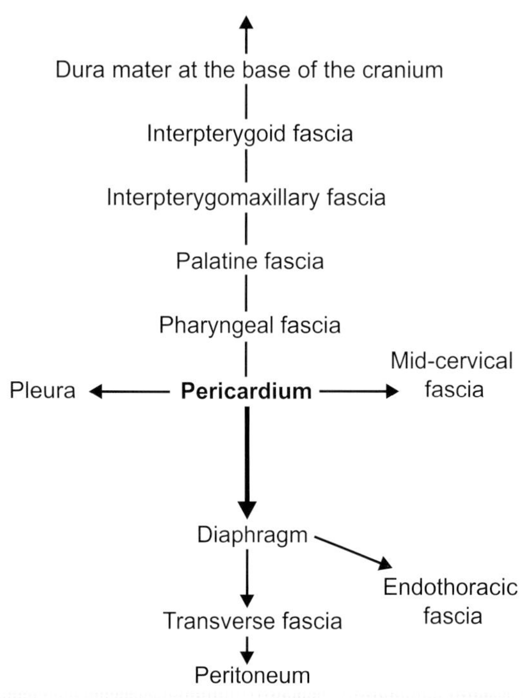

Fig 4.19

The fascial connections of the pericardium.
(After Paoletti.) ©Sully Editions.

and not just the part that reflects symptoms. In this holistic approach to the pregnant patient, osteopathy anticipates changes and encourages physiological adaptations within the cardiovascular and respiratory systems to take place, reducing any adverse physiological states that may arise at this time.

High-Velocity, Low-Amplitude Techniques

High-velocity, low-amplitude (HVLA) or high-velocity thrust (HVT) techniques are perfectly acceptable to patients during pregnancy. They should all be short-lever or minimal-lever techniques done within the mid-range, and never at the end of range, because the actions of the pregnancy hormones on the muscles and ligaments can weaken them. Adverse reactions to treatment include muscle spasm and soreness as the tissue reacts by contracting or even bruising. A simple way to avoid this is always to listen to the tissues you are treating. If there is unexpected resistance as you build your levers, then stop and unwind the tissue. Never force the issue, thinking that it is tight just because she is nervous. Tissues change rapidly during pregnancy, and if you lose your concentration and go onto automatic pilot you will miss the change and overtreat.

In the last trimester, especially, it is best practice to treat the cervical and thoracic spine and ribs in the sitting position.

Warning

A word of caution is needed here. The vertebral arteries run in the canal inside the cervical vertebrae. In both the pregnant and the non-pregnant patient, the usual clinical tests for vertebral artery compression are mandatory before applying the techniques. These involve extension and rotation maneuvers, which are provocation tests to stress the vertebral artery in the canal before the technique is applied. Any vertigo or discomfort felt by the patient when the head is held in this position for just a few seconds means that there is an absolute contraindication to an HVT technique. If need be, the patient should be referred for appropriate imaging of the upper cervical spine, including a computed tomographic (CT) scan, when she has had her baby. From the history, if the patient reports episodes of vertigo with her head held in extension, then again it is wise to proceed only with extreme caution, in order to avoid damaging the vulnerable vertebral artery. If there is any doubt as to safety, an HVT technique is never the technique of choice.

The thrust techniques can be applied to the upper cervical, mid-cervical and lower cervical spine by changing the hand position and the contact point.

Position of the patient

The patient sits with her legs over the side of the treatment table spine, holding them in a neutral position.

Position of the osteopath

The osteopath stands facing her, by her side.

Ambition of the technique

The aim is to break facet fixation which is causing muscular hypertonia and stasis. Also, any viscerosomatic reflex restrictions are dealt with in this way.

Application of the technique

For a right-sided lesion, the applicator is the left index finger behind the right transverse process at the level concerned (Fig 4.20).

As the cervical spine is primarily a rotation column, most of the HVT techniques will be done in a rotation direction.

The maneuver proceeds, with the vectors leading to a minimal lever build-up. The thrust is given with the smallest force and minimal amplitude needed to achieve mobilization of the joint in a rotation direction. It is poor technique to pull the transverse process or the patient's head into rotation. The rotation is used along with other vectors and levers to focus the attention down to the level of the applicator, and thus the lesion, with the minimum use of force. The thrust is a shockwave through the

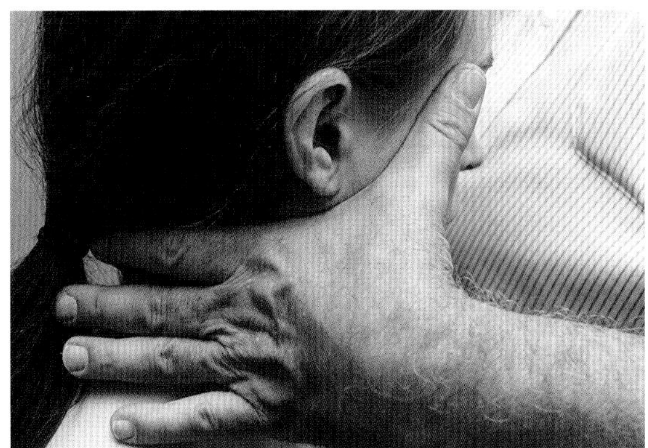

Fig 4.20
A high-velocity, low-amplitude (HVLA) thrust technique with the patient sitting.

tissues in the direction of the primary lever, rotation, to produce the effect of cavitation. The force comes from a momentary contraction of the osteopath's pectoral muscles, using a simultaneous isometric contraction of his diaphragm.

Variation of the angle of force means that this technique is suitable for most levels in the cervical spine down to and including C6.

Beyond this, it involves more of a side-bending maneuver or a force directed downwards towards the cervicodorsal junction.

Cradle Hold Technique for the Cervical Spine

Position of the patient

The patient is supine, with her head resting on two pillows. She will not be supine for very long, and therefore this technique is considered safe in pregnancy.

The cradle hold (Fig 4.21) is a very useful variation on the usual chin hold, which can be difficult to

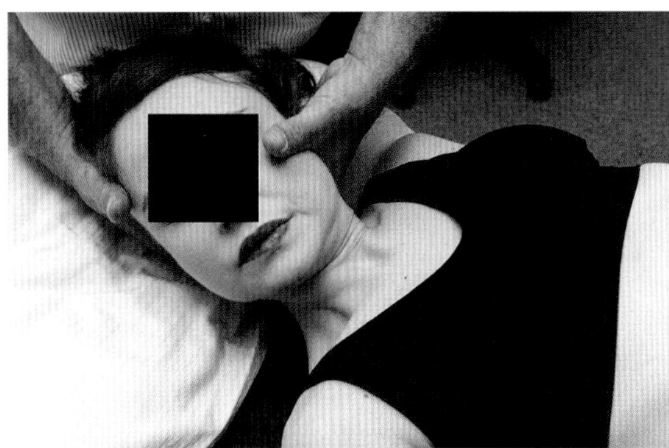

Fig 4.21
The cradle hold technique for the cervical spine.

stabilize in pregnancy due to the action of the hormone relaxin, which makes ligaments softer. This gives a false impression of hypermobility. Keeping the chin flexed on the chest opens the posterior structures, including the foramina where the cervical nerves exit and the space available for the spinal cord. This avoids any undue compression on these neurological structures.

Position of the osteopath

The osteopath stands at the head of the table.

Ambition of the technique

The aim is to break facet fixation at one segment in the cervical spine, using the minimum of force and leverage for safety.

Application of the technique

The osteopath puts the patient's head onto his abdomen, with her chin almost touching her chest, allowing his fingertips to contact the articular pillars behind the sternocleidomastoid muscle on each side.

Using a lateral gliding motion of his hips and knees, he palpates some movement at each segment as it descends down the cervical column, feeling for restriction in motion and tissue tension. He is feeling for a blocking of motion caused by facet joint restriction. If he finds this restriction, he slides the index finger of the applicator hand down behind the articular pillar until the contact point, which is the first metacarpophalangeal joint, behind the joint. If this is on the right side of the patient's neck, he will be using his right hand to apply thrust.

He contacts the occipital bone with the palm of his hand and supports the weight of the head with his other hand by cupping the opposite ear. It is poor technique to cover the ear, as patients dislike this feeling.

Keeping these vectors, the osteopath takes a broad step to the side, almost sitting on the corner of the table. Thus, his center of gravity is in the center of the technique, creating sufficient lever to do the job, but not excess lever which will block the joint. He should aim to keep her chin on her chest throughout the technique to maintain her cervical flexion and to ensure that it is safe to open the vertebral artery. Therefore, this is a minimal lever technique. The thrust is performed as a combination of rapid pronation of the operator's contact point hand, and a similar supination of the supporting hand.

Sitting Technique for the Cervicodorsal Spine

Position of the patient

The patient sits with her legs over the side of the treatment table, as before (Fig 4.22).

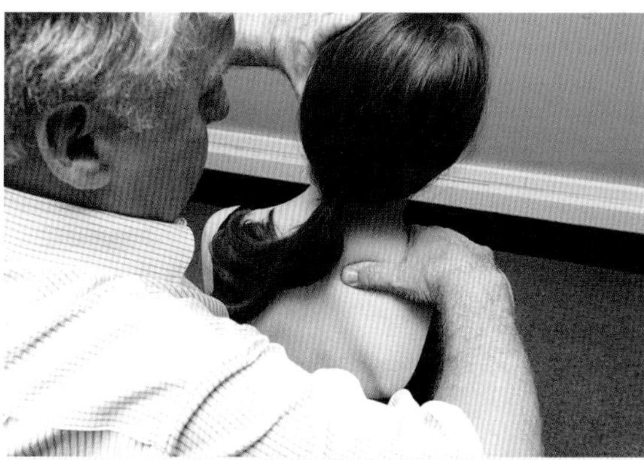

Fig 4.22
HVLA technique to the cervicodorsal junction, with the patient sitting.

Position of the osteopath

He stands behind her.

Ambition of the technique

The aim is to break facet fixation at the cervicodorsal junction or the first rib.

Application of the technique

The osteopath's left hand produces side-bending reverse rotation and some compression, as before. The right thumb is applied to the spinous process of the lesioned segment and the impulse is towards the patient's left axilla. A variation involves placing the thumb so as to contact the transverse process of T1 for the first rib lesion.

Sitting "Lift-Off" Technique

This technique has been part of the osteopath's range since manipulation was first used therapeutically. It is gentle yet specific, designed to break the facet fixation at the point of the lesioned segment on the side concerned.

Position of the patient

The patient sits with her legs over the side of the treatment table (Fig 4.23).

Position of the osteopath

The osteopath stands behind her, with feet apart and one foot behind the other.

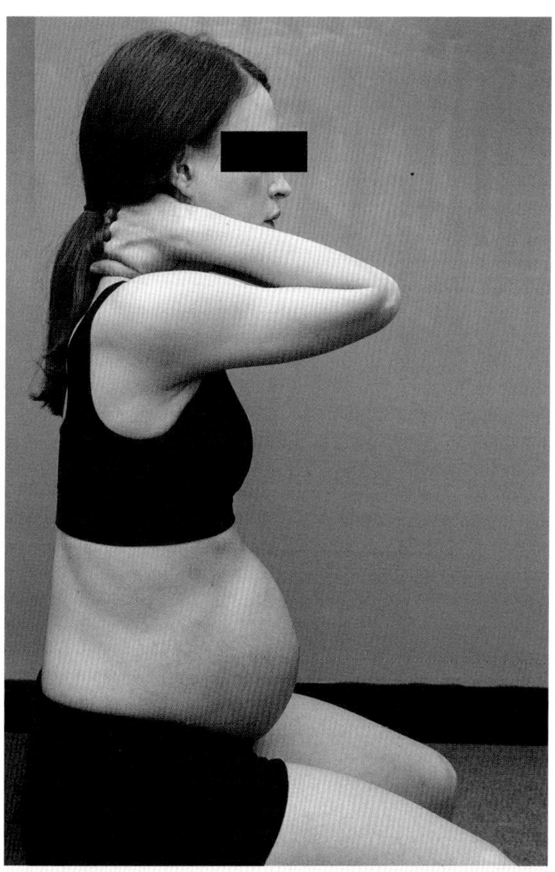

Fig 4.23
Classic position for the "lift-off" technique.

Ambition of the technique

The aim is to "lift" the vertebra above away from the vertebra below, releasing the lesioned facet joint on the side where it has been restricted.

Application of the technique

A number of modifications are necessary because of the patient's pregnancy.

Classically, either the patient has her hands interlaced behind her neck, crossing the elbows together, or the palms of the hands are on the shoulders. The problem here is that the enlarging breast tissue is tender and she will not like compression of the breasts towards her own chest wall. Also, if her breast expansion is sizeable, then it might be difficult for her to interlace her fingers behind the neck, especially for the upper thoracic vertebrae.

Students are traditionally taught to bring the elbows together, so that any force will drive the impulse through the arms and shoulders to the lesioned segment. In pregnancy, the tissues are relatively hypermobile due to the hormonal influences of estrogen and relaxin. The technique can therefore be modified by gently pulling the elbows apart and placing the hands high on the shoulders. From the front, a "W" shape can be seen, not a "V" (Figs 4.24 and 4.25). This has the added advantage of distracting the scapulae and, as she moves into flexion, bringing the vertebra to the point of tension and further stabilizing the technique.

The osteopath uses a pad over his sternum or angle of his rib (Fig 4.26). This does two things: firstly, it helps to focus the force on a specific level of the thoracic spine in lesion, and secondly, in the case of female osteopaths, it protects their own breast tissue from repeated trauma and thus the potential for injury.

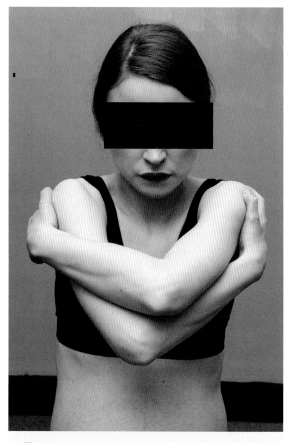

Fig 4.24
The "V" of the elbows.

Taking hold of the bottom elbow by cupping it with his interlaced fingers, the operator applies the vectors of compression, a small amount of traction, and small amounts of side-bending and reverse rotation to localize the forces to the point of application (Fig 4.27).

He asks the patient to move gently counter-clockwise in a circular fashion, from flexion into extension and side-bending. This is easier if he takes a very small step to the side simultaneously. If she bends to the left, he will move to the right, and vice versa. As she comes around the circle,

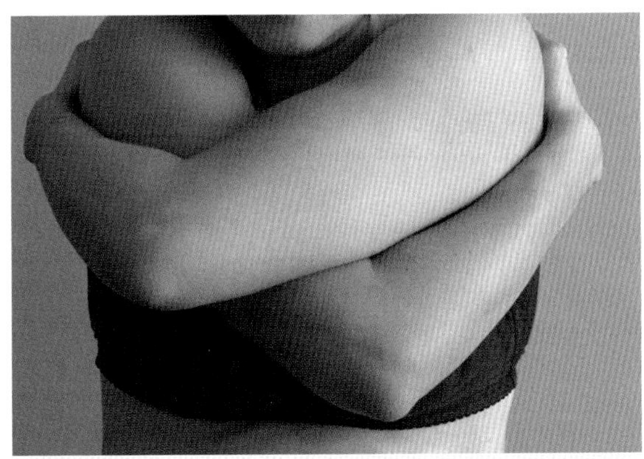

Fig 4.25
The "W" of the elbows.

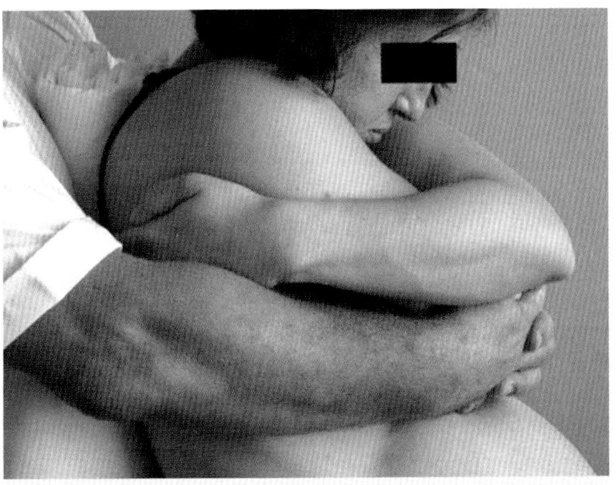

Fig 4.26
Use of a pad between the osteopath and the patient helps to focus the tension, as well as protecting the osteopath from injury.

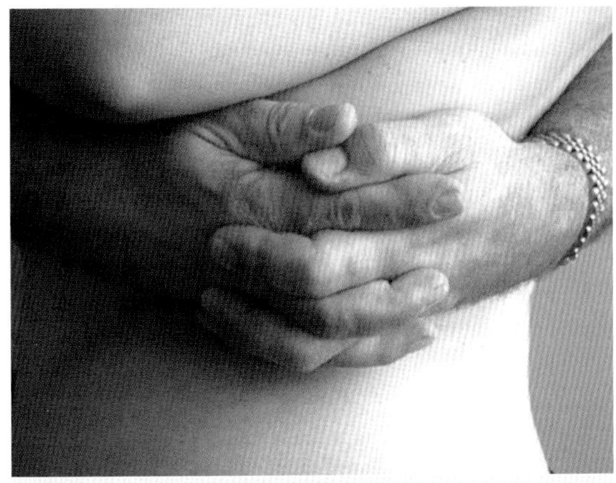

Fig 4.27
Cupping the bottom elbow.

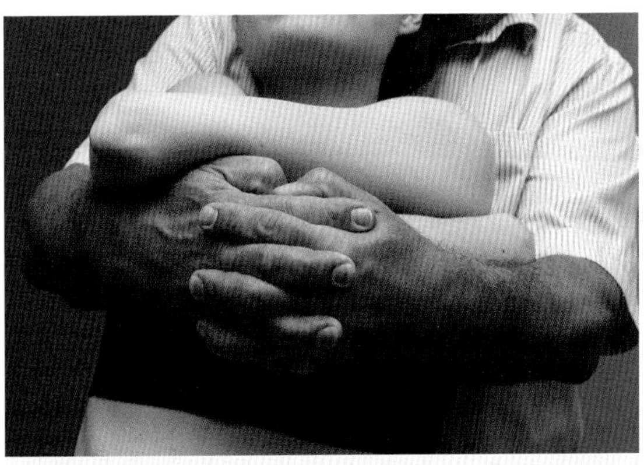

Fig 4.28
Palpating through the pad to find the point of maximum tension between all of the vectors before applying the impulse.

moving into extension, he will feel the tension under the pad (Fig 4.28). He allows her to drop into flexion and neutral side-bending as she moves back into flexion. The whole process therefore involves flexion, side-bending, and reverse rotation, moving back into the start position two or three times. The circle, by nature, is quite small. As the movements are repeated and the momentum builds, so the osteopath applies a force through the elbows directly towards his chest with impulse and into extension (Fig 4.29). The timing is essential because the thrust is applied exactly as the movement into extension brings the force to his pad.

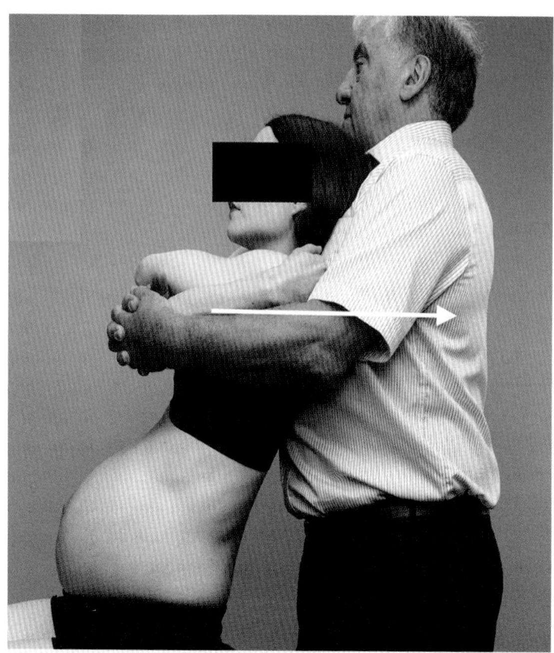

Fig 4.29
The force is directed straight back towards the osteopath with a bilateral pectoral contraction.

For first rib lesions, the process is very similar, save that the lesion will be at the level of the relevant costotransverse joint, and so the applicator will be more lateral over this joint and not at the facet joints.

Modification of the Supine Dorsal Thrust Technique (Dog Technique)

Position of the patient

The patient lies supine, with the head resting on pillows. She has her hands and arms crossed, with the elbows separated as before.

Position of the osteopath

The osteopath stands at the side of the treatment table, on the opposite side to the lesion.

Ambition of the technique

The aim is to break facet fixation between vertebral segments in the thoracic spine.

Application of the technique

Once again, this is a classic element in the osteopath's armory, which needs to be modified in light of the pregnancy.

Firstly, because of the action of her pregnancy hormones on the lower esophageal sphincter, she will invariably suffer gastric reflux. Any undue pressure on her chest will push down on the abdomen and may well provoke reflux, so it should be avoided. Secondly, there is a problem with tender breast tissue, as mentioned earlier. Thirdly, the hand position of the osteopath must be adapted: classically, the "fist" grip is used and is very effective at localizing pressure where you want it. Here, we use an open hand technique with the wrist held in slight extension, to minimize the uncomfortable pressure against the spinous processes (Fig 4.30).

The open hand is placed under the patient, with the wrist in extension and the thenar eminence over the transverse process of the joint in lesion. If the lesioned segment is on the right, he will be on the left, facing towards her head, and vice versa.

The upper hand rests on her forearms. A pillow can be placed under her arms to limit the pressure on her breasts. Once again, female osteopaths may use a pillow placed between the patient's

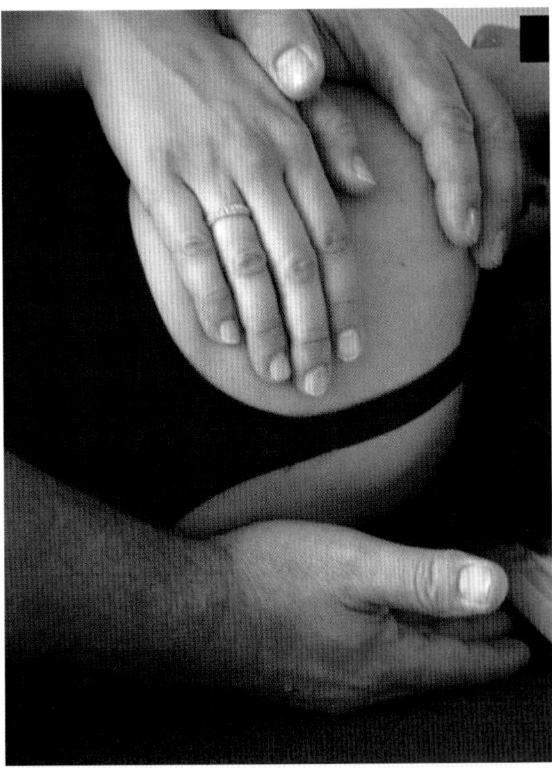

Fig 4.30
The open hand variation for the dog technique.

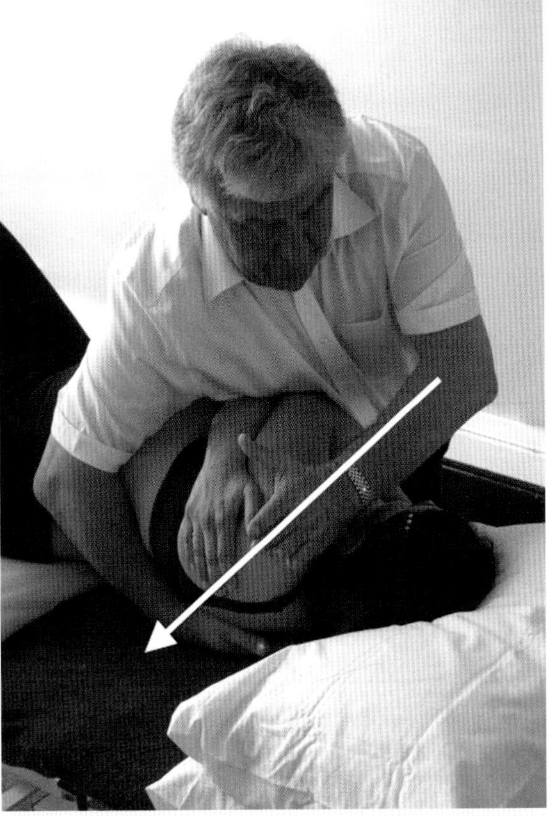

Fig 4.31
The cephalad forearm. The arrow shows the direction of the force applied. It passes through the shoulder and does not compress the patient's chest.

elbows and their own breasts to minimize any potential trauma. Hydraulic tables can be adjusted to be a little lower to help accommodate the extra height.

The osteopath uses his cephalad forearm to apply the vectors of flexion and extension and reverse rotation, which are held by his chest (Fig 4.31). Then, as he moves the patient's spine into extension, he uses the patient's shoulder to gently apply the downward impulse towards the table in flexion and compression, at the same time as the hand under the patient applies a gentle impulse towards her head.

The two impulses need to be timed exactly to occur together, one from above and one from below, and thus gap the facet joint with the minimum possible but maximum effective force. Certainly, because the force is applied through the shoulder instead of straight down through the chest, it is much better tolerated by the patient.

References

1. Clark Kennedy AE. *The Patient and His Disease*, vol. 1. 1945.
2. Hartman L. *A Handbook of Osteopathic Technique*. Nelson Thornes, 2006.
3. Greenman P. *Principles of Manual Medicine*. Lippincott, Williams and Wilkins, 2003.
4. Upledger J, Vredevoogd J. *Craniosacral Therapy*. Eastland Press, 1983.
5. Milnes K, Moran R. Physiological effects of a CV4 cranial osteopathic technique on autonomic nervous system function: a preliminary investigation. *Int J Osteopathic Med*. 2007 Mar;10(1):8–17.
6. Chaitow L. *Cranial Manipulation: Theory and Practice*. Churchill Livingstone, 1999.
7. Chaitow L. *Positional Release Techniques*. Churchill Livingstone, 1996.
8. St-Louis J, Brochu M. The cardiovascular paradox of pregnancy. Med Sci (Paris). 2007 Nov;23(11):944–9.
9. Chesnutt AN. Physiology of normal pregnancy. Crit Care Clin. 2004 Oct;20(4):609–15.

Below the Diaphragm: Changes in Anatomy and Physiology During Pregnancy

5

Life is Motion and Motion is Life

The diagnosis and treatment of motion occur at a macro- and micro-level, and are the essence of the osteopathic contact. In every system, we try to understand the difference between healthy tissue and tissues that are different from normal by perceiving change that comes with palpating altered physiology and comparing it to that which we perceive as normal. According to Caroline Stone, motion relates to physiology.[1]

The presence or absence of motion is often used as a defining characteristic within medicine, as, for example, when pediatricians apply the APGAR score after a child is born. They assess the heart rate via the pulse, the breathing rate and effort via motion in the chest, and the degree of activity or motion in the baby in general, together with muscle tone. All of these factors use motion as an indicator of normality in that child.

The process of autoregulation ensures that the organism minimizes cell damage by allowing motion only within preset physiological parameters.

All pathology of the viscera results in visceral restrictions. When this happens, the viscera in question are no longer freely mobile in their cavity but are partially fixed to another structure. The body is forced to compensate for this situation, which leads to a functional problem and, eventually, if compensation is inadequate, to a structural problem. Treatment consists of stimulation of the viscera in order to restore primary physiological mobility and motility.[2]

In a paper published in 2002, Chegini stated that, whether they are induced by infection, inflammation, ischemia, or surgical injury, peritoneal adhesions are the leading cause of pelvic pain, bowel obstruction, and infertility.[3] He said at the time that the mechanisms underlying the predisposition to peritoneal adhesions, as well as their site specificity, were completely unknown. In 2008, Wiseman published a paper that looked at the etiology of adhesion formation in relation to other diagnosed pathologies.[4] In a survey of 687 women in the USA, he found that 85% of patients reviewed had abdominal or pelvic adhesions, 69% chronic abdominal or pelvic pain, 55% irritable bowel syndrome (IBS), 44% recurrent bowel obstruction, 40% endometriosis, and 29% interstitial cystitis. The relationship of these pathologies to visceral adhesions showed that these diseases or dysfunctions are such that normal mobility of the organs is profoundly disturbed. Liakakos et al. looked at the etiology, pathophysiology, and clinical significance of peritoneal adhesions.[5] Unfortunately, there is no available marker to predict the occurrence or the extent and severity of adhesions preoperatively. Ischemia has been thought to be the most important insult that leads to adhesion development.

Little work has been done to determine the effect of adhesions on the ability of the subdiaphragmatic organs to move away from the advancing, rising uterus during pregnancy. If there are any scars or adhesions pre-pregnancy, do they tear and cause visceral bleeding or pain? Do they prevent normal organ displacement and thus lead to compression and venous drainage compromise? One thing is for sure: the rise of the growing uterus will simply push the organs to one side as it attempts to create space for itself and for the growing fetus. In 2008, Sulaiman et al. looked at the growth of nerve fibers into peritoneal adhesions in mice, providing the first direct evidence for the growth of sensory nerve fibers within abdominal visceral adhesions.[6] They postulated, in other words, that if the adhesions are profound, they will be painful in themselves, as well as causing visceral pain because of the damage they can do.

In each of the visceral systems to be found below the diaphragm, changes have to take place. Pregnancy is a physiological state, not a pathological one; therefore, these changes are usually reversible once the baby is born. Some of the changes are silent, while others will cause symptoms in themselves. A thorough grasp of the adaptations in organ systems demanded by pregnancy is essential if we are to understand what a normal pregnancy entails. When we are taking the medical part of the pregnancy case history, an understanding of normal and abnormal physiology will give us an appreciation of what is normal below the diaphragm in pregnancy. A cognizance of normality starts with an understanding of the potential symptoms in each system.

The Gastrointestinal System and Diet in Pregnancy

Unlike in liver disease, there are no gastrointestinal diseases specifically caused by pregnancy. However, pregnancy may complicate most gastrointestinal dysfunctions, particularly gastro-esophageal reflux and irritable bowel syndrome. In addition, gastro-intestinal symptoms are extremely common in the pregnant patient. Symptoms such as nausea, vomiting, and dyspepsia occur in 52–90% of all patients.[7] Most of these symptoms are a manifestation of normal altered physiology and occur both functionally and anatomically. These changes may cause new symptoms, make pre-existing disease worse, or may mask potentially serious disease. The osteopath must be able to distinguish whether the symptoms are those of normal pregnancy or potentially stem from a life-threatening complication, such as peptic ulcer.

Changes in Physiology of the Gastrointestinal Tract during Pregnancy

Pregnancy has many effects on digestion, and not all of them are positive. Progesterone relaxes smooth muscles in the gut walls. Gastric emptying and peristalsis are slowed in order to maximize the absorption of nutrients. The slow emptying of the stomach can, in consequence, lead to gastro-esophageal reflux. Constipation, if severe, can lead to referred pain to the lumbar spine or to the iliac fossa on one side or the other.

Appetite, diet, and weight gain

During pregnancy, nutritional requirements, including those for vitamins and minerals, are increased, and several maternal alterations take place to meet this demand. The mother's appetite usually increases, so that food intake is greater, although some women have a decreased appetite or experience nausea and vomiting. These symptoms may be related to relative levels of human chorionic gonadotrophin (HCG), which peak during the first trimester, but the exact mechanisms are unclear.

Appetite is stimulated in early pregnancy by the action of progesterone on the hypothalamus. In early pregnancy, the intake of food exceeds needs, which means that the excess is laid down as fat, to be used later as the fetus grows at the end of the pregnancy.

A woman's weight gain in pregnancy is ideally 2 kilos (4.4 pounds) in the first 20 weeks, followed by 0.5 kilos (1 pound) per week thereafter. This totals approximately 12 kilos (26.5 pounds) but that will depend on many factors, including pre-pregnancy weight, metabolism, pre-existing health, and morphology. Weight gain tends to be made up of the elements shown in Box 5.1.

The pregnant patient's food intake is important to maintain a healthy balanced diet during pregnancy.

BOX 5.1

The distribution of weight gain in pregnancy

Increased blood volume	1.3.kg	(2.9 lb)
Interstitial fluid	1.4–4.5 kg	(3.1–10 lb)
Breasts	0.4 kg	(0.9 lb)
Fat	3.5 kg	(7.7 lb)
Placenta	0.7 kg	(1.5 lb)
Fetus	3.4 kg	(7.5 lb)
Amniotic fluid	0.8 kg	(1.8 lb)
Uterus	1.0 kg	(2.2 lb)

BOX 5.2

Dietary changes needed in pregnancy

Calcium	+140%
Folate	+100%
Zinc	+30%
Iodine	+25%
Protein	+1%
Iron	+8%

She will need to radically alter the amounts of various foods, such as calcium, to counter the parasitic action of the fetus.

Suggested dietary changes needed to maintain a healthy pregnancy include the additions listed in Box 5.2.[8]

New technologies have reduced the need to prescribe specific diets for our patients during pregnancy. The author suggests to every patient that she conducts an internet search for diets that suit her during pregnancy. There are hundreds of internet sites that provide this information and she can look for ones that show which foods contain particular nutrients – calcium or iron, for example. In this way, she will eat what she herself wants, rather than trying to stick to a diet made up of foods that she does not like.

Nausea and vomiting

Nausea and vomiting are common in the first trimester of pregnancy and may be the first signs of pregnancy. Characteristically, they occur in the morning, but can go on all day. They usually peak between weeks 10 and 15 of gestation and resolve at approximately 20 weeks.

One theory suggests that they are caused by an imbalance in the glucose metabolism of early pregnancy because they usually disappear after week 18. Many of this author's patients have found it useful to take a glass of cola or any other sweet, fizzy drink to bed with them and leave it on the bedside table. Pregnant women usually need get up at night to urinate, so the suggestion is that they take the glass of sweet drink before they go back to sleep, when it will gone flat. When they wake up, their blood sugar will be higher, and they tend to feel less discomfort.

Nausea in pregnancy is more common among women who are primigravid, younger, less educated, and overweight.[9] In general, it is harmless to the mother and the fetus. When vomiting is prolonged and intractable, and interferes with nutrition and fluid intake, it is called hyperemesis gravidarum.[10] Vomiting may be severe enough to cause weight loss, which can lead to electrolyte abnormalities and acid–base disturbances requiring hospitalization. While nausea and vomiting occur in 50–90% of all pregnancies, hyperemesis gravidarum is not common and has an incidence ranging from 0.5–10 per 1000 pregnancies. Hyperemesis gravidarum is more common in nulliparous patients, twin pregnancies, and women younger than 25.[9] Nausea and vomiting in pregnancy can be secondary to other diseases, including appendicitis, pancreatitis, cholecystitis, and peptic ulcer disease. These disorders must not be overlooked because a delay in diagnosis could be serious.

The reason why nausea and vomiting are so common in pregnancy is still not understood, although many believe the hormonal changes that occur during pregnancy are most likely involved.[11] Estrogen may play a key role because patients with higher levels have more nausea and vomiting. However, nausea and vomiting are more prevalent in the first trimester, when estrogen levels are lower, compared with the third trimester, when estrogen levels are higher. Progesterone has also been implicated in slowing transit time in the bowel. The pathophysiological significance of progesterone inducing nausea and vomiting is limited by the fact that symptoms improve as term approaches and progesterone levels increase. Another hormone, HCG, which is present in its highest concentration during the first trimester, may be a more likely cause.

Morning sickness or nausea is still the subject of much debate in medicine. As irritating as morning sickness may be for pregnant women, it may protect embryos. Some doctors believe that the morning sickness of pregnancy is actually a sign of a healthy pregnancy, despite the discomfort that it brings.[12]

However, it is still unclear from the research whether morning sickness actually does help pregnancies succeed. If morning sickness were just the by-product of a healthy pregnancy, then it should accompany all healthy pregnancies, but it does not: while two-thirds of pregnant women experience morning sickness, the rest do not seem to suffer very much at all.

Morning sickness is usually triggered in specific circumstances, such as after eating certain meats and strong-tasting vegetables, which were historically likely to contain food-borne microbes or birth defect-inducing chemicals. It may also be sparked by alcohol and cigarette smoke. All this suggests that morning sickness serves a useful function, evolving to protect mothers and embryos from things that may be dangerous. Also, in women who experience morning sickness, symptoms peak precisely when embryonic organ development is most susceptible to chemical disruption, between week 6 and week 18 of pregnancy.

The relationship between *Helicobacter pylori* infection and increased vomiting has been extensively investigated in pregnancy, but the results again are inconclusive.[13]

The treatment of nausea and vomiting in pregnancy depends on the severity of the symptoms and ranges from changes in dietary habits to hospitalization. For mild nausea and vomiting, a change of diet may be all that is needed. Conventionally, antiemetics should be avoided in the first trimester. Because of its relative safety, vitamin B6 has frequently been used. Vitamin B6 administered at a dose of 25 mg orally every 8 hours improved severe nausea and decreased vomiting significantly in a double-blind, placebo-controlled study. Ginger and acupressure may also be effective; however, if the symptoms continue, the patient needs consultant care.[14]

The Mouth, Esophagus, and Stomach

The mouth and esophagus are dealt with here as they form part of the digestive system, though they are not, of course, situated below the diaphragm.

There is increased vascularity and a tendency to bleeding, as well as hypertrophy of the interdental papillae. The gums may become hyperemic and soft, and may bleed when mildly traumatized, as with a toothbrush.

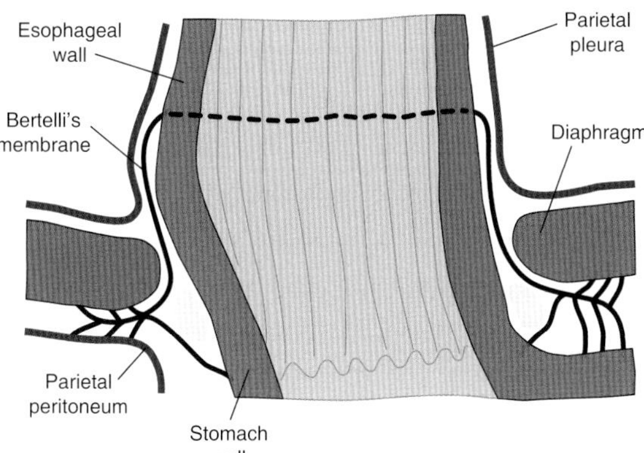

Fig 5.1
The attachments of the diaphragm and the esophagus.

Increased salivation, or ptyalism, is common. Some patients experience changes in their sense of taste, leading to strange food cravings.

The upper gastrointestinal tract (Fig 5.1) is commonly affected by pregnancy. The enlarging uterus displaces the stomach, pushing it towards the left axilla, and may anatomically alter the pressure gradient between the abdomen and thorax. Increased pressure within the stomach causes reflux of the gastric contents into the esophagus, which lies in the negative pressure of the intrathoracic cavity. The pressure gradient may even accentuate an anatomical defect, causing a hiatus hernia and contributing to gastro-esophageal reflux.[15] It is for these reasons that the symptoms of heartburn increase as term approaches. Contributing to the increased incidence of gastro-esophageal reflux are the motility changes that occur with pregnancy. Lower esophageal sphincter tone is decreased secondary to increased levels of progesterone and relaxin, and decreased levels of the peptide hormone motilin.[16] These changes may also delay gastric emptying and further aggravate the upper gastrointestinal symptoms associated with pregnancy.

Gastric emptying has been partially studied in pregnancy. Non-dyspeptic asymptomatic women have normal solid gastric emptying in early pregnancy, and gastric emptying does not lengthen in the third trimester or postpartum.[10,17] Patients with hyperemesis gravidarum, however, do demonstrate prolonged gastric emptying.

Gastro-esophageal reflux and peptic ulcer disease

Heartburn and reflux are common in pregnancy, occurring in 50–90% of cases, but typically are mild, becoming severe in only a very small percentage of women.[15] The peak incidence of heartburn is in the third trimester and the condition resolves with delivery. The risk of symptomatic gastro-esophageal reflux disease (GERD, or GORD) is related to increased gestation age, the presence of heartburn before pregnancy, and parity.[16] Heartburn is not caused by reflux itself, but is the effect of the refluxed gastric contents on the lower esophageal sphincter mucosa.

Progesterone seems to cause lower esophageal sphincter relaxation, but estrogen levels would have to be high first. An expanding uterus and increased intra-abdominal pressure have been assumed to be important factors in promoting GERD, especially late in pregnancy. The effects of the hormone relaxin in lowering sphincter tone have also been suggested as being important.[18]

Lifestyle modification certainly has a role to play in treating GERD. Dietary measures, such as limiting oral intake within 3 hours of bedtime, increasing fruit consumption, reducing the volume of meals, cutting down on dietary fat, and eliminating caffeine, chocolate, and mint are measures that have some effect in controlling symptoms. Alcohol and smoking should be eliminated. Advice about elevating the head of the bed and avoiding lying flat for too long may provide some benefit.

It is not a bad idea to suggest to a pregnant woman that her main calorific intake should be at midday. This means that they do not sit slumped after a heavy evening meal but remain more upright, allowing the gastric contents to drain. Small meals, taken more often, is another key piece of advice. Avoiding challenging foods, such as salad ingredients, can make a difference: steering clear of raw foods, such as uncooked tomato, onion, and cucumber, which have been shown to take longer to digest, means that food flows faster through the stomach and is less likely to reflux. Avoiding gassy drinks, even sparkling water, is another part of the equation.

Peptic ulcer disease is no more common in pregnancy than in normal populations.[8] There is evidence, however, to suggest that pregnancy aggravates the symptoms of peptic ulcer disease. One study interviewed 313 pregnant patients with peptic ulcer and noted that 44% became asymptomatic, 44% had improved symptoms, and 75% had recurrent symptoms postpartum.[19] Many physiologists believe that increased levels of progesterone reduce both basal and stimulated acid production, thus decreasing acid-related symptoms. It is also understood that increased levels of histamine produced by the stomach contribute to decreased acid secretion.

Although it is clear that *H. pylori* plays a pivotal role in peptic ulcer disease, the relationship of *H. pylori* to pregnancy continues to be investigated.

The Small Intestine, Large Intestine and Appendix

The small intestine

The small intestine exhibits a decrease in motility during pregnancy. One study noted that the mean small bowel transit time increased significantly in each trimester and decreased back to normal levels postpartum. The increased transit time is related to elevations in progesterone levels during normal pregnancy and may contribute to the increased symptoms of constipation in late pregnancy.[20]

The duodenum and the small intestine are attached to the mesocolon, the liver, and the hepatic flexure. Most of the attachment is at the sphincter of Oddi or at the junction of the duodenum and jejunum. This leaves the jejunum and ileum free to move almost anywhere in the abdomen, being fixed at the mesentery but free along their other surfaces. At the distal end of the small intestine, where the ileum and the cecum meet at the iliocecal valve, there is an attachment via the root of the mesentery. Contraction along the root of the mesentery will pull the cecum towards the midline, closing the hepatic angle and leading to a slowing of food transit in the gut.

The large intestine

The many changes that pregnancy exerts on the large intestine, particularly the colon, lead to increased symptoms of constipation. The colon may be subject to the same decrease in motility that affects the other portions of the gastrointestinal tract. Progesterone has been shown to alter colonic transit time in rats,[21] but this effect has not been demonstrated in humans, and there are many studies that have generated conflicting data. The functional changes that occur with the enlarging uterus may mechanically limit colonic emptying and probably are the main reason for symptomatic constipation in late pregnancy. The uterus undergoes dextrorotation and the pressure on the right side of the bowel causes pressure over the cecum that can inhibit transit time. The uterus moves to the right because the sigmoid colon, full of solid fecal matter, is on the left. There is also a significant increase in water and sodium absorption secondary to higher levels of the hormone aldosterone during pregnancy, leading to a dry stool volume and prolonged colonic transit time.

Constipation due to reduced gut motility and mobility is another common problem. If severe, it can lead to referred pain to the lumbar spine, or to the iliac fossa on one side or the other. The constipation will exacerbate hemorrhoids if they pre-exist or may produce them for the first time. This is because venous stasis causes the smooth muscles in the large venous vessels to become slack and expand, and also because of reduced venous return to the heart as the gravid uterus compresses the abdominal vena cava. This results in back-pressure in the veins of the lower extremity, causing venous distension and varicosities. If these occur in the anal canal, they present as hemorrhoids; in the vagina, they are known as vulval varicosities. Once again, these stem from the effect of progesterone levels in pregnancy on smooth muscle.

The slower transit of food materials enhances the absorption of iron and calcium in the upper part of the intestine, which can lead to constipation, too. The action of the hormone calcitol adds to this effect, so that by the 6th month of pregnancy calcium absorption is twice that of non-pregnant women. Physiologically, this is a good thing, as the parasitic action of the fetus can often lead to weakness of the teeth and nails. Dietary calcium should be increased by 140% during pregnancy. (It is for this reason that women in some countries, like the UK, are entitled to free dental care during pregnancy.)

Gastrointestinal bleeding

The most common cause of lower gastrointestinal bleeding in pregnancy is hemorrhoids. Hemorrhoids are caused by prolapse of the anal canal cushions, which are rich in blood vessels. The increased circulating blood volume, increased abdominal pressure, and venous stasis caused by the enlarging uterus during pregnancy are contributing factors. It is not surprising that bleeding may occur with straining at defecation. Coupled with the frequent constipation of late pregnancy, this can be very distressing. External hemorrhoids occur distal to the anal margin and rarely bleed unless they are thrombosed.[20]

Bleeding from a gastrointestinal ulcer is the second most common form of upper gastrointestinal bleeding in a pregnant patient. The Mallory–Weis syndrome is a lesion characterized by mucosal ulceration just below the gastro-esophageal junction that is due to increased abdominal pressure and the shearing forces on the lower part of the esophagus caused by vomiting.[22] Clearly, this is a surgical complication and should be dealt with in hospital.

Inflammatory bowel disease

The term inflammatory bowel disease is frequently used to describe two entities: ulcerative colitis and Crohn's disease. Ulcerative colitis is a chronic recurrent disease characterized by diffuse mucosal inflammation occurring in the colon. It usually begins in the rectum and spreads continuously throughout the colon. Crohn's disease is also a chronic recurrent inflammatory condition, but may affect the whole alimentary canal. The incidence of Crohn's disease is 5 per 100,000 whereas that of ulcerative colitis is slightly more common at 15 per 100,000. The peak age of onset for both conditions during the child-bearing years ranges from 15 to 30 years.[21]

Inflammatory bowel disease, particularly ulcerative colitis, accounts for lower gastrointestinal bleeding in some women. Patients with mild ulcerative colitis that exists pre-pregnancy often pass blood and mucus with normal stools. As the colitis becomes more severe and spreads proximally, diarrhea can occur. Profuse hemorrhage is one of the complications of Crohn's colitis and requires emergency surgery.

Regional enteritis of the small intestines rarely causes profuse hemorrhage but may lead to iron deficiency anemia; this is difficult to differentially diagnose in pregnancy.[21]

The outcome of pregnancy in inflammatory bowel disease, as well as the influence of pregnancy on inflammatory bowel disease, has been extensively studied, and much of the research has shown that most women with these diseases will proceed to have normal, full-term pregnancies. Patients with these problems should be seen by a consultant obstetrician or a gastroenterologist, as the bleeding does need to be controlled and the inflammatory process dealt with.

Irritable bowel syndrome in pregnancy

Irritable bowel syndrome (IBS) is the most common gastrointestinal disorder, accounting for nearly 50% of referrals to a gastroenterologist. Female patients outnumber male patients by 3 to 1.[23] The diagnosis of IBS depends on the presence of specific symptoms: abdominal discomfort for 12 weeks or longer, which need not be continuous, together with relief of discomfort with defecation, an association of discomfort with altered stool frequency, and an association of discomfort with altered stool form.

Other manifestations include abdominal bloating, passage of mucus, sense of incomplete evacuation, and temporary resolution of pain with bowel movements. Patients may demonstrate constipation predominance or diarrhea predominance, or they may fluctuate between the two with alternating constipation and diarrhea. Fever, weight loss, and rectal bleeding are not commonly associated with IBS.[24]

The pathophysiology of IBS is not clear but disturbances in colonic motility and alteration in colonic emptying are frequently noted.[25] There is some evidence that IBS patients may have visceral hypersensitivity, making them more sensitive to motility-induced internal spasm and distension.[26]

IBS rarely begins during pregnancy and typically will have been present for many years. Functional bowel disease usually improves during pregnancy, especially after the first trimester. In those patients with dyspepsia and nausea, the hormonal changes creating nausea in pregnancy may trigger a worsening of symptoms, and possibly may even lead to a picture resembling hyperemesis gravidarum (see earlier).

Constipation, diarrhea, and pregnancy

Between 11% and 38% of healthy women report constipation during pregnancy, most commonly in the third trimester, and 34% report increased stool frequency.[27] The average frequency of bowel movements ranges from three times per day to once every 3 days. Unfortunately, most patients define constipation as infrequent bowel movements; thus they become concerned if their bowels fail to open for a certain number of days. This change in bowel habit is perfectly normal during pregnancy and is partly due to dextrorotation of the uterus, which presses on the ascending colon, as mentioned earlier. The uterus is forced to the right as it grows by the bulk of the left-sided sigmoid colon. If the pregnant patient does not move her bowels every day, this should not be taken as a serious sign. Laxatives are not generally a good idea in pregnancy; instead, encourage the patient to eat a compote made with soft fruit such as prunes and apricots, and to increase the fiber in her diet.[20]

Diarrhea is not a real problem of pregnancy, when compared to constipation. It may occur in pregnant women, as in non-pregnant women, and the differential diagnosis is the same.[28] It could be a component of IBS or be caused by an infection. If it continues for more than a couple of days, she should be referred to the family physician/GP for investigation.

Appendicitis

Appendicitis is the most common non-obstetric surgical emergency in pregnancy, occurring in approximately 1 in 1000 pregnancies.[29] Symptoms are similar to those in the non-pregnant patient; however, the location of the abdominal tenderness may be different, depending on the size of the uterus. The enlarging uterus may shift the appendix from the right lower quadrant to the right upper quadrant, causing confusion in the diagnosis. In addition to the change in location, other factors during pregnancy may delay diagnosis. Symptoms such as anorexia, nausea, and vomiting are common in pregnancy. Abdominal ultrasound imaging is important in helping to diagnose appendicitis.

The Liver, Gallbladder, and Pancreas in Pregnancy

The Liver

Portal hypertension or a cirrhotic liver can cause varicose veins to develop around the esophagus (esophageal varices; Fig 5.2). Pregnancy slightly increases the risk of massive bleeding from these veins, especially during the last 3 months.

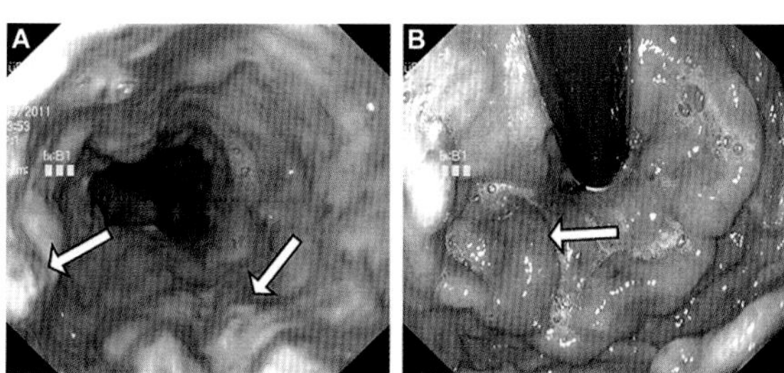

Fig 5.2
Esophageal varices due to portal hypertension in pregnancy.

Liver or gallbladder problems may result from hormonal changes during pregnancy. Some changes cause only minor, transient symptoms.

The normal hormonal effects of pregnancy can slow the movement of bile through the bile ducts, producing cholestasis. The most obvious symptom is itching all over the body (usually in the last few months of pregnancy) but no rash develops. The disorder usually resolves after delivery but tends to recur in subsequent pregnancies.

Pregnant women can experience spider angiomas and palmar erythema. Spider angiomas (Fig 5.3) are found only in the distribution of the superior vena cava, and are thus commonly found on the face, neck, upper part of the trunk, and arms.

About 65% of white women but only 10% of black women experience symptoms relating to the liver. In

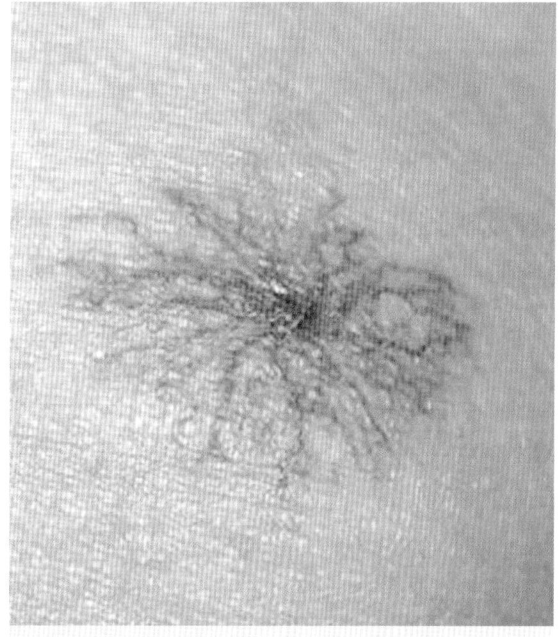

Fig 5.3
Spider angioma.

addition, women may have reduced serum albumin concentration, elevated serum alkaline phosphatase activity, and increased cholesterol levels. These are common symptoms of liver disease, but they are not evidence of liver disease if they occur during pregnancy.[30]

Pregnant women who develop gallstones are closely monitored. If a gallstone blocks the gallbladder or causes an infection, surgery may be necessary. This surgery is usually safe for pregnant women and the fetus.

The Gallbladder

Acute cholecystitis

Pregnancy increases the risk of gallstones (cholelithiasis). Gallbladder emptying and gallbladder motility are decreased during pregnancy, providing the necessary environment for an increased risk of gallstone formation.

Along with these functional changes, the chemical components of the bile are altered during pregnancy. The bile is more saturated and becomes very thick and muddy. It is surprising that, even though the gallbladder is altered in so many ways, gallstones and their complications are still uncommon during pregnancy.

The incidence of gallbladder disease during pregnancy is approximately 0.2–0.3% and does not exceed that in non-pregnant women. Cholecystitis (inflammation of the gallbladder) occurs in approximately 1 in 1000 pregnancies and approximately one-third of cases require surgical intervention.[28] The clinical presentation is similar to that in the non-pregnant patient, consisting of persistent right upper quadrant pain, nausea, vomiting, fever, and raised white blood cells. Fortunately, the diagnosis can be confirmed accurately and safely during pregnancy by abdominal ultrasound.

Gallstones and pregnancy

There is an increased risk of gallstone formation in pregnancy. The risk is related to parity: two pregnancies double the risk, and four quadruples it. Some 2% of women followed during pregnancy will develop gallstones.[30,31] Although biliary colic may occur in up to 28% of women, acute cholecystitis is rare. Although many studies support the higher risk of gallstones, it is still unclear why they occur. Bile stasis within the gallbladder, leading to the supersaturation of cholesterol, is an important factor in the formation of gallstones.[32] The condition is characterized by itching, known as pruritus, which generally appears in the last 3 months of pregnancy (though it can arise sooner). It is of variable severity and can be extremely distressing for the mother. Both the raised bile salts and the pruritus completely disappear soon after the birth and generally do not seem to cause long-term health problems for mothers.

Some studies have shown a link between intrahepatic cholestasis and still birth, and it for this reason that your patient might be offered early delivery if her clinicians feel that she or her baby might be at risk.

The liver and gallbladder undergo compression from the rising uterus. The liver is pushed towards the right axilla and there is a decrease in diaphragmatic excursion, which means that there is less pumping of the liver; again, this can contribute to gallbladder stasis. Pregnancy has been shown to affect biliary motility and cholesterol secretion. The fasting volume and residual volume in the gallbladder are increased during pregnancy, promoting bile stasis. Gallbladder stasis progresses during the first 20 weeks of pregnancy and seems to level off until delivery, when gallbladder emptying normalizes. These effects are most likely secondary to high levels of progesterone during pregnancy.

Although estrogens have not been shown to alter biliary motility, they do have a role in promoting gallbladder disease. In a study looking at the effects of estrogen supplementation in the non-pregnant population, it was shown that biliary secretion of cholesterol was increased by 40%.[33]

The Pancreas

Acute pancreatitis

Acute pancreatitis is rare during pregnancy, usually occurring in the third trimester or even postpartum. Presentation is similar in character to that in the non-pregnant patient. Diagnosis relies on clinical presentation and blood analysis.[30] Classically, patients present with mid-epigastric pain, which radiates to the back. Nausea and vomiting may be early symptoms. Serum amylase may be lower during pregnancy, secondary to increased renal clearance. Gallstones are the most common cause of pancreatitis in pregnancy, accounting for 75–90% of cases: approximately twice the rate in the non-pregnant patient.[31]

The Kidney in Pregnancy

Changes in Renal Physiology During Pregnancy

Like the heart, the kidneys work harder throughout pregnancy. They filter the increasing volume of blood, which reaches a maximum between 16 and 24 weeks, and remains at this maximum until immediately before delivery. At that point, pressure from the enlarging uterus may slightly decrease the blood supply to the kidneys.

Both kidneys grow in size by 1–1.5 cm (0.4–0.6 inches) during pregnancy.[34] Kidney volume increases by up to 30%, primarily due to a rise in renal vascular and interstitial volume. There are no histological changes or alterations in the number of nephrons, but the glomerular filtration rate is also increased.

The renal pelvises and caliceal systems may be dilated due to the effects of progesterone and mechanical compression of the ureters at the pelvic brim. Dilatation of the ureters and renal pelvis (hydroureter and hydronephrosis) is more prominent on the right than the left and is seen in up to 80% of pregnant women These changes can be visualized on ultrasound examination by the second trimester and may not resolve until 6–12 weeks postpartum.[35]

The uterus presses on the bladder, reducing its size so that it fills with urine more quickly than usual. This pressure also makes a pregnant woman need to urinate more often and more urgently.

After the 12th week of gestation, progesterone can induce dilatation and weak tone of the renal calyx and ureters. With advancing gestation, the enlarging uterus can compress the ureters as they cross the pelvic brim and cause further dilatation by obstructing flow (Fig 5.4). These changes may contribute to the frequency of urinary tract infections (UTIs) during pregnancy.[36]

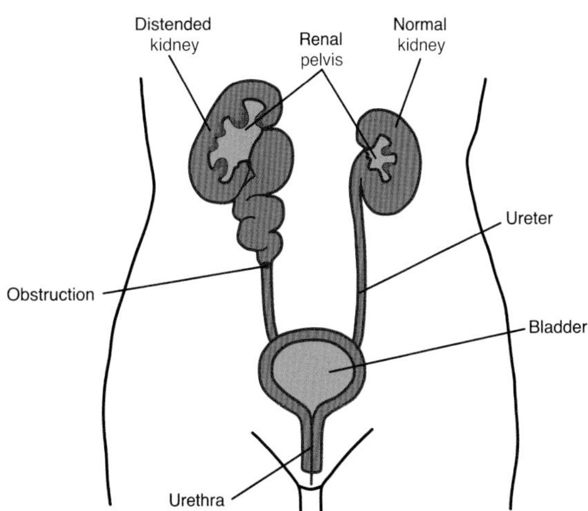

Fig 5.4
Urinary tract obstruction showing kidney hypertrophy.

Activity of the kidneys normally increases when a person lies down and decreases when a person stands. The difference is amplified during pregnancy and this can be one reason why a pregnant woman needs to urinate frequently and can be disturbed at night. Another factor is the progesterone effect on the walls of the bladder. Late in pregnancy, lying on the side, particularly the left side, increases kidney activity more than lying on the back. Lying on the left side relieves the pressure that the enlarged uterus puts on the venous plexuses carrying blood from the legs. As a result, blood flow improves and kidney activity increases.

Renal plasma flow and glomerular filtration rate begin to increase progressively during the first trimester. At term, both are 50–60% higher than in the non-pregnant state. This parallels the increases in blood volume and cardiac output. The elevations in plasma flow and glomerular filtration result in a rise in creatinine clearance. Blood urea and serum creatinine are reduced by 40%. The increase in glomerular filtration may overwhelm the ability of the renal tubules to reabsorb, leading to glucose and protein losses in the urine. Thus, mild glycosuria (1–10 g/day) and/or proteinuria (to 300 mg/day) can occur in normal pregnancy.

Renal Complications of Pregnancy

Pre-eclampsia is an important clinical syndrome and anyone dealing with pregnant patients should be aware of it (Box 5.3). Its precise origins are not known but the relationship between the kidney and pre-eclampsia is unequivocal.

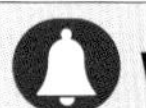

Warning

The triad of hypertension, edema, and proteinuria must never be ignored, and patients should be immediately referred to their doctor or midwife for evaluation.

BOX 5.3

Clinical features of pre-eclampsia

- Historical:
  - Nulliparity
  - Multiple gestations
  - Family history
  - Pre-existing renal or vascular decrease
- Hypertension:
  - 140/90 mmHg after 20 weeks *or*
  - 30 mmHg increase in systolic pressure *or*
  - 15 mmHg increase in diastolic pressure
- Sudden appearance of edema, especially in hands and face
- Rapid weight gain
- Headache and visual disturbances

Changes to kidney physiology can often produce urinary symptoms in pregnant women. They include urinary frequency, nocturia, dysuria, urge incontinence, and occasionally an inability to pass urine. It is important to identify whether these symptoms are reflections of normal physiological changes in pregnancy, or whether they represent an underlying pathological cause.

There is a small increase in urine output due to the increased renal perfusion and glomerular filtration rate.

These changes can occur in up to 80% of pregnancies and are commonly asymptomatic. They can result in an increase of the volume of urine in the collecting system and then an increased risk of UTI, which is more frequent in pregnancy. Pregnancy predisposes women to bacteriuria, which in the non-pregnant state is usually self-limiting, but which in pregnancy can predispose to development of UTIs.

Normal pregnancy-related physiological changes contribute to UTIs, including dilatation of the upper collecting systems, hypotonic renal pelvises, increases in urinary tract dead space and vesico-ureteral reflux, and reductions in natural antibacterial activity in the urine and in phagocytic activity of leukocytes at the mucosal surfaces. UTIs in pregnant women usually do not present with typical symptoms, and may even be asymptomatic. All these factors increase the likelihood for infections to ascend to the kidneys; pyelonephritis is a serious complication of UTI.

Higher progesterone levels mean that the bladder wall relaxes and increases the capacity of the bladder. There is compression from the enlarging uterus, however, which causes displacement and reduces capacity. There can be some reflux along the ureters back up to the kidney, caused by increased pressure within the bladder and decreased pressure within the wall of the ureters.

Biochemically, there is a fall in serum creatinine and urea due to increased renal plasma flow.

Symptoms of urinary frequency are common, especially in the first trimester. There are many causes, as mentioned earlier. Sometimes women have to get up at night more frequently, and this can increase as the pregnancy continues. It is probably caused by greater excretion of sodium and water at night, compared with non-pregnant women.

Urination can be burning or painful in pregnancy, either as water is passed or straight after. This symptom should not be ignored, as it can be the sign of a urinary infection.

Incontinence is not usually a problem during pregnancy; however, many women do feel that they involuntarily pass a few drops of urine due to pressure on the bladder from the rising uterus. This occurs in coughing, sneezing, or laughing.

The differential diagnosis of acute cystitis or acute pyelonephritis is always based on a urine dipstick test. If there is any doubt, the patient should be referred to the midwife, so that any pathology can be identified and dealt with.

Renal calculi or stones occur during pregnancy as they do in the non-pregnant population. They present with acute renal colic. There is intense loin pain on the presenting side and the differential diagnosis will be based on an ultrasound scan and biochemical analysis. It is important to make a differential diagnosis in osteopathic practice from a rib lesion or facet joint or muscular pain associated with the change in lateral plane curve at the thoracolumbar junction or 12th rib.

The Musculoskeletal System in Pregnancy

Review of the Biomechanics of the Lumbar Spine

The lumbar spine is a massive bony pile of vertebrae that becomes thicker and heavier as the sacrum approaches. The disc spaces of the lower lumbar spines are thicker than those of any other segments; they are more vascular and contain more nuclear material. Some authorities believe that this is the reason why they commonly fail and give rise to disc degeneration, herniation, and prolapse.

The lumbosacral angle, lying between the axis of L5 and the axis of the sacrum, averages 140 degrees (Fig 5.5). The angle of pelvic tilt formed by the horizontal and the line joining the sacral promontory to the superior border of the pubic symphysis averages 60 degrees. This is particularly important during pregnancy when the lumbar lordosis has to change in order to accommodate the growing uterus and fetus, more of which later.

The ligaments of the spine will change in the same way as any other ligamentous structure during pregnancy. The hormone relaxin, secreted by the

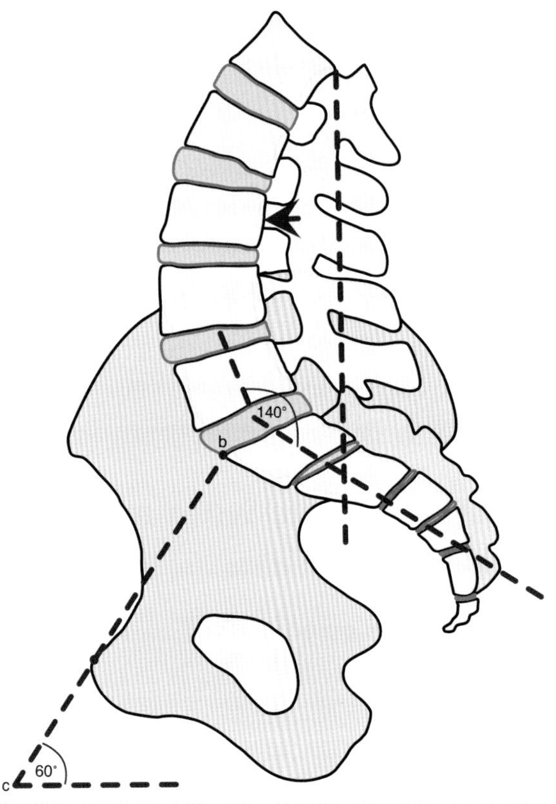

Fig 5.5
The lumbosacral angle in lordosis.

corpus luteum of pregnancy, is not very specific. Its function is to weaken the cross-bridges in collagen structures and allow for unwinding of the connections between the supporting bony structures. The main structures to be affected are the pelvic ligaments holding the bones of the pelvis together. This occurs mainly during the last trimester of pregnancy but can start earlier in women whose spines are very stiff. However, other structures, such as the lumbar and thoracic spines and the thoracolumbar junction, will change, too. Even though relaxation of the pelvic ligaments has been thought to be responsible for pelvic pain during pregnancy, it now seems that the whole subject is much more complex than was first thought because some studies have shown the opposite to what until now has been quoted as fact. It may not be just ligamentous relaxation alone that gives women back pain in pregnancy.[37,38,39]

The main ligaments of the lumbar spine are the anterior and posterior longitudinal ligaments and the annulus fibrosus of the disc spaces. The architecture of the spine is such that there is no point of separation between these structures. It is analogous with a river and the sea, in that it is a continuous flowing structure. The important point is that the main nerve and venous supply to the disc arrives via the posterior and anterior longitudinal ligaments, and therefore a central disc prolapse is painful while a lateral prolapse need not be.

These structures are augmented by the supraspinous and interspinous ligaments, which run between the spinous processes and transverse processes of respective vertebrae throughout the spine.

Apart from the ligaments mentioned above, there is the thick and powerful ligamentum flavum, which reaches between the laminae of adjacent vertebrae and the ligamentous capsular apparatus of the intervertebral joints.

Physiological Movements of the Spine

During flexion movements, the capsules and ligaments of the individual vertebrae are maximally stretched, as well as the long ligaments of the spine and the posterior fibers of the annulus fibrosus and the vertebral arch, as mentioned above. These stretched ligaments finally limit flexion.

During extension, the anterior fibers of the annulus and the anterior longitudinal ligament are on stretch. The articular processes of the lower and upper vertebrae come together, and the spinous processes can actually touch one another. This is what finally limits extension.

During lateral flexion or side-bending, the intertransverse ligament on one side is stretched and the one on the other side relaxes. When seen from behind, the articular processes slide relative to each other, rising on one side and lowering on the other, leading to stretch of the ligamentum flavum and the capsules on one side, and a relaxation on the other.

The ranges of motion for the cervical, thoracic, and lumbar spines are shown in Box 5.4.

Low back pain and pregnancy: evidence and theories

The incidence of low back and pelvic pain among our pregnant patients is nothing new; in fact, if you treat women in pregnancy, the commonest presenting symptom will be back pain in one form or another. For the last hundred years, researchers have noted that back pain in pregnancy has been associated with ligamentous laxity and an increase in joint mobility.[40,41] The number of patients who suffer in this way varies according to the quoted sources (Box 5.5). In figures from 2011,[42] 1 patient in 2 experienced lumbopelvic pain.

The search for pain generators has considered various structures as being potentially responsible. Certainly, weight gain[49] and ligamentous instability, both inherent to pregnancy, should be high on the list of anyone seeking to understand why this patient has this problem at this time. Weight gain during

BOX 5.4

Comparison of ranges of motion (in degrees) for the cervical thoracic and lumbar spines

	Flexion (F)/ extension (E)	Lateral flexion	Axial rotation
Cervical spine	F40/E75	20	45–50
Thoracic spine	F105/E60	20	35
Lumbar spine	F60/E35	35–45	5

BOX 5.5

The incidence of low back pain in pregnancy

Researcher	Year	Incidence
Orvieto[43]	1994	54.8% of 449 patients
Middleditch and Oliver[44]	1997	51% of 335 patients
Mogren[45]	2005	72% of 891 patients
Mousavi[46]	2006	49.5% of 395 patients
Mota, et al.[47]	2015	67.6% of 105 patients
Shijagurumayam, et al.[48]	2019	34% of 1,384 patients

pregnancy, pregnancy length, and neonatal weight have often been thought to be factors of importance here, but one study showed that there were no differences between two groups of pregnant patients studied.[50] Not surprisingly, previous episodes of back pain while non-pregnant or pregnant have been found to be of importance. The occurrence of back pain during pregnancy did not affect the pregnancy outcome. Also, if a woman puts a lot of weight on during pregnancy and suffers low back pain, the pain can persist and still be present at 24 months, unless she reduces her weight to pre-pregnancy levels. The fact that women increase their body weight by up to 12.5 kilos (28 pounds) by the end of a physiological pregnancy[51] means that, as the weight goes up, so does the physical stress placed on the supporting structures.

One study from 1995 felt that weight gain could explain part of the increase in lordosis during pregnancy, but the effect was not very strong.[52] Posture will also change during pregnancy so as to adapt to the increasing weight, and this too has been identified as one of the factors causing back pain. [52,53] The development of a deep lordosis could mean extra weight on the pars interarticularis and the development of spondylolysis (degeneration of the facet joints) or spondylolisthesis (anomalous development or trauma that causes fracture of the pars interarticularis and forward slip of the vertebral bodies) during a pregnancy, and thus again lead to low back pain.[54,55]

The literature relating to ligamentous or non-bony structures as a cause of back pain is very strong. Facet joints, muscles, ligaments, and fascia have all been reported as etiologies of acute and chronic low back pain.[56] Lumbar apophyseal joints are not usually weight-bearing, but with the developing lordosis of the progressing pregnancy they can become so; if the rising levels of hormones cause a temporary laxity in the joints, the instability will produce a stretch in the joint capsules, rich in nociceptive pain fibers, and thus lead to low back pain.[57]

The diagnosis of facet joint pain has been made by diagnostic facet joint or median nerve branch injections with a local anesthetic. This standard technique is used to discover the source of local pain. (It is most unlikely to be used during pregnancy, where the case history questioning and clinical testing are usually deemed sufficient.) The results of one study demonstrated that local anesthetic injections are useful for the diagnosis of non-radicular low back pain but may yield false-positive results with respect to lumbar facet pain, depending on the technique utilized. In a radiographic study of the non-discal locations of degeneration and back pain, findings in symptomatic subjects which departed from the normal anatomic features of the posterior spinal elements in asymptomatic volunteers included: rupture of the interspinous ligament(s), degeneration of the interspinous space with perispinous cyst formation, posterior spinal facet (zygapophyseal joint) arthrosis, related central spinal canal, lateral recess, and neural foramen stenosis, and posterior element alterations associated with various forms of spondylolisthesis , and perispinal muscle rupture/degeneration.[58] These findings indicate that the posterior elements are major locations of degenerative spinal and perispinal disease that may accompany, or even precede, degenerative disc disease. Although not yet proven as a reliable source of patient signs and symptoms in all individuals, because these observations may be made in patients with radicular, referred, and/or local low back pain, they should be considered in the evaluation of the symptomatic patient presenting with a clinical lumbosacral syndrome. This is especially so in pregnancy, when loading on the posterior elements of the vertebral segments is so much greater due to the development of the deep lordosis.

The development of a spondylolisthesis during pregnancy has also been identified as part of pregnancy back pain syndrome.[54] Pregnancy is a risk factor for those with an existing problem, as well as those whose condition is as yet unidentified. A risk analysis published in 1986 found that pregnancy did not constitute a major risk for the progression of an existing spondylolisthesis, but it was felt to be a contributing factor to early degeneration.[59] A later paper examined the evidence from 949 women and 120 men, and discovered that women who had borne children had a significantly higher incidence of degenerative spondylolisthesis than nulliparous women (28% versus 16.7%), therefore concluding that pregnancy was an important factor in the development of a degenerative spondylolisthesis.[60] The importance of these pieces of work is the contribution they make to an understanding of the etiology of the problem.

There are several reasons why there is a forward slip of one vertebra on another. It may be caused by a congenital defect of the pars interarticularis or it may be a fracture of the pars. If there is excessive wear of the L4/5 disc, accompanied by either a change in facet joint angles or degeneration of those facet joints at that level, this too can lead to a forward slip of one vertebra on another. In all cases, the stability of the segment is controlled by the integrity of the ligaments of the spine holding bones together. If the ligaments are weakened, or if there is an increase in body weight, then, logically, the risk of segment failure must be increased. In pregnancy, the ligaments are weakened.[61] In 2007, a study that looked at ligamentous laxity in pregnancy showed that all the women measured underwent an increase in joint laxity and that they changed in the middle of the pregnancy.[62] One area of future research might be to devise a questionnaire to establish whether this also corresponds with the onset of back pain in pregnancy.

In an unpublished cohort analysis of patients presenting for treatment at the Expectant Mother's Clinic at the British School of Osteopathy, back pain was a common symptom. The data analysis in that study reveals that the back pain came on as early as 12 weeks in some subjects, but it took a further 10 weeks for them to seek help. This poses a question as to the relationship between the onset of the pain, the time it takes to report the pain, and the woman's pregnancy laxity. She might be exhibiting early laxity change and, therefore, may start to experience back pain earlier than someone whose rate of change, and therefore ligamentous laxity, is lower.[63]

The Postural Changes of Pregnancy

The normal pre-pregnant antero-posterior spinal curves

In Figures 5.6 and 5.7 we can see the normal spinal curves from the side: the antero-posterior curves. It shows the cervical and lumbar lordoses and the thoracic and sacral kyphoses. The center of gravity line should ideally run from the mastoid process, down through the center of the shoulder joint and hip joint, towards the front of the knee joint, and through the lateral malleolus of the ankle.

It is important to state that this is the ideal posture, as commonly found in textbooks but only rarely seen in practice. Humans are constantly evolving and so the way that their bodies react to their internal and external environments changes from one generation to the next. Our children are better fed and have a more nutritionally balanced diet than at any other time in history, and hopefully they are more active and take part in more sporting activities too. (In recent times, however, we are witnessing children who spend many hours each day in front of games consoles or computer and TV screens, and we shall soon see the effects of these sedentary pastimes on their health.)

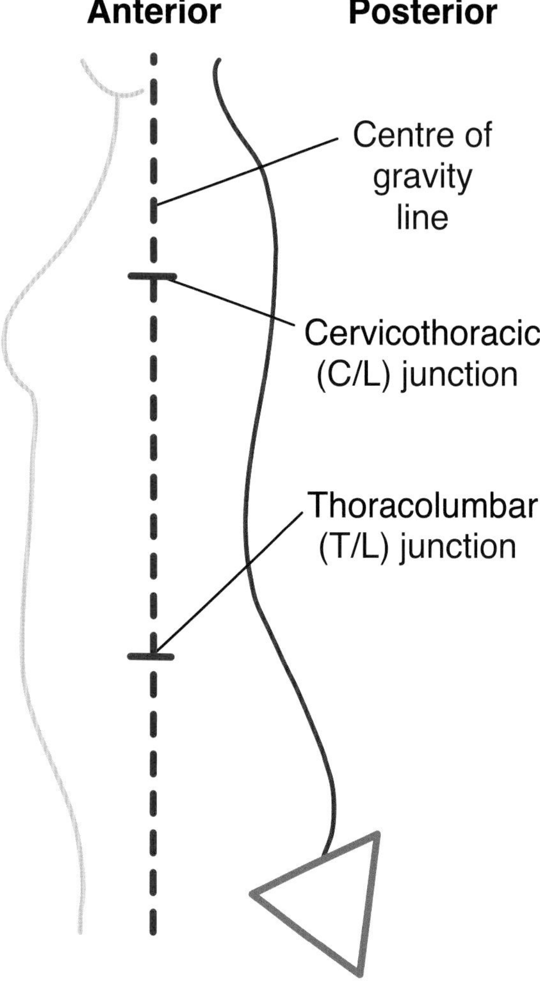

Fig 5.6
The "normal" antero-posterior pre-pregnancy posture.

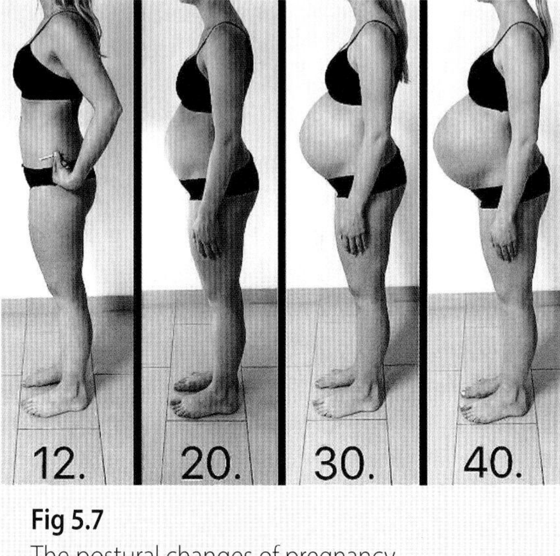

Fig 5.7
The postural changes of pregnancy.

The chairs we sit in and the beds we sleep in are designed by ergonomists to reduce the stresses and strains of daily living. Yet when we look at posture studies, it soon becomes apparent that pure posture is a myth. Therefore, the descriptions of posture that are provided here, and the account of the changes that take place during a pregnancy and the timings of those changes, should be taken as guidelines and not golden rules. Individuals will always adapt according to individual circumstances, but in pregnancy, every individual does undergo change.

Changes in the first trimester

By the end of the 12th week, the expanding uterus is seen above the pelvic brim. This causes a stretch and a reactive contraction in the rectus abdominis muscle due to the pressure from within. The rectus abdominis is attached between the xiphoid process of the sternum and the pubic symphysis. This will cause the pubic symphysis to rise and the pelvis to rotate posteriorly, causing a flattening of the lumbar lordosis (Figs 5.8 and 5.9). There is, in effect, a shortening of the abdominal muscles.

Most of this movement will be controlled by a good range of motion at the thoracolumbar junction. However, Scheuermann's disease (also called Scheuermann's kyphosis or spinal osteochondrosis; see Chapter 3) is a very common finding at this level, and if it interferes with the change in spinal

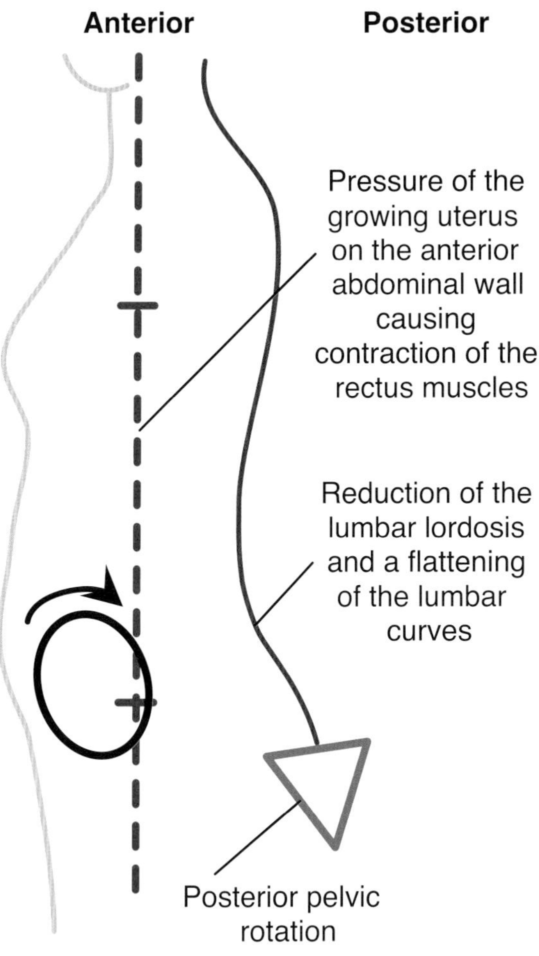

Fig 5.8
Antero-posterior curves at the end of the first trimester.

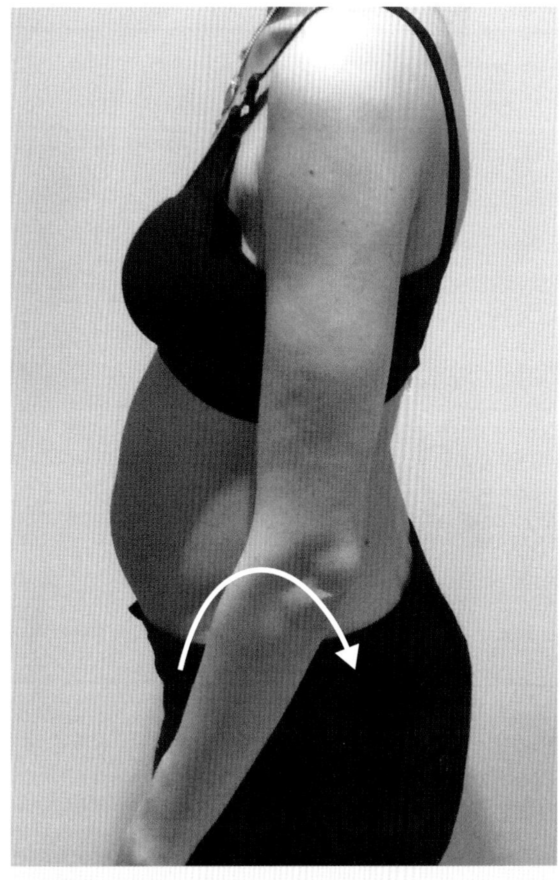

Fig 5.9
Antero-posterior spinal curves at the end of the first trimester.

movements and curves, it can be one of the factors leading to ligamentous back pain at the end of the first trimester. Multiparous women whose abdominal muscles have been stretched in a previous pregnancy may develop a deeper lordosis at this stage because of the relative weakness of the muscles if they did not regain good tone and form between pregnancies. As the expanding uterus pushes against the weak muscles, they cannot easily contract, leading to a sagging of the abdomen and a deepening of the lumbar curve, with all that entails. She will appear to be more pregnant than she actually is.

Other factors are important in relation to pre-pregnancy posture. For example, there may be previous trauma and injury to the area, causing very early degenerative changes.

Women with different shapes will develop and change differently, such that thin, slender individuals

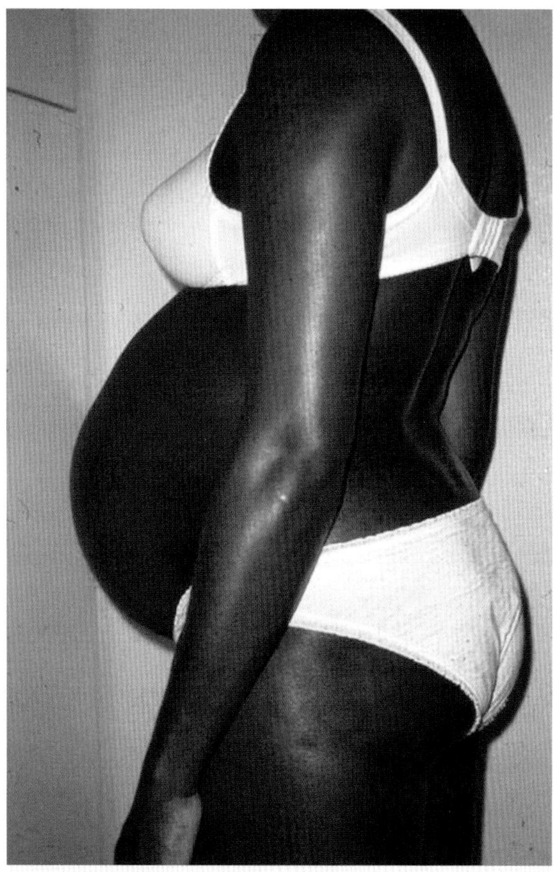

Fig 5.10
The classic kypholordotic posture commonly seen in Afro-Caribbean women.

will develop a different lumbar curve compared to those who have a pre-existing deep lumbar lordosis. This can be governed by genetics, such as in the case of familial patterns or twins, or even by racial characteristics, as seen in short, slender women who have southern Indian origins, or Afro-Caribbean women who may have developed a deep lumbar lordosis (Fig 5.10).

A deeper lordosis may predispose to lumbar facet weight-bearing. The facet joints of the spine are designed to guide motion, not to support the body weight, and if subjected to this force they will undergo early degeration or spondylarthrosis. With the laxity of pregnancy affecting the collagen of the capsules of the facet joints, they can become painful and go through inflammatory changes as early as the end of the 12th week.

Studies in the US have shown different outcomes for delivery of African–American patients when compared to white women, depending on morphology and body type. One study concluded that white women have a wider pelvic inlet, wider outlet, and shallower antero-posterior outlet than African–American women. In addition, after vaginal delivery, white women demonstrate less pelvic floor mobility. These differences may contribute to observed racial differences in obstetric outcomes and to the development of pelvic floor disorders.[56,64]

Breast development will vary from individual to individual, and from pregnancy to pregnancy. As the pelvis begins to rotate backwards between the end of the first and the end of the second trimesters, so the scapulae will start to rotate around the chest wall as the thoracic kyphosis develops at this time, too. If the breasts have already started to develop, in terms of both cup size and in strap size, their weight will exert an extra pull on the thoracolumbar junction.

This increased breast heaviness can lead to entrapment syndromes involving the upper extremities and the brachial plexus. Thoracic outlet syndromes, pectoralis minor syndrome, and first rib syndromes all need to be differentially diagnosed from each other and from spinal entrapment syndromes. Parasthesia in the hands and fingers is often misdiagnosed as carpal tunnel syndrome caused by a build-up of water within the tissue spaces at the wrist. Tinel's sign needs to be positive, and the distribution of the numbness examined carefully to ensure that it lies in a C8/T1 distribution.[65,66,67,68]

The rising uterus displaces the lower ribs, which can cause pain at the costotransverse articulations, even early on. This will produce spinal pain on lateral or rotational movement or deep inspiration, and is often missed when diagnosing the cause of lateral spinal pain.

The key to understanding the condition lies in the history, including respiration as a focus of questioning, and then in examination lateral to the facet joints with active and passive movements.

Changes in the second trimester

By the time the pregnant patient reaches the end of the 24th week, the weight of the gravid uterus lies posterior on the structures of the lumbar spine and the sacroiliac joints. The sacroiliac joints are designed to be weight-bearing structures; the facet joints are not, and as mentioned earlier, will commonly become painful and inflamed at this time.

The stretch on the anterior abdominal muscles can produce sharp pain as layers of muscle tissue tear and separate, causing a diastasis recti. One theory relating to the stretch marks of pregnancy that appear at this time is that they are due to seperation of fascial planes, and damage to the superficial layers of the skin and superficial muscles over the abdomen.[56,64,69,70]

Other structures required to stretch to adopt this new posture include the quadratus lumborum muscles, the psoas muscles, and the thoracolumbar fascia.

The woman's center of gravity now lies posterior to the normal line, giving space for the baby to grow in the expanding uterus (Figs 5.11 and 5.12). She should feel movement and kicking, usually from 20 weeks, and this can cause rib pain and intercostal spasms.

The low lumbar spines, particularly L4/5 and S1, are notoriously anomolous segments.[71] A lumbarized sacrum or a sacralized lumbar, where the lumbar spine has an extra vertebra or may be missing one, will interfere with the changing spinal mechanics of pregnancy. Figure 5.13 shows a sacralized lumbar vertebra between L5 and the sacrum. Normal easy movement at this level will be affected by the bone restriction.

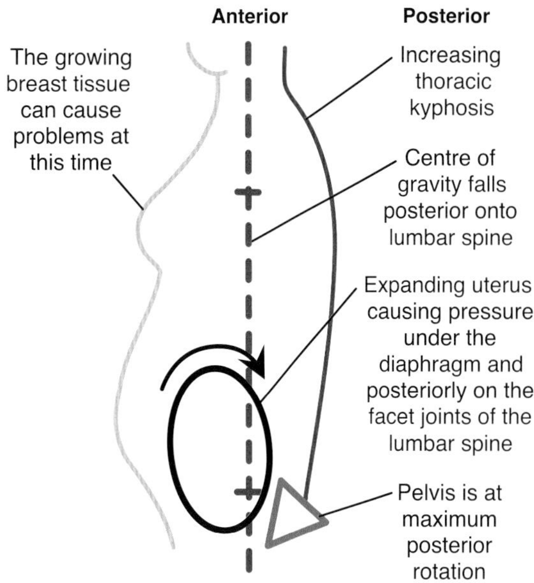

Fig 5.11
Antero-posterior curves at the end of the second trimester.

Changes in the third trimester

Towards the end of the pregnancy, as the patient approaches her 40th week, the changes in her posture are maximal. Approximately 80% of women will develop a "lordotic" posture with an exaggerated thoracic kyposis and a deep lumbar lordosis (Figs 5.14 and 5.15).

This is because her weight-bearing changes, due to pelvic rotation anteriorly through an axis of rotation via the hip joints, encouraging increased weight and

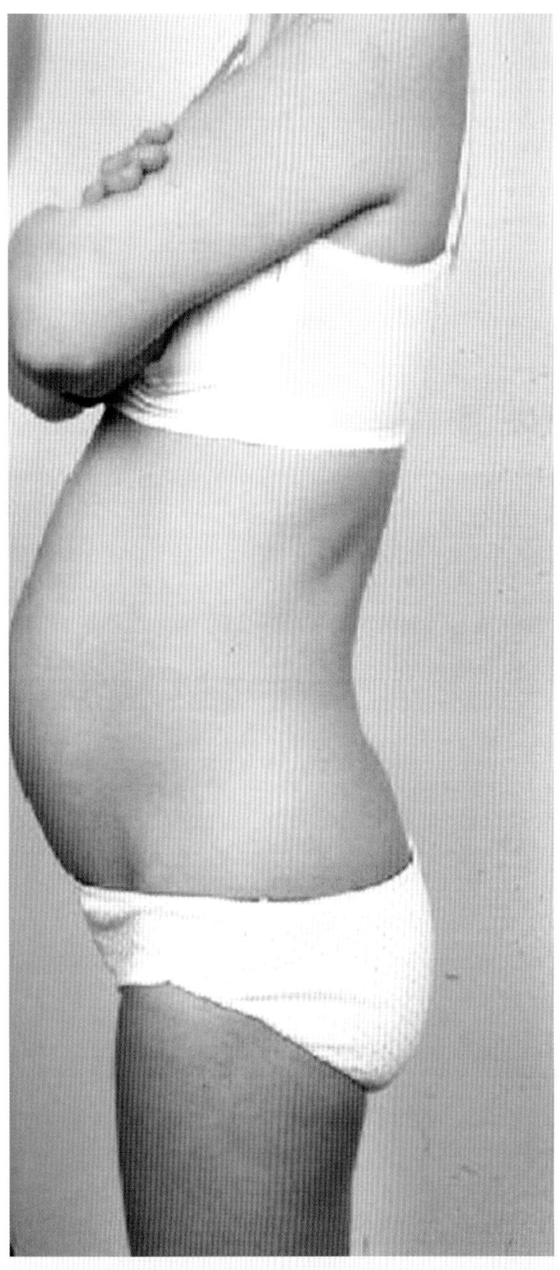

Fig 5.12
Antero-posterior spinal curves at the end of the second trimester.

demand on the anterior abdominal muscles and the pelvic floor, and due to the weight of the baby presenting down into the pelvis as the head comes to engage (more so in primaparous women).

Patients with a "lordotic" posture certainly suffer more from symphysis pubis dysfunction (SPD) when compared to the "sway-back" group.

A smaller number of pregnant patients, around 20%, will develop a "sway-back" posture, where the center of gravity stays posterior. Figure 5.16 was taken by the author to illustrate a sway-back posture at the end of a pregnancy! It shows that the pelvis has rotated anteriorly a little but most of the weight is still posterior to the center of gravity line. These are typically tall, asthenic women, who are hypermobile compared to the general population. There is no evidence to suggest that their labors are any different or more difficult when compared to the lordotic group. They tend to need fewer high-velocity, low-amplitude (HVLA) techniques, as the facets are not greatly compromised, but in this group the sacroiliac joints and the sacrum between the iliac bones can develop problems.

They are also more likely to suffer from hypermobile syndromes where the ligaments are too lax, causing spasm of the small postural muscles and locking of the apophyseal joints as the body attempts to compensate. These patients respond very much better to indirect or functional unwinding techniques than they do to direct soft tissue massage techniques, which tend to fatigue the tissues if the osteopath is not very careful. HVLA techniques are possible in this group but the most minimal of leverage techniques should be chosen, and applied with the absolute minimum of force and strain.

At the end of the pregnancy, as the lordosis develops, the lumbar spine facet joints must take the weight of the body directly. Compression of the facet joints and

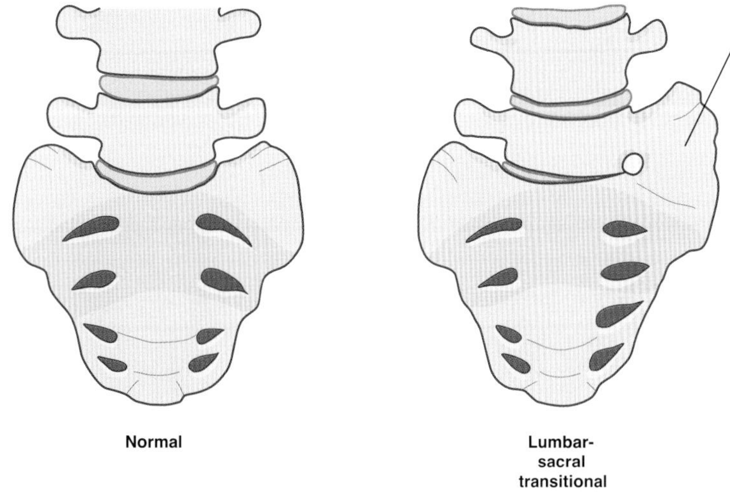

Fig 5.13
Anomolous development at the base of the lumbar spine.

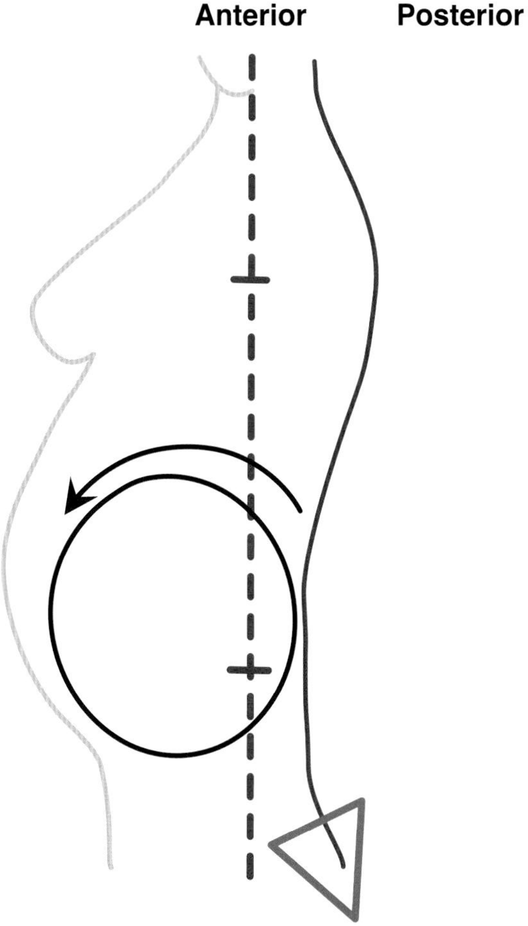

Anterior Posterior

Fig 5.14
Antero-posterior posture at the end of the third trimester.

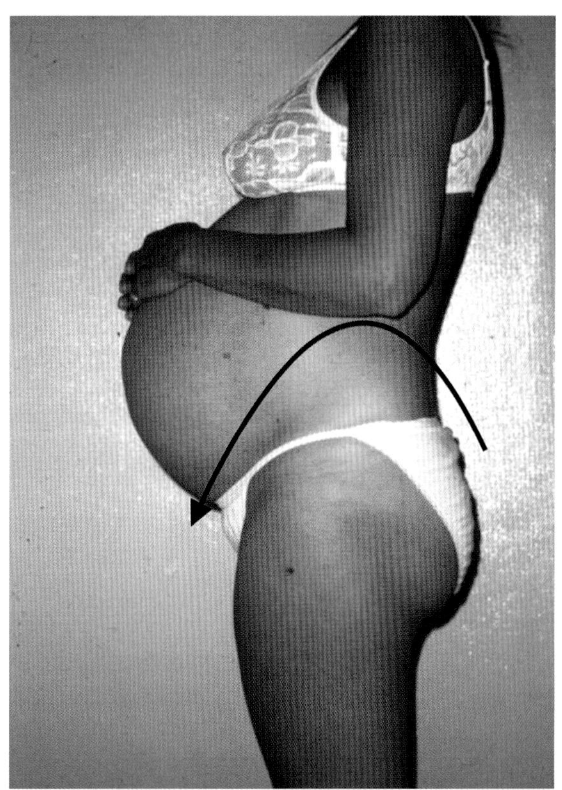

Fig 5.15
Antero-posterior spinal curves at the end of the third trimester in a patient with a "lordotic" posture.

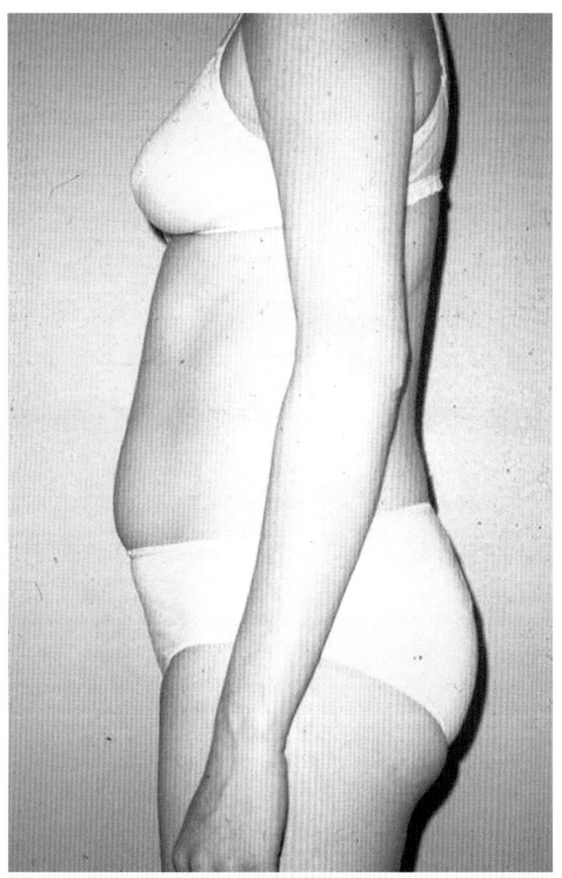

Fig 5.16
A "sway back" posture during the third trimester.

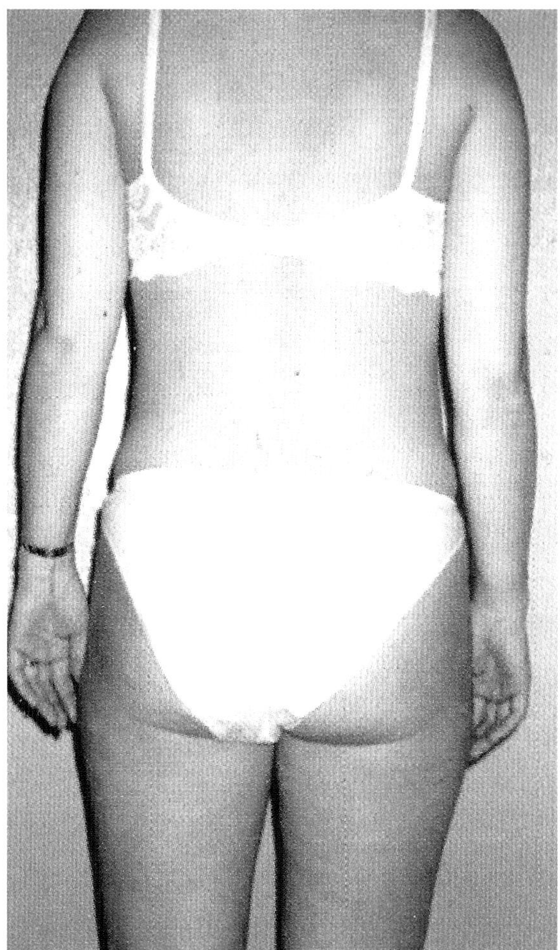

Fig 5.17
Lateral plane curve changes.

strain on the ligamentous capsular apparatus leads to non-specific back pain and postural muscle fatigue. Muscles are designed for movement and rest, but if they are made to contract and hold the weight of the expanding abdomen for too long, ischemic and congestion pain syndromes will develop. This can present as a bilateral muscular ache that can peak to spasm if extension or rotation movements provoke it. It is worse with weight-bearing and bending and lifting, all of which challenge the intersegmental and interspinous postural muscles. Locking of the facets, causing unilateral back pain, is not uncommon at this time.

Changes in the lateral plane

Changes to posture also occur in the lateral plane (Fig 5.17). It is very rare in any population anywhere in the world to find a straight spine. The presence of a minor lateral plane curve or scoliosis is common.[72,73,74,75] By the time children become adults, they have finished their growth phases and the morphology of their spines does not change very much. (Incidentally, it is for this reason that, when student osteopaths examine each other during their training, the presence of minor lateral plane curves is so frequently noted!) The curves in the lateral plane have many origins. They might be the result of a primary short leg on one side, a smaller hemipelvis, anomalous development at the lumbar spine, as mentioned earlier, or trauma to the long bones as a child. Whatever the cause of the curve – and in many cases the real cause is never found – the changes to the lateral plane curves take place at the junction areas of the L5/S1 segments, the thoracolumbar and cervicodorsal junctions, and the junction between the occiput and C1/2.

An important law of nature is that the eyes and the ears must line up with the horizon for normal balance of the special senses. The presence of a short leg, for example, will throw this off balance, and so the body develops a series of lateral plane curves to try to support the weight either side of the midline in as balanced and non-traumatic a way as possible.

During pregnancy, these otherwise controlled and asymptomatic lateral plane curves can become disturbed, giving rise to symptoms.

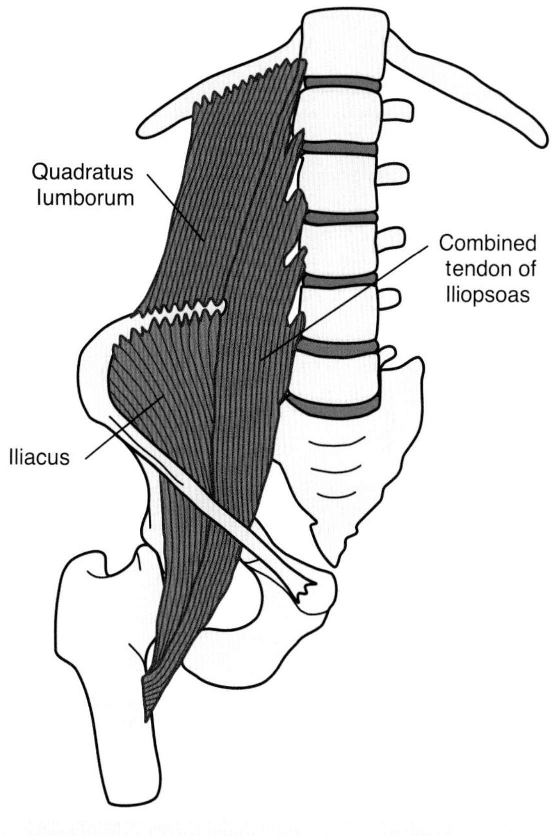

Fig 5.18
The psoas muscles.

The importance of the thoracolumbar junction

This lumbar spine change is also governed by the mobility at the thoracolumbar junction and by the activity of the psoas muscles anterior to the lumbar spine. Psoas, acting bilaterally, stabilizes the spine, encourages lumbar flexion, and, when acting from above, flexes the hips on the trunk (Figs 5.18 and 5.19). As the axis of rotation is through the hip joints, the integrity and good function of the psoas muscles is of paramount importance at the end of a pregnancy. It has been said, somewhat poetically, that the psoas muscles are the rails on which the baby train runs when it leaves the pelvis!

At the thoracolumbar junction, the function of the psoas muscles during the last trimester and during labor, as the descent of the uterus is guided into the pelvis, is important, too; however, if one muscle is chronically shortened due to a lateral plane abnormality, this can theoretically lead to a delay or an increase in the time it takes for the baby to transit the birth canal.

It certainly produces thoracolumbar pain anteriorly, which might be mistaken for renal pain,

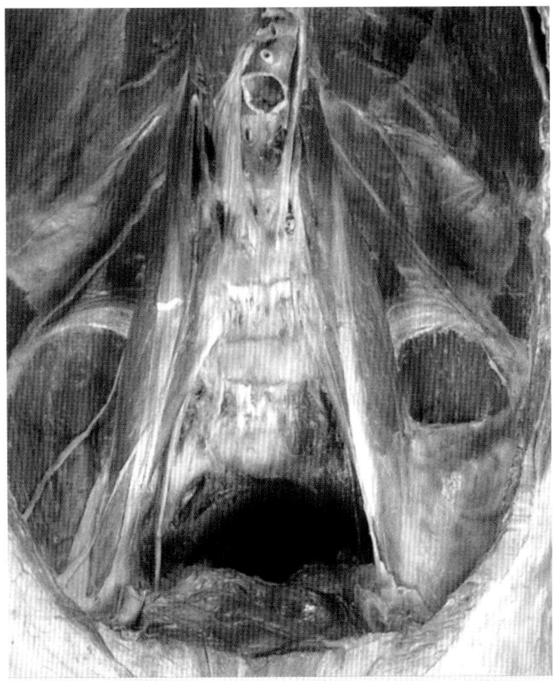

Fig 5.19
The psoas muscles.

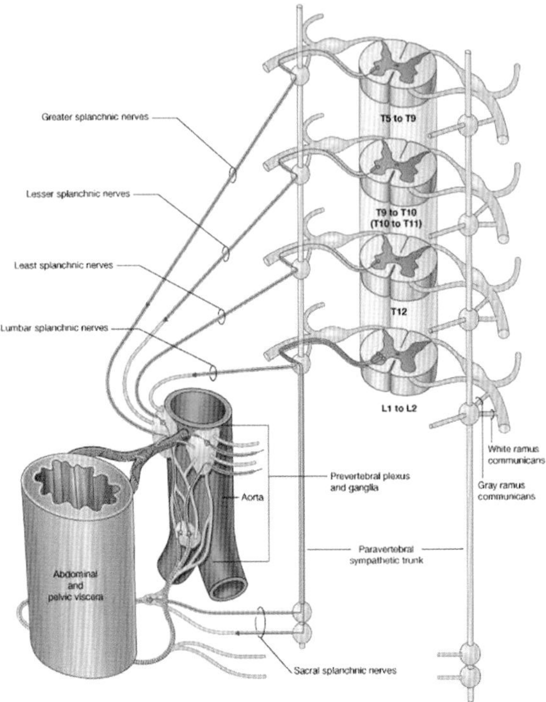

Fig 5.20
The splanchnic nerves.
From Gray's Anatomy for Students, 4th edn, Richard Drake, A. Wayne Vogl, Adam Mitchell. Copyright Elsevier, 2019. Reproduced by kind permission of the publishers.

and it will cause lateral pelvic pain if the iliac part of the muscle goes into spasm. Osteopathic treatments are indicated here to balance the two psoas tensions and maybe stretch the shortened side before the patient goes into labor.

The sympathetic ganglia are situated at the thoracolumbar junction and these control neural impulses relating to the vasculature of the pelvis, control of dilatation of the cervix, and pain pathways. All of these functions are important obstetrically and should be in the forefront of the mind of the osteopath who is working with pregnant patients.

This region is where the named splanchnic nerves come in (greater, lesser, least, and lumbar; Fig 5.20). The pre-ganglionic fibers enter the sympathetic trunk and exit as splanchnic nerves, instead of forming synapses in the sympathetic ganglia. The synapses occur in prevertebral ganglia (celiac, superior mesenteric, inferior mesenteric, and aortico-renal; Box 5.6).

Lastly, the 11th and 12th ribs and the crura of the diaphragm are related to function in the pelvic and abdominal organs. Any change in the lateral plane will cause a change in breathing mechanics because of these attachments.

There is little change in the curves through the thoracic spine because of the stabilizing function of the ribs. Studies have found that pregnancy does not increase the risk of curve progression in the thoracic spine after skeletal maturity. The risk of curve

BOX 5.6

The sympathetic ganglia and innervation

Named ganglia	Region supplied	Named nerve
Celiac ganglia	Foregut	Greater splanchnic nerves (T5/6–T9)
Superior mesenteric ganglia	Midgut	No named splanchnic nerve
Inferior mesenteric ganglia	Hindgut	Lumbar splanchnic nerves (L1–L2/3)
Aortico-renal ganglia	Kidney	Lesser (T9–10,11) and least (T12) splanchnic nerves

progression during pregnancy is unaffected by the age at first pregnancy, the number of pregnancies, and the stability of the curve at skeletal maturity. In addition, the pregnancy itself is rarely affected by scoliosis.[76]

At the cervicodorsal spine, changes in the angles between the 1st rib and the thorax can be compromised by the need for change in upper rib breathing mechanics (see Chapter 3). Costochondral pain anteriorly can also occur for the first time during a pregnancy.

At the occiput, tension headaches are common during pregnancy, as are pains and spasms in the trapezius muscles, and the muscles linking the whole of the neck and shoulder complex. The imbalance does not end there. The whole of the cranial skeleton is working hard to keep the special senses in alignment and this can cause strains into the cranial base and subsequent craniofacial symptoms.

In summary, examination and treatment of the lateral plane curves are as important as treatment of postural changes in the antero-posterior plane but are often neglected.

Visceral Osteopathy in Pregnancy

As far as visceral techniques are concerned, a revision of the ligamentous supports and fascial connections that control the mobility of the abdominal and pelvic organs can reveal potential strain patterns. However, there is a change in surface anatomy because of the fact that the organs move out of the way as they are compressed and forced around the abdominal wall by the expanding uterus. The landmarks that signal the position of the organs can change from individual to individual anyway in the non-pregnant state, and so identifying the exact position of the liver or the duodenojejunal junction can be almost impossible to do with accuracy and precision during and at the end of a pregnancy. The use of functional and myofascial release techniques globally to the abdominal mass will relax and release any strains that might be evident and causing pain, but to describe the effects of your techniques with certainty is just not possible in late pregnancy.

The excellent work of Finet and Williame[77] demonstrates the effect of the descending diaphragm on the abdominal organs. They suggest specific treatment regimes based on their work, but these do not necessarily translate well into the treatment of the pregnant patient because of the limitations outlined above.

Organ Attachments Below the Diaphragm and Potential Changes in Mobility

No organ exists alone: they all lie on or adjacent to other organs, and where they touch they should be able to slide. Sometimes the pressure of one organ against another is very strong and this can leave grooves marks or impressions, as does the heart within the mediastinum on the lung surfaces, for example, or the hepatic flexure of the colon on the liver. These are the visceral articulations; they are governed by the shape and size of each organ and guided in their motion by fascial attachments in sheets or chains. If these movements are restricted, the flow of fluid within the organs can be restricted, too, and this can lead to edema, congestion, and eventually dysfunction.[78,79,80]

During pregnancy, when the growing and expanding uterus pushes the other abdominal organs away to allow room for the fetus to grow, these fascial attachments need to be stretched and relaxed, which is another function of the hormone relaxin during pregnancy. Osteopathic visceral manipulations at this time, to release adhesions and to facilitate changes, can be very beneficial for the mother's changing structure and function, and can have a part to play in organ function and dysfunction.[4,77,81,82]

As the gravid uterus rises, it turns to the right, guided by the mass of the sigmoid colon; this is known as dextrorotation, and it causes a displacement and a compression of the organs in the abdomen and the pelvis (Fig 5.21). The normal anatomy is arranged for them to slide on each other, but they are anchored to the bony skeleton or to fascial attachments, and obviously the movement of the organs will be limited by the muscles of the abdominal walls, the diaphragm and ribs, and the pelvic floor. A clear understanding of normal pre-pregnant relationships and anatomy is important to be able to work out just where these organs move to, and how the potential movement is limited and compromised. The morphology of the patient and the amount of fat in the abdomen, together with previous pregnancies and how they affected the tone of the abdominal walls, are the final factors that need to be taken into account.

The Effect of the Visceral Ligaments During Pregnancy

Figure 5.22 shows the connections between the organs themselves and the bony attachments. These visceral ligaments are described in *Gray's Anatomy* as thickenings or folds of the peritoneum, and they contain collagen and fibrin in different quantities, according to location. Ligaments that are named, such as Toldt's fascia or the lienorenal ligament, appear to have a greater proportion of collagen to elastin in their make-up. The ligaments anchor the organs, allowing mobility around a fixed point. The

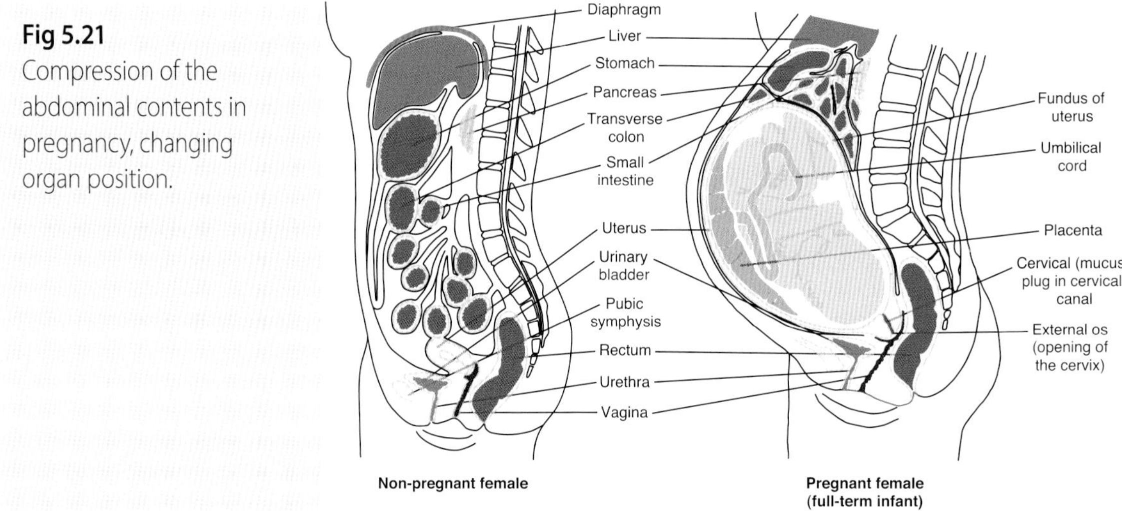

Fig 5.21
Compression of the abdominal contents in pregnancy, changing organ position.

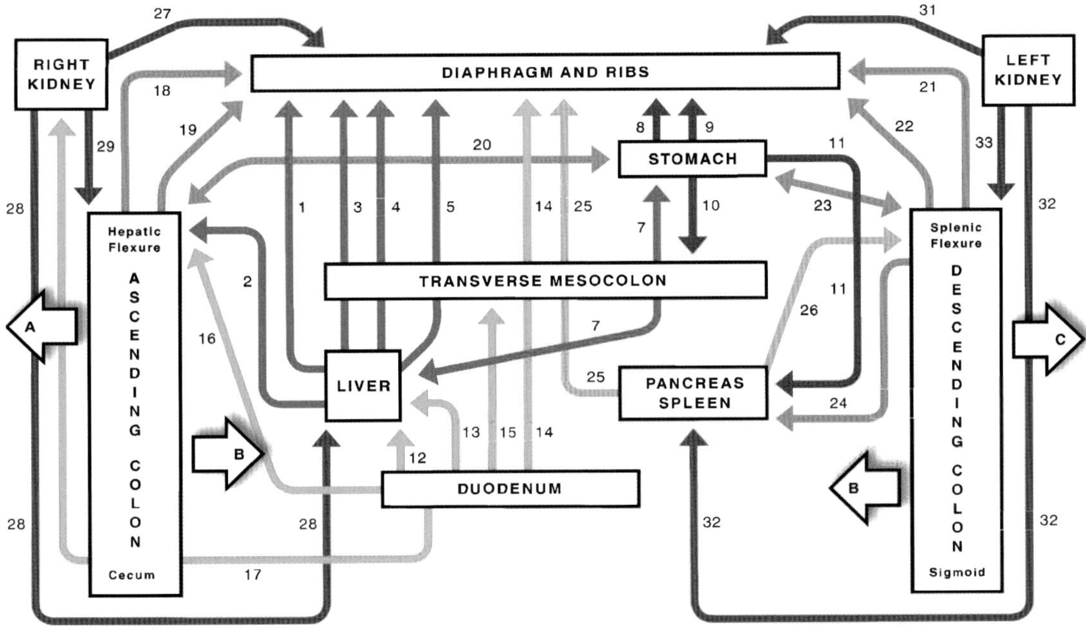

Fig 5.22

The visceral map: connections between the organs via the visceral ligaments. © Dr Stephen Sandler

Key:

LIVER

1. To the diaphragm via the right triangular ligament
2. To the colon/duodenum via the cysticoduodenocolic ligament
3. To the diaphragm via the falciform ligament
4. To the diaphragm via the left triangular ligament
5. To the diaphragm via the central tendon to the sternum
6. To the umbilicus and pelvis (not shown)
7. To the stomach via the gastrohepatic ligament

STOMACH

8. To the diaphragm via the gastrophrenic ligament
9. To the diaphragm via the attachment at the lower esophageal sphincter
10. To the transverse colon via the mesocolon and the greater omentum
11. To the spleen via the gastrosplenic ligament
20. To the right colon via the gastrocolic ligament
23. To the left colon via the gastrocolic ligament

DUODENUM

12. To the liver via the hepatoduodenal ligament
13. To the gall bladder via the cysticoduodenal ligament
14. To the diaphragm via the ligament and muscle of Treitz
15. To the transverse mesocolon
16. To the right colon via the duodenocolic ligament
17. To the right kidney via the duodenorenal ligament

RIGHT COLON

18. To the diaphragm via the phrenicocolic ligament
19. To the 10th rib
20. To the stomach via the gastrocolic ligament

LEFT COLON

21. To the diaphragm via the phrenicocolic ligament
22. To the 9th rib
23. To the stomach via the gastrocolic ligament
24. To the spleen via the gastrosplenic ligament

PANCREAS AND SPLEEN

25. To the diaphragm via the phrenicosplenic ligament
26. To the transverse left colon via the splenicocolic ligament

RIGHT KIDNEY

27. To the diaphragm via the posterior renal fascia
28. To the liver via the hepaticorenal ligament
29. To the right colon at the hepatic angle via Toldt's fascia
30. To the blood vessels entering and leaving the kidney via the fascia of Treitz (not shown)

LEFT KIDNEY

31. To the diaphragm via the posterior renal fascia
32. To the pancreas via the pancreaticorenal ligament
33. To the colon at the splenic flexure via Toldt's fascia
34. To the blood vessels entering and leaving the kidney via the fascia of Treitz (not shown)

most important bony structures for this process are the ribs, along with the diaphragm. Directly or indirectly, all of the abdominal organs are guided in this way. The mesocolon and Toldt's fascia guide and support the intra-abdominal organs in a similar fashion. How the supporting structures change during pregnancy, either in position or in action, is fundamental to understanding just what happens to the abdominal contents at this time.

If we take the ascending and descending colons as an example, they are anchored by the transverse mesocolon medially and by Toldt's fascia laterally (Fig 5.23). The lateral attachments are much stronger. The mesocolon itself is attached to several other organs, as can be seen; however, the attachments to the organs are thinner and more elastic, and the mesentery, being full of blood, is naturally more mobile.

The transverse mesocolon is attached to the ribs and diaphragm, and as the diaphragm is pushed up during pregnancy (Fig 5.24), so the transverse mesocolon and all that is attached to it are pushed up, too. The diaphragm becomes increasingly more dome-shaped as the pregnancy continues. At the end of the pregnancy, the patient will engage in more upper rib breathing than diaphragm or abdominal breathing.

Under normal respiration, the diaphragm descends and the ribs flare as a person breathes in. With the progression of the pregnancy, the descent of the diaphragm is greatly restricted but the ribs flare more, due to the uterine bulk and the fat in the mesentery, so that organs beneath the ribs are displaced. The liver cannot ascend more than the diaphragm allows and is therefore forced around the right abdominal wall so that, at the end of the pregnancy, it lies high up and lateral, and its usual mobility is greatly restricted.

The stomach is compressed and rotates to the left around the abdominal wall, and the increased pressure, together with relaxation of the lower esophageal sphincter under the influence of the pregnancy hormones, means that the compression from below and the restriction in the diaphragm above result in a squeezing of the stomach; this is thought to be responsible for the symptoms of gastro-esophageal reflux (Fig 5.25).

The position of the pancreas and spleen are uncertain during pregnancy. These organs are normally attached to the left kidney via the pancreaticorenal ligament, to the diaphragm via the phrenicosplenic ligament, and to the transverse left colon via the splenicocolic ligament. They are thin and mobile, compared to the bulkier stomach or liver, and so their displacement will be all the greater.

The kidneys are retroperitoneal and slide superiorly and inferiorly with each breath taken. There appears to be little change in their position or respiratory-induced motion during pregnancy, and they slip and slide around the rib cage very much as before.

The ureters, however, can be lengthened as the elastic tissue within their walls relaxes, and entrapment of the ureters against the brim of the pelvis can lead to ureteric stasis, spasms, and maybe even a UTI or hydronephrosis.[83] The absolute cause of hydronephrosis and hydroureter in pregnancy is unknown: there may be several contributing factors, including the dextrorotation of the uterus, which may explain why the right ureter is usually more dilated than the left, and hyperplasia of smooth muscle in the distal one-third of the ureter may cause a reduction in luminal size.

As described earlier, the duodenum and the small intestine are, again, attached to the mesocolon, liver and hepatic flexure, mostly at the sphincter of Oddi or the duodenojejunal junction. The jejunum and ileum are therefore free to move almost anywhere in the abdomen, being fixed at the mesentery but free along the other surfaces. At the distal end of the small intestine, where the ileum and the cecum meet at the

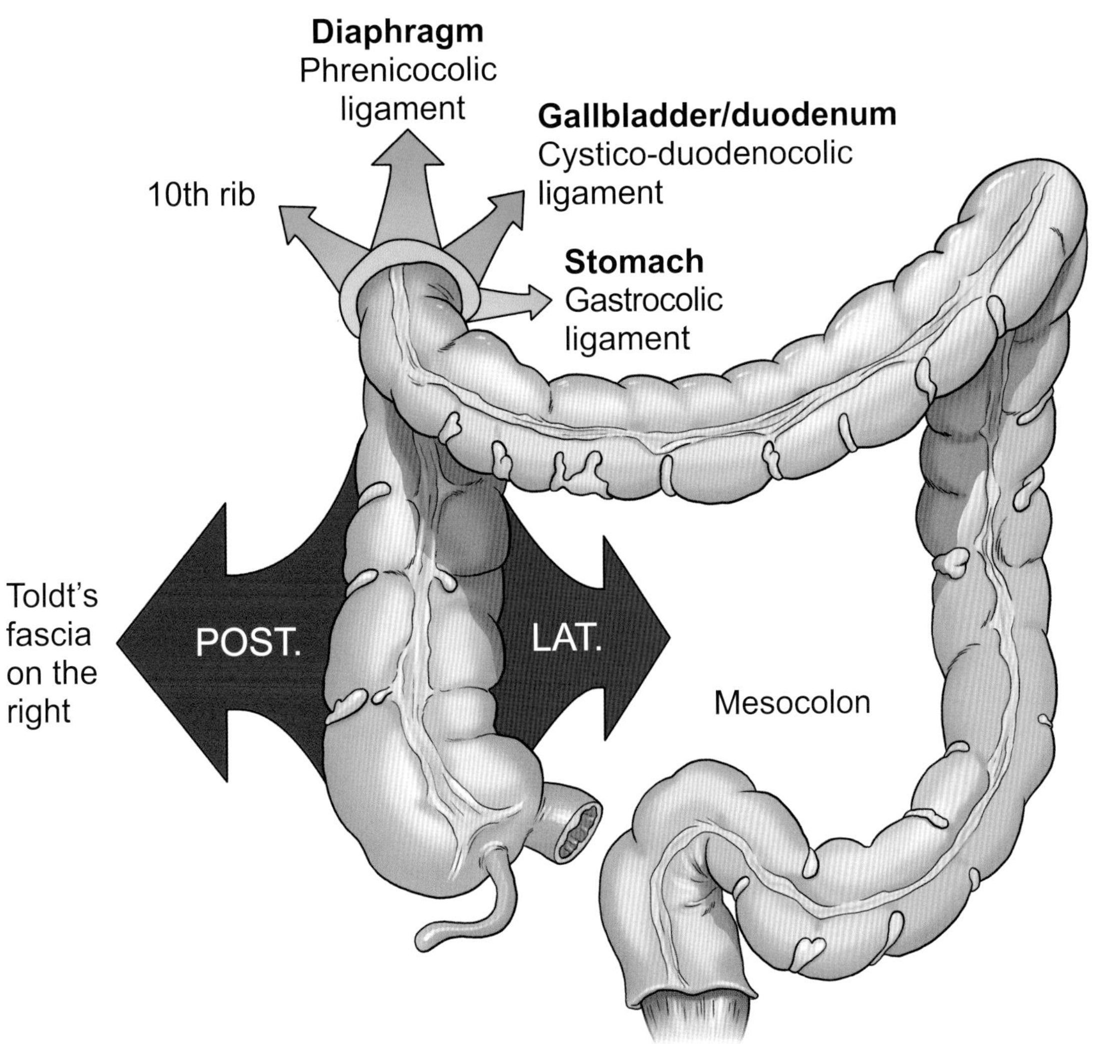

Fig 5.23
The attachments of the gut to the ascending colon.
©François Ricard.

iliocecal valve, there is an attachment via the root of the mesentery. Contraction along the root of the mesentery will pull the cecum towards the midline, closing the hepatic angle and leading to a slowing of food transit in the gut. The cecum has a difficult job in non-pregnant women, lifting a semifluid mass with the consistency of wet sand up against gravity, but if the hepatic angle is closed or reduced, the stool mass is going to stay in the ascending colon for longer and thus becomes drier and more solid than usual.

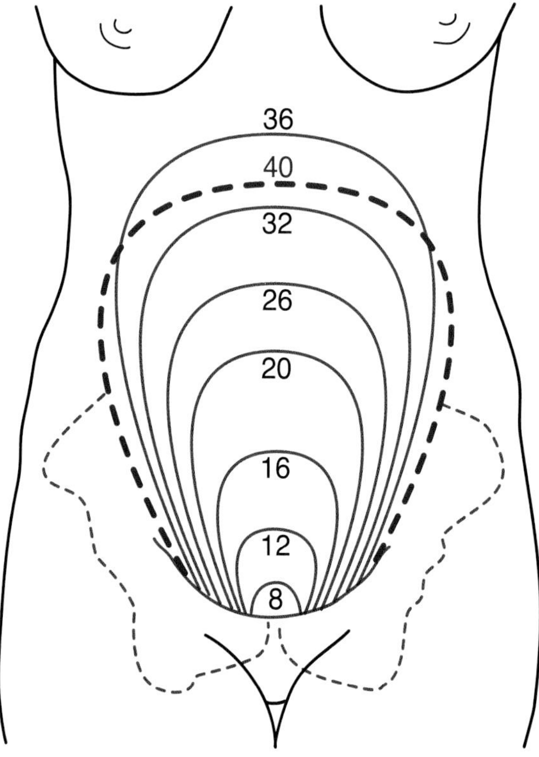

Fig 5.24
The height of the fundus at different stages of pregnancy.

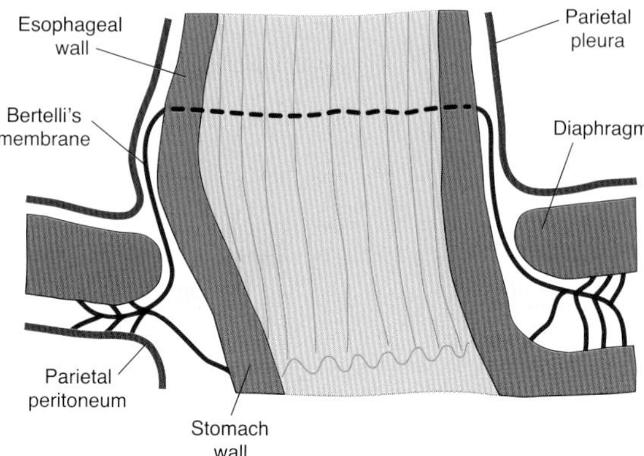

Fig 5.25
The attachments of the diaphragm and the esophagus.

However, as the colon is attached laterally by Toldt's fascia and as the growing uterus pushes the colon more laterally, this closure mechanism is negated; this is why constipation, although common in pregnancy, is by no means a universal complaint.

Osteopathic visceral techniques rely on a sound knowledge of the surface anatomy and the relations between the sliding surfaces of the organs. In pregnancy, all of this will change as the organs move and are compressed. The normal specific visceral motility techniques are more difficult to apply, especially at the end of the pregnancy, because of the imprecise palpation of the abdominal organs. Mobility techniques acting on the ribs and diaphragm supports, or techniques around the pelvic brim, are better and more accurate. In fact, as a rule during pregnancy, if you want to treat the abdominal organs, treat the ribs and diaphragm, and thus ensure that there is good movement of whatever is attached to them; in this way, you will give them the best possible chance of efficient function. Specific visceral motility and mobility techniques in the absence of specific visceral landmarks will not be possible with any degree of accuracy.

References

1. Stone C. *Science in the Art of Osteopathy: Osteopathic Principles and Practice*. Nelson Thornes, 1999.
2. Barral JP, Mercier P. *Visceral Manipulation*. Eastland Press, 1988.
3. Chegini N. Peritoneal molecular environment, adhesion formation and clinical implication. Front Biosci. 2002 Apr 1;7:e91–115.
4. Wiseman DM. Disorders of adhesions or adhesion related disorder: monolithic entities or part of something bigger--CAPPS (complex abdomino pelvic and pain syndrome). Semin Reprod Med. 2008 Jul;26(4):356–68.
5. Liakakos T, Thomakos N, Fine PM, Dervenis C, Young RL. Peritoneal adhesions: etiology, pathophysiology, and

clinical significance: recent advances in prevention and management. Dig Surg. 2001;18(4):260–73
6. Sulaiman H, Gabella G, Davis C, Mutsaers SE, Boulos P, Laurent GJ et al. Growth of nerve fibres into murine peritoneal adhesions. J Pathol. 2000 Nov;192(3):396-403.
7. O'Brien B, Zhou Q. Variables related to nausea and vomiting during pregnancy. Birth. 1995;22(2):93–100.
8. Cappell MS. Gastric and duodenal ulcers during pregnancy. Gastroenterol Clin North Am. 2003 Mar;32(1): 263–308.
9. Depue RH, Ross RK, Bernstein L, Judd HL, Henderson BE. Hyperemesis gravidarum in relation to estradiol levels, pregnancy outcome, and other maternal factors: a seroepidemiologic study. Am J Obstet Gynecol. 1987 May;156(5):1137.
10. Maes BD, Spitz B, Ghoos YF, Hiele MI, Evenepoel P, Rutgeerts PJ. Gastric emptying in hyperemesis gravidarum and non-dyspeptic pregnancy. Aliment Pharmacol Ther. 1999;13(2):237–43.
11. Walsh JW, Hasler WL, Nugent CE, Owyang C. Progesterone and estrogen are potential mediators of gastric slow-wave dysrhythmias in nausea of pregnancy. Am J Physiol. 1996;270(3Pt1):G506–14.
12. Choi CQ. Causes of morning sickness revealed. Despite the misery, nausea and vomiting actually serve a useful purpose. Live Science, May 18, 2008; https://www.livescience.com/2531-morning-sickness-revealed.htm.
13. Goldberg D, Szilagy A, Graves L. Hyperemesis gravidarum and Helicobacter pylori infection: a systematic review. Obstet Gynecol. 2007 Sep;110 (3):695–703.
14. Sahakian V, Rouse D, Sipes S, Rose N, Niebyl J. Vitamin B6 is effective therapy for nausea and vomiting of pregnancy: a randomized, double-blind placebo controlled study. Obstet Gynecol. 1991 Jul;78(1):33.
15. Baron TH, Richter JE. Gastroesophageal reflux disease in pregnancy. Gastroenterol Clin North Am. 1992 Dec;21(4):777.
16. Bainbridge ET, Temple JG, Nicholas SP, Newton JR, Boriah V. Symptomatic gastro-oesophageal reflux in pregnancy. A comparative study of white Europeans and Asians in Birmingham. Br J Clin Pract. 1983 Feb;37(2):53–7.
17. Wong CA, Loffredi M, Ganchiff JN, Zhao J, Zhao W, Avram ML. Gastric emptying of water in term pregnancy. Anesthesiology. 2002 Jun;96(6):1395–400.
18. Koch KL. Gastrointestinal factors in nausea and vomiting of pregnancy. Am J Obstet Gynecol. 2002;186(5 Suppl 2):S198–203.
19. Clark DH. Peptic ulcer in women. Br Med J. 1953 Jun;1(4822):1259.
20. Wald A. Constipation, diarrhea, and symptomatic hemorrhoids during pregnancy. Gastroenterol Clin North Am. 2003 Mar;32(1):309–22.
21. Willoughby CP, Truelove SC. Ulcerative colitis and pregnancy. Gut 1980 Jun;21(6):469–74.
22. Byrne JJ, Moran MM. The Mallory-Weiss syndrome. N Engl J Med. 1965;272:398.
23. Everhart JE, Renault PF. Irritable bowel syndrome in office-based practice in the United States. Gastroenterology. 1991 Apr;100(4):998–1005.
24. Whitehead WE, Cheskin LG, Heller BR, Robinson JC, Crowell MD, Benjamin C, et al. Evidence for exacerbation of irritable bowel syndrome during menses. Gastroenterology. 1990 Jun;98(6):1485–9.
25. Galati JS, McKee DP, Quigley EM. Response to intraluminal gas in irritable bowel syndrome. Motility versus perception. Dig Dis Sci. 1995 Jun;40(6):1381–7.
26. Mayer EA, Gebhart GF. Basic and clinical aspects of visceral hyperalgesia. Gastroenterology. 1994 Jul;107(1):271–93.
27. Hasler WL. The irritable bowel syndrome during pregnancy. Gastroenterol Clin N Am. 2003 Mar;32(1):385–406.
28. Kilpatrick CC, Monga M. Approach to the acute abdomen in pregnancy. Obstet Gynecol Clin N Am. 2007 Sep;34(3):389–402.
29. Tracey M, Fletcher HS. Appendicitis in pregnancy. Am Surg. 2000 Jun;66(6):555–60.
30. Present DH. Diseases of the biliary tract and pregnancy. In JJ Rovinsky, AF Guttmacher, SH Cherry (eds), *Medical, Surgical and Gynecologic Complications of Pregnancy*, p. 215. Lippincott, Williams and Wilkins, 1985.
31. Hiatt JR, Hiatt JC, Williams RA, Klein SR. Biliary disease in pregnancy: strategy for surgical management. Am J Surg. 1986 Feb;151(2):263–5.
32. Henriksson P, Eriksson A. Estrogen-induced gallstone formation in males. J Clin Invest. 1989 Sep;84(3):811–16.
33. Xiao ZL, Chen Q, Biancani P, Behar J. Mechanisms of gallbladder hypomotility in pregnant guinea pigs. Gastroenterology. 1999 Feb;116(2):411–19.
34. Bailey RR, Rolleston GL. Kidney length and ureteric dilatation in the puerperium. J Obstet Gynaecol Br Commonw. 1971 Jan;78(1):55.
35. Rasmussen PE, Nielsen FR. Hydronephrosis during pregnancy: a literature survey. Eur J Obstet Gynecol Reprod Biol. 1988 Mar;27(3):249.
36. Ciliberto CF, Marx GF, Johnston D. Physiological changes associated with pregnancy. Update Anaesthes. 2008 Dec;24(2):72-6.
37. Albert H, Godskesen M, Westergaard JG, Chard T, Gunn L. Circulating levels of relaxin are normal in pregnant

women with pelvic pain. Eur J Obstet Gynecol Reprod Biol. 1997 Jul;74(1):19–22.
38. MacLennan AH. The role of the hormone relaxin in human reproduction and pelvic girdle relaxation. Scand J Rheumatol Suppl. 1991;88:7–15.
39. Stone C. *Visceral and Obstetric Osteopathy*. Churchill Livingstone, 2007.
40. Hisaw FL. Experimental relaxation of the pubic ligament of guinea pig. Proc Soc Exp Biol Med. 1926 May;23:661–3.
41. Abramson D, Roberts SM, Wilson P. Relaxation of pelvic ligaments in pregnancy. Surg Gynae Obstet. 1934;58:595.
42. Katonis P, Kampouroglou A, Aggelopoulos A, Kakavelakis K, Lykoudis S, Makriginnakis A, et al. Pregnancy related low back pain .Hippokratia. 2011 Jul;15(3):205–10.
43. Orvieto R, Achiron A, Ben-Rafael Z, Gelernter I, Achiron R. Low-back pain of pregnancy. Acta Obstet. Gynecol. Scand. 1994 Mar;73(3):209–14.
44. Middleditch A, Oliver J. Functional Anatomy of the Spine, 2nd edn, p 220. Elsevier, 2005.
45. Mogren IM. Does caesarean section negatively influence the post-partum prognosis of low back pain and pelvic pain during pregnancy? S.Eur Spine J. 2007 Jan;16(1):123.
46. Mousavi SJ, Parnianpour M, Vleeming A. Pregnancy related pelvic girdle pain and low back pain in an Iranian population. Spine (Phila Pa 1976). 2007 Feb;32(3):E100–4.
47. Mota MJ, Cardoso M, Carvalho A, Marques A, Sá-Couto P, Demain S. Women's experiences of back pain in pregnancy. J Back Musculoskelet Rehabil. 2015;28(2):351-7.
48. Shijagurumayam Acharya R, Tveter AT, Grotle M, Eberhard-Gran M, Stuge B. Pregnancy and severity of low back- and pelvic girdle pain in pregnant Nepalese women. BMC Pregnancy Childbirth. 2019 Jul;19(1):247.
49. Ramachenderan J, Bradford J, McLean M. Maternal obesity and pregnancy complications: a review. Aust N Z J Obstet Gynaecol. 2008 Jun;48(3):228–35.
50. Garshasbi A, Faghih Zadeh S. The effect of exercise on the intensity of low back pain in pregnant women. Int J Gynaecol Obstet. 2005 Mar;88(3):271–5.
51. Bennett VR, Brown LK. *Myles Textbook for Midwives*. Churchill Livingstone, 1993.
52. Dumas GA, Reid JG, Wolfe LA, Griffin MP, McGrath MJ. Exercise posture and back pain during pregnancy. Clin Biomech. 1995 Mar;10(2):98–103.
53. Sihvonen T, Huttenen M, Makkonen M, Airaksinen O. Functional changes in back muscle activity correlate with pain intensity and prediction of low back pain during pregnancy. Arch Phys Med Rehab. 1998 Oct;79(10): 1210–12.
54. Lansac J, Nelken S, Gaja J, Dumont M. Spondylolisthesis and pregnancy. Rev Fr Gynae Obstet. 1969;64(12):689–93.
55. Elliott JM, Fleming H, Tucker K. Asymptomatic spondylolisthesis and pregnancy. J Orthop Sports Phys Ther. 2010 May;40(5):324.
56. Hoyte L, Damaser MS. Magnetic resonance-based female pelvic anatomy as relevant for maternal childbirth injury simulations. Ann N Y Acad Sci. 2007 Apr;1101:361–76.
57. Nadaud MC, McClure S, Weiner BK. Do facet joint capsular ligaments contain estrogen receptors? Application to pathogenesis of degenerative spondylolisthesis. Am J Orthop. 2001 Oct;30(10):753–4.
58. Jinkins JR. Acquired degenerative changes of the intervertebral segments at and suprajacent to the lumbo sacral junction. A radioanatomic analysis of the nondiscal structures of the spinal column and peri spinal soft tissues. Eur J Radiol. 2004 May;50(2):134–58.
59. Saraste H. Spondylolisthesis and pregnancy–a risk analysis. Acta Obstet Gynaecol Scand. 1986;65(7):727–9.
60. Sanderson PL, Fraser RD. The influence of pregnancy on the development of degenerative spondylolisthesis. J Bone Joint Surg Br. 1996 Nov;78(6):951–4.
61. Mogren IM. Previous physical activity decreases the risk of low back pain and pelvic pain during pregnancy. Scand J Public Health. 2005;33(4):300–6.
62. Van De Pol G, Van Brummen HJ, Bruinse HW, Heintz AP, Van Der Vaart CH. Pregnancy-related pelvic girdle pain in the Netherlands. Acta Obstet Gynecol Scand. 2007;86(4):416–22.
63. Sandler SE. The Association between Joint Laxity and Female Hormones Associated with the Menstrual Cycle, Pregnancy, with the Post Partum and with the Menopause. PhD Thesis. VDM, 2009.
64. Hoyte L, Thomas J, Foster RT, Shott S, Jakab M, Weidner AC. Racial differences in pelvic morphology among asymptomatic nulliparous women as seen on three-dimensional magnetic resonance images. Am J Obstet Gynecol. 2005 Dec;193(6):2035–40.
65. Smith MW, Marcus PS, Wurtz LD. Orthopedic issues in pregnancy. Obstet Gynecol Surv. 2008 Feb;63(2):103–11.
66. Mondelli M, Rossi S, Monti E, Aprile I, Caliandro P, Pazzaglia C, et al. Long term follow-up of carpal tunnel syndrome during pregnancy: a cohort study and review of the literature. Electromyogr Clin Neurophysiol. 2007 Sep;47(6):259–71.
67. Ablove RH, Ablove TS. Prevalence of carpal tunnel syndrome in pregnant women. WMJ. 2009 Jul;108(4):194–6.
68. Tupković E, Nisić M, Kendić S, Salihović S, Balić A, Brigić K, et al. Median nerve: neurophysiological parameters in

third trimester of pregnancy. Bosn J Basic Med Sci. 2007 Feb;7(1):84–9.

69. Mallol J, Belda MA, Costa D, Noval A, Sola M. Prophylaxis of striae gravidarum with a topical formulation: a double-blind trial. Int J Cosmetic Sci 1991;3:51–7.
70. 70. Wierrani F, Kozak W, Schramm W, Grunberger W. Attempt of preventive treatment of striae gravidarum using preventive massage ointment administration. Wien Klin Wochenschr 1992;104(2):42–4.
71. Mahato NK. Association of rudimentary sacral zygapophyseal facets and accessory and ligamentous articulations: implications for load transmission at the L5-S1 junction. Clin Anat. 2010 Sep;23(6):707–11.
72. Ostojić Z, Kristo T, Ostojić L, Petrović P, Vasilj I, Santić Z, et al. Prevalence of scoliosis in school-children from Mostar, Bosnia and Herzegovina. Coll Antropol. 2006 Mar;30(1):59–64.
73. Wong HK, Hui JHP, Rajan U, Chia HP. Idiopathic scoliosis in Singapore schoolchildren: a prevalence study 15 years into the screening program. Spine (Phila PA 1976). 2005 May;30(10):1188–96.
74. Leaver JM, Alvik A, Warren MD. Prescriptive screening for adolescent idiopathic scoliosis: a review of the evidence. Int J Epidemiol. 1982 Jun;11(2):101–11.
75. Sipko T, Grygier D, Barczyk K, Eliasz G. The occurrence of strain symptoms in the lumbosacral region and pelvis during pregnancy and after childbirth. J Manipulative Physiol Ther. 2010 Jun;33(5):370–7.
76. Betz RR, Bunnell WP, Lambrecht-Mulier E, MacEwen GD. Scoliosis and pregnancy. J Bone Joint Surg Am. 1987 Jan;69(1):90–6.
77. Finet G, Williame C. *Treating Visceral Dysfunction*. Stillness Press, 2000.
78. Hackethal A, Sick C, Brueggmann D, Tchartchian G, Wallwiener M, Muenstedt K, et al. Awareness and perception of intra-abdominal adhesions and related consequences: survey of gynaecologists in German hospitals. Eur J Obstet Gynecol Reprod Biol. 2010 Jun;150(2):180–9.
79. Senthilkumar MP, Dreyer JS. Peritoneal adhesions: pathogenesis, assessment and effects. Trop Gastroenterol. 2006 Jan–Mar;27(1):11–18.
80. Healy JC, Reznek RH. The peritoneum, mesenteries and omenta: normal anatomy and pathological processes. Eur Radiol. 1998;8(6):886–900.
81. Keltz MD, Peck L, Liu S, Kim AH, Arici A, Olive DL. Large bowel-to-pelvic sidewall adhesions associated with chronic pelvic pain. J Am Assoc Gynecol Laparosc. 1995 Nov;3(1):55–9.
82. Alpay Z, Saed GM, Diamond MP. Postoperative adhesions: from formation to prevention. Semin Reprod Med. 2008 Jul;26(4):313–21.
83. Nielsen FR, Rasmussen PE. Hydronephrosis during pregnancy: four cases of hydronephrosis causing symptoms during pregnancy. Eur J Obstet Gynecol Reprod Biol. 1988 Mar;27(3):245–8.

Treatment Techniques for the Diaphragm and Below During Pregnancy 6

As always, it is important to emphasize that it is not good practice to treat pregnant patients prone, as any undue pressure on the abdomen at any stage in pregnancy is an absolute contraindication. Patients may find it more comfortable to lie in a half-prone, half-side-lying position, where the weight of the baby is not compressed, but it is still better to have them sitting or side-lying if possible. If the pregnant patient is supine, the weight of the gravid uterus on the ascending blood vessels – in particular, the inferior vena cava – can have the unwanted effect of reducing venous return from the lower limbs and lowering her blood pressure. If she is going to be treated in the supine position, have her propped up at 45 degrees with lots of pillows, and put pillows under her knees, too, so that her legs are supported. It is still probably best practice to limit this patient position to no more than 10 minutes or so.

Soft Tissue Relaxation Techniques with the Patient Sitting

On average, women will put on 12 kilos (29 pounds) of extra weight during pregnancy. This consists of an extra 2 kilos (4.4 pounds) in the first 20 weeks and then 0.5 kilos (1 pound) per week thereafter.

The weight of the developing breast tissue, and the increasing weight generally during the middle and final trimesters, together with the change in the antero-posterior postural curves, mean that the long spinal muscles running from the sacrum to the occiput can easily become chronically hypertonic during pregnancy; they will thus be liable to congestion syndromes and will fatigue easily (see Box 5.1).

Longitudinal Stretch Technique

A longitudinal stretch technique will encourage fluid exchange from the lumbar spine and sacrum back towards the heart.

Position of the patient

The patient sits on a stool or a chair and leans over the treatment table, with her head supported by pillows. Her arms are crossed, supporting the head, and her spine is held in a fairly neutral position (Fig 6.1).

Position of the osteopath

The osteopath stands, kneels, or sits behind her (Fig 6.2). You may not be familiar with working in this position, but it affords you the opportunity to use both hands in a sweeping motion over the superficial muscles and fascia, so that fluid moves up towards the heart from the congested lumbar spine and pelvis.

Ambition of the technique

The aim is to create a wave of fluid in advance of the osteopath's hands and fingers as he moves from below upwards.

Application of the technique

The technique is performed from the superficial tissues to the deeper ones. The osteopath's hands (and, in particular, his thumbs) push gently up the back, one on either side of the spinous processes, encouraging a wave of fluid to move in front of them

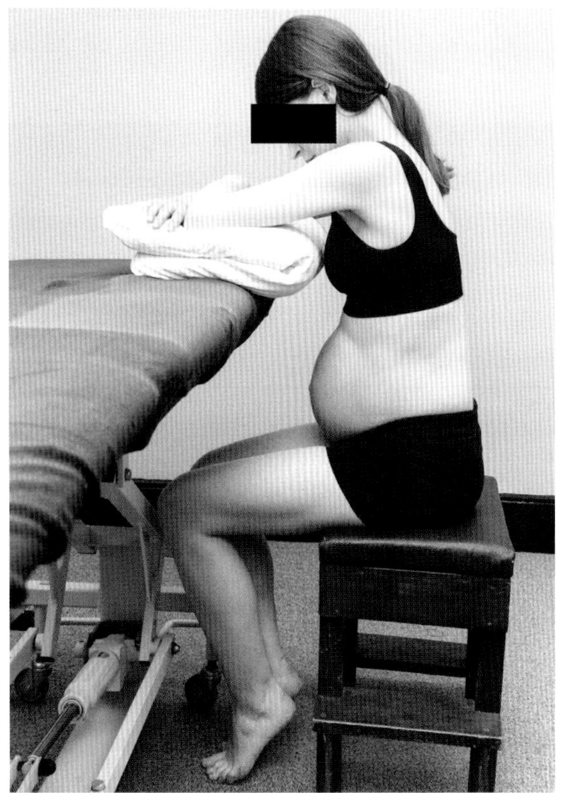

Fig 6.1
Patient sitting in a leaning position over the treatment table.

and draining the muscles longitudinally (Fig 6.2). As an analogy, it is helpful to imagine that you are treading on a hosepipe full of fluid and walking the fluid up the pipe, so that it empties out at the end. At the level of the shoulder blades the two hands separate, passing laterally over the latissimus dorsi muscles before returning via the flank muscles to the start position.

This very gentle and relaxing "massage" technique is particularly enjoyed by patients during pregnancy, and it can be one of many techniques that you can teach to partners for use at home.

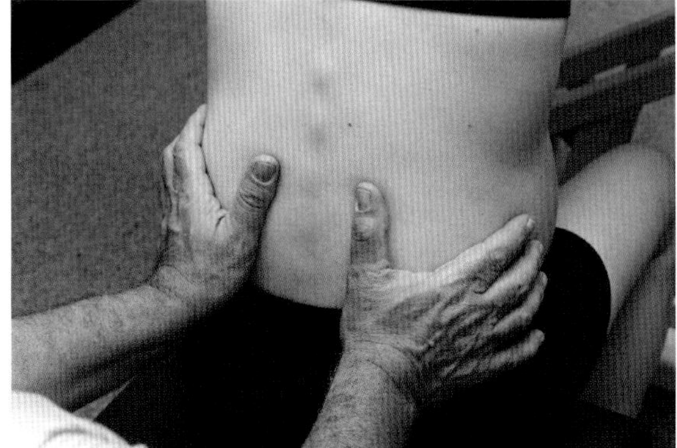

Fig 6.2
The osteopath sitting behind the patient. Note that his thumbs are parallel with the patient's spine.

Soft Tissue Techniques with the Patient Side-lying

Side-lying Eight-fingers Stretch Technique for Lumbar Spinal Muscles

Position of the patient

The patient lies on either side in the form of a three-sided square (Fig 6.3), with her neck supported by pillows. The shoulders and hips are maintained in the vertical position with respect to the treatment table, her knees are bent at 90 degrees, and her head is well supported. Her spine should be parallel with the back of the table so that she is lying square. A small pillow or a folded towel is used under her waist so that the abdominal muscles are relaxed.

Position of the osteopath

The osteopath stands facing the patient, with his forearms resting on her iliac crests and thorax.

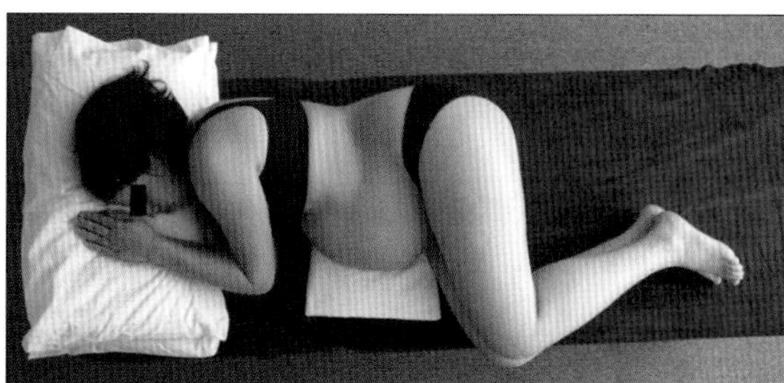

Fig 6.3
The patient lying in a "three-sided square" position.

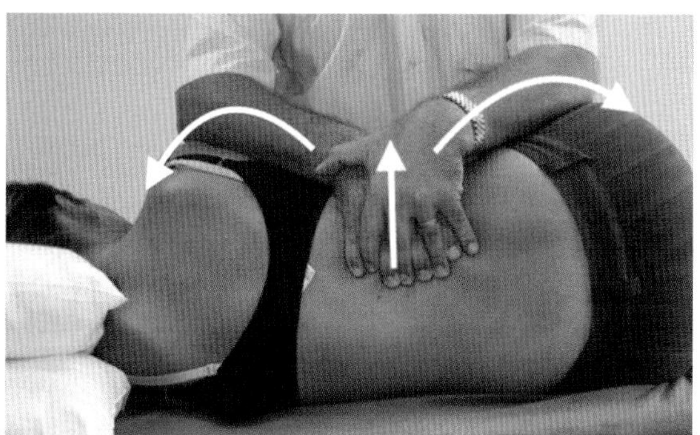

Fig 6.4
The eight fingers stretch technique for the erector spinae muscles.

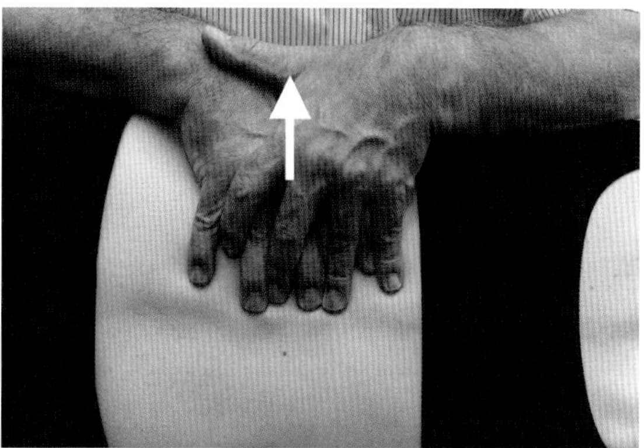

Fig 6.5
The hands in close-up for the soft tissue technique.

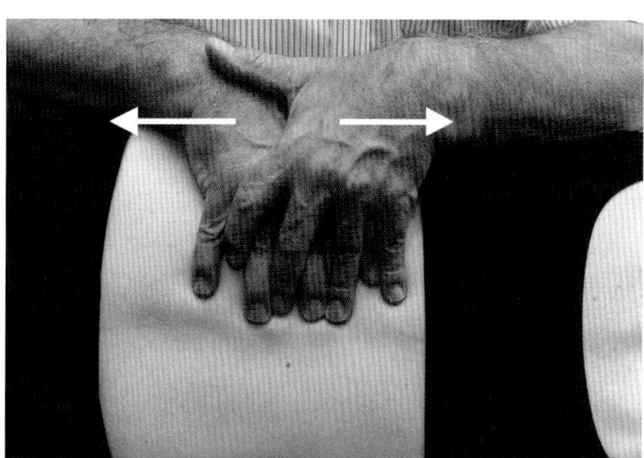

Fig 6.6
The elbows move towards the head and the sacrum to impart a lateral motion to the technique.

Ambition of the technique

This cross-fiber, soft-tissue stretch technique is used to release the smaller, deeper postural muscles if there is somatic dysfunction over an area or if there is tension due to postural stress.

Application of the technique

In Figures 6.4 and 6.5 we can see that the osteopath's fingers are interlinked and gently push down to the treatment table to buckle or gather the muscle bulk; then, with the fingertips, they pull up, away from the treatment table, stretching the muscle bulk as it bows towards him.

A gentle lateral motion towards the head and the feet from each arm will encourage bowing of the spine and gap the foraminal spaces between the vertebrae (Fig 6.6).

This technique can also be used to stretch a tight quadratus lumborum muscle between the 12th rib and the iliac crest.

Ligamentous Articulation Techniques with the Patient Side-lying

Articulation into Flexion/Extension

Position of the patient

The patient lies on her side in a three-sided square, as before.

Position of the osteopath

The osteopath stands to face her, as before.

Ambition of the technique

The technique has several roles to play in pregnancy. It can be used as a pumping technique to clear blood away from the deep lumbar veins in cases of pelvic congestion. It can impart a longitudinal soft tissue stretch. It can also gently stretch ligamentous tissues and joint capsules if they are shortened.

Application of the technique

This is a variation on the usual lumbar flexion technique, except that, as the patient is pregnant, the osteopath uses only one of her legs to avoid any abdominal compression (Fig 6.7). He flexes and extends her spine by placing her lower legs across his thighs as he moves his pelvis into rotation left and right around his vertical axis. He compares each segment's motion, looking for the segment that is painful or restricted. He is assessing the quality, as well as the quantity, of restriction. A normal end feel to the motion that comes before it is expected may indicate a shortened ligament, while a more bouncy or elastic feeling at the end of the range of motion is more likely to indicate motion restricted by muscular tension. A complete block to the motion, often accompanied by pain, indicates a facet restriction or a bone anomaly. By holding back on the spinous process below, he can stretch the tissues between the two spinous processes as he moves the vertebra above away from the vertebra below (Fig 6.8).

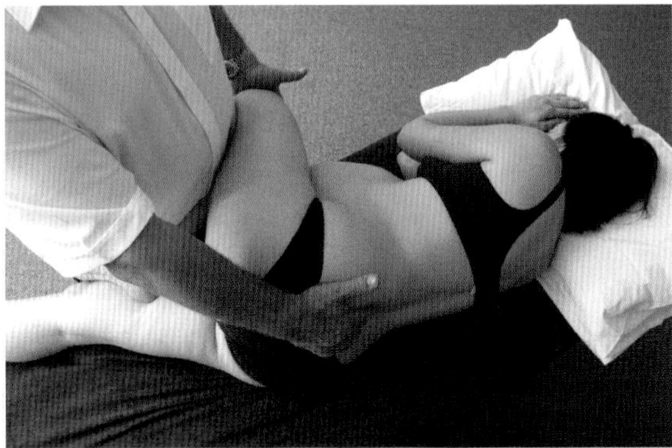

Fig 6.7
The use of a single leg is sufficient in pregnancy to avoid compression of the abdomen.

The technique can be reinforced with the patient lying on her side with her knees together, and the osteopath's caudal forearm applying an element of traction to the lumbar spine along the long axis of the spine via the sacrum (Fig 6.9). The other hand is used to palpate the interspinal spaces, and to modify the technique and limit it to a specific segment if desired.

Articulation into Side-bending or Lateral Flexion

Position of the patient

The patient lies in a side-lying position on the treatment table, as before.

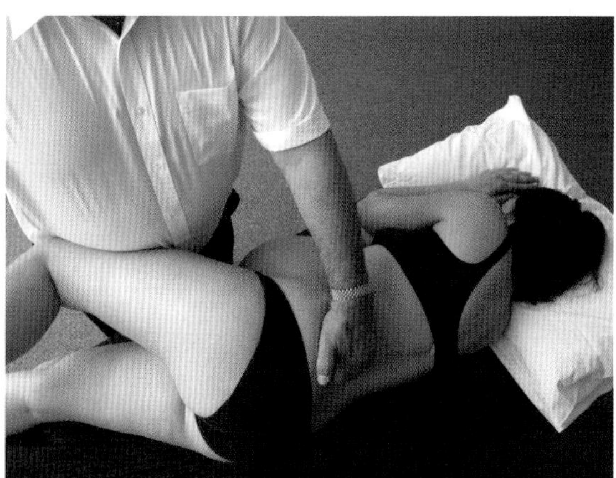

Fig 6.8
Single leg flexion and extension as an articulation technique to stretch the spinal ligaments and capsules.

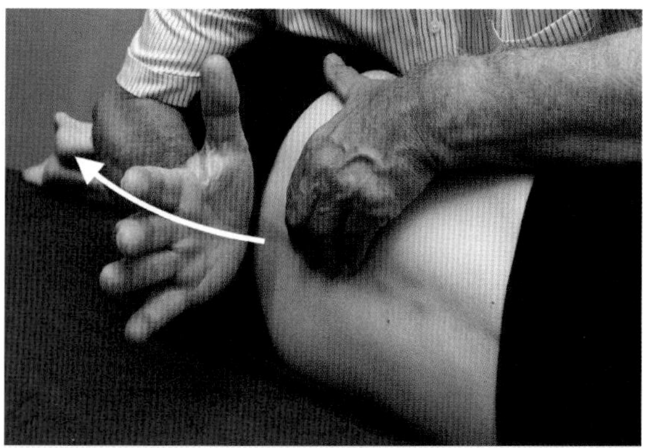

Fig 6.9
Reinforced sacral flexion to stretch the L5/S1 interspace.

Position of the osteopath

The osteopath sits on the treatment table behind the patient's pelvis, turning to face her lumbar spine (Fig 6.10).

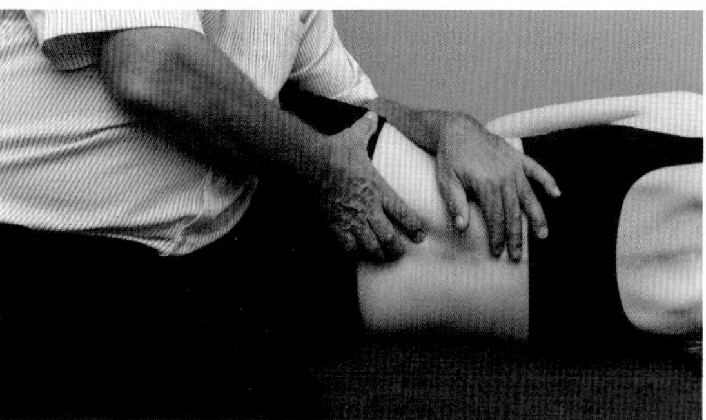

Fig 6.10
Articulation into lateral flexion or side-bending.

Ambition of the technique

The technique is used to open the facet joints and the intervertebral foramina in cases such as sciatic nerve impingement at the level of the foramen.

Application of the technique

The osteopath uses his cephalad forearm to hook around the crest of the patient's iliac spine. His other hand monitors at the spinal interspaces, as before. He uses a gentle rocking motion of his body into side-bending or lateral flexion to open and close the upper and lower facet joints into a side-bending or lateral flexion movement (Fig 6.11). This is an example of using short levers to be very specific during pregnancy and to make use of the fact that, under the actions of the ovarian hormones, notably relaxin, the ligaments will stretch very easily at this time.

Circumduction of Figure of Eight Articulations to the Lumbar Spine with the Patient Side-lying

Position of the patient

The position of the patient is as before.

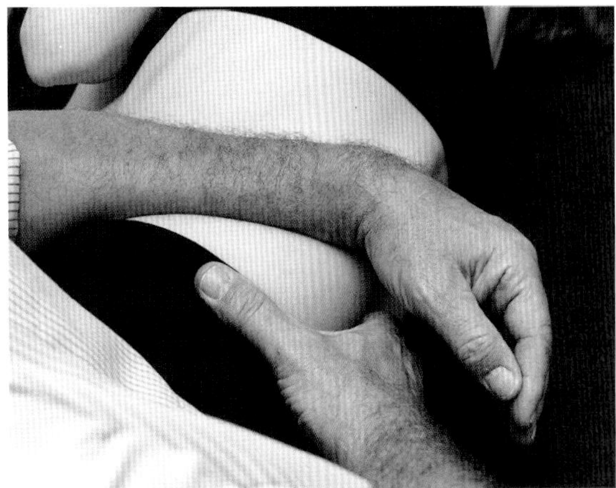

Fig 6.11
Lumbar side-lying or lateral flexion articulation.

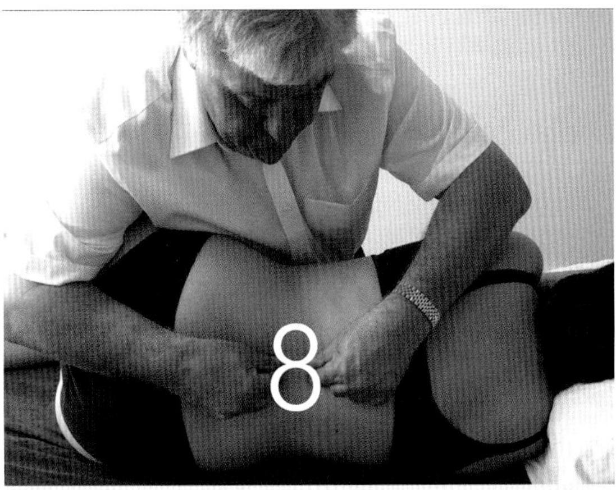

Fig 6.12
The figure of eight articulation is done with the fingers of both hands working in the lateral plane.

Position of the osteopath

The osteopath is in front of the patient as before. He gently rests his arms on the patient's thorax and pelvis, then grasps two adjacent spinous processes with his fingers (Fig 6.12).

Ambition of the technique

The aim is to increase the range of motion, specifically at restricted segments, by stretching short ligaments and capsules at the individual facet joints.

Application of the technique

In Figures 6.12 and 6.13, we can see the figure of eight in two planes.

The center of the eight will be at the spinal interspace of the lesioned segment, which will generally be restricted by ligamentous tightness.

Thinking of his fingertips, the osteopath moves his hips and shoulders such that he induces the parameters of side-bending and reverse rotation to and from the center of the eight in a vertical plane to stretch the capsules of the facet joints by fixing the spinous processes as he moves (Fig 6.14).

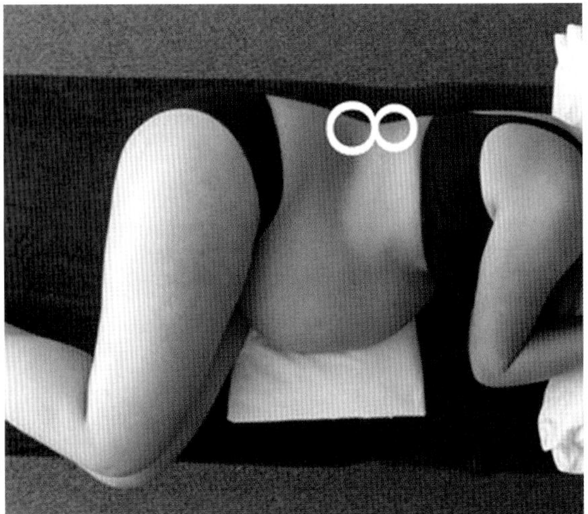

Fig 6.13
The figure of eight articulation is done with the fingers of both hands working in the antero-posterior plane.

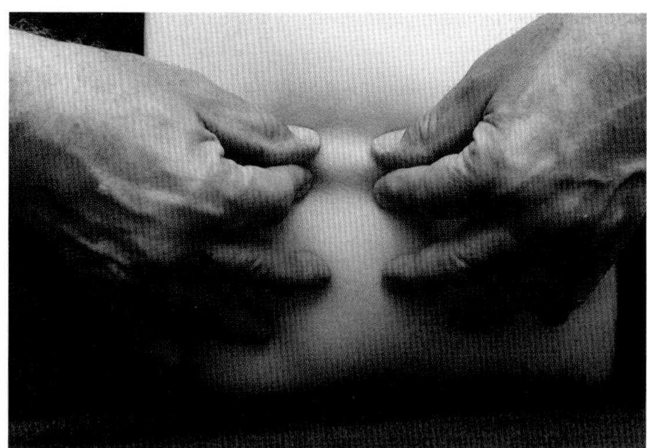

Fig 6.14
The movement is controlled by palpation with the fingertips at the spinous processes.

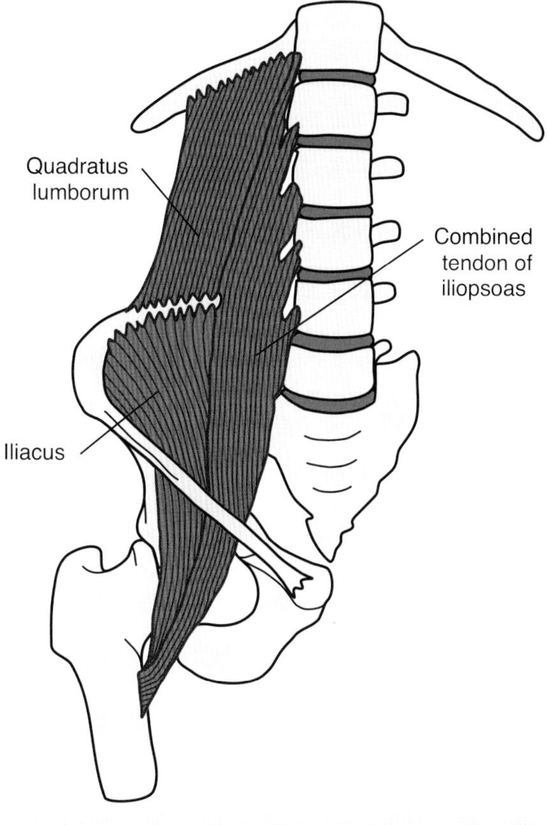

Fig 6.15
The iliopsoas muscles.

The process can be repeated in the horizontal plane using a flexion and extension movement of the osteopath's spine, again restricting the motion to the lesioned segment only. The technique can be repeated up and down the lumbar spine so as to give a segmental localized stretch and mobilization of each ligamentous capsular apparatus in turn. Very short levers and very specific articulation techniques are extremely effective in pregnancy. It goes without saying that the short erector spinae muscles, such as the postural muscles of multifidus and the segmental rotators, are likewise encouraged to move and release.

Technique for Psoas Muscle Stretch with the Patient Side-lying

The psoas or iliopsoas muscle lies on the front of the spine, originating from the lateral surfaces of the vertebral bodies of T12 and L1–L4, and their associated intervertebral discs (Fig 6.15). They unite with the iliacus muscles at the level of the inguinal ligament and cross the hip joint to insert on the lesser trochanter. They are hip flexors, acting from above, and spine flexors, acting from below.

Position of the patient

The patient lies her side, as before.

Position of the osteopath

The osteopath stands behind her at the level of the thoracolumbar junction.

Ambition of the technique

The aim is to stretch overtight, and thus dysfunctional, muscle states in the psoas muscles. These muscles are particularly important in pregnancy.

Application of the technique

The patient takes the bottom leg and holds her bottom knee in flexion (Fig 6.16). This limits the flexion/extension movement of the top leg and the spine, preventing a hyperlordosis. For greater specificity, the osteopath can fix his cephalad hand at the thoracolumbar junction, limiting movement to this level. His other hand holds the patient's top knee, supporting the calf and avoiding separating her legs. He gently swivels around his own vertical axis into rotation, bringing the top leg back into extension. This induces a stretch along the length of the psoas which is uppermost. The technique continues as the muscle increases in length.

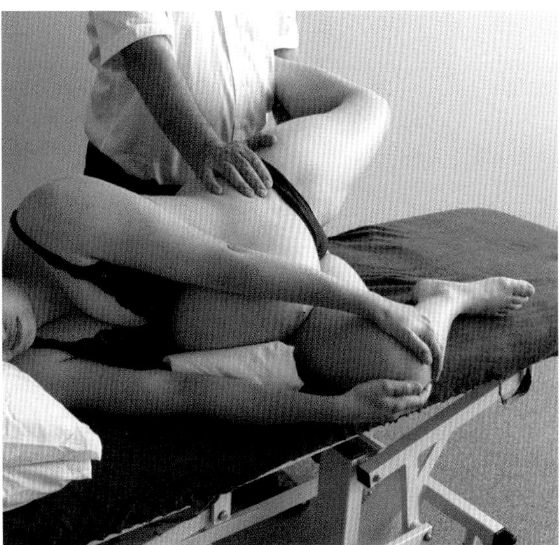

Fig 6.16
The psoas stretch technique.

Techniques for the Ribs and Diaphragm with the Patient Sitting

Position of the patient

The patient sits at the end of the treatment table or with her feet over the side of the table. It is important for her to sit very upright for the next two techniques. There is a natural tendency for the patient to slump into flexion, which should be avoided.

Position of the osteopath

The osteopath stands side-on to the patient. For the patient's right middle ribs, her right arm is draped over his right shoulder (Fig 6.17). For the left, it is reversed.

In Figure 6.18, showing the osteopath in front of the patient, we can see that his wrist and forearm are contacting the anterior part of the patient's pectoral region. As the technique proceeds, it is a common error for the arm to be hyperextended at the shoulder, risking damage to the anterior part of the shoulder capsule. In the later stages of pregnancy, the shoulder ligaments are weaker due to the action of the hormone relaxin. Firm contact with the front of the shoulder in this way will minimize risk.

The osteopath's left hand contacts the interspace between the ribs (Fig 6.19), as shown earlier in the side-lying position. The aim is to hold down on the rib below while the rib above moves away from it. This is similar to the side-lying technique for rib stretching above the diaphragm, as seen in Chapter 4.

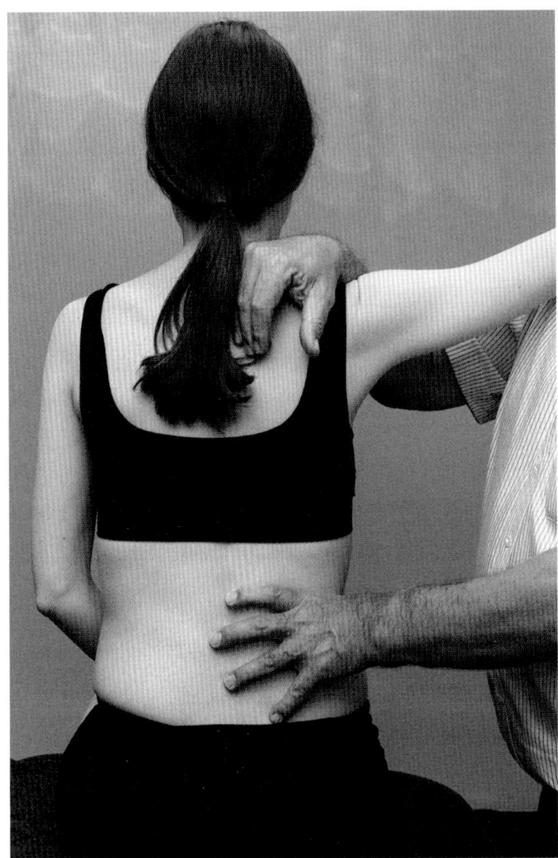

Fig 6.17
Sitting rib stretch technique.

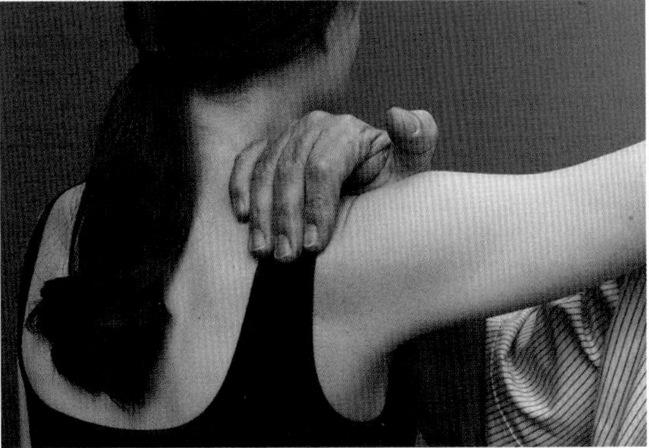

Fig 6.18
The osteopath's hand and forearm prevent the patient's shoulder from moving forwards.

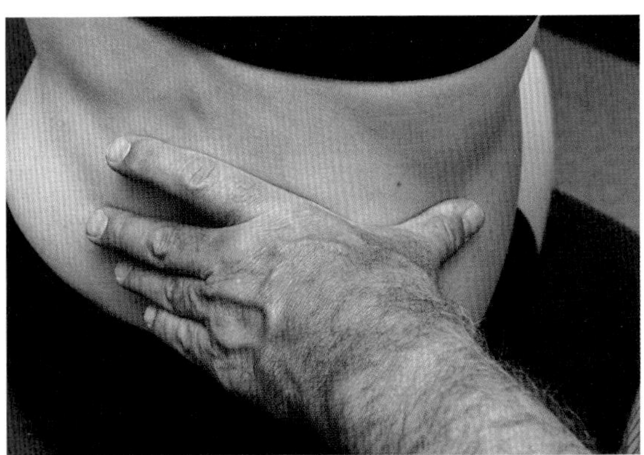

Fig 6.19
Hand position fixing the rib below and allowing the interspace to be stretched.

Ambition of the technique

These next two techniques are very helpful at the end of the pregnancy in the third trimester, when the rising gravid uterus compresses the abdominal contents below the diaphragm, restricting the ability of the diaphragm to descend in full inspiration. Patients often complain of having no space to breathe, with dyspnea being a common symptom. They become upper rib breathers only, and so, once again, the importance of the upper rib articulations and "pump handle" movements are important.

Application of the technique

The osteopath moves from his front foot to his back foot, while fixing the shoulder and pushing down on the rib below as his weight is transferred backwards. This will have the effect of separating the two ribs and stretching the intercostal muscles and the diaphragm.

Sitting Extension Articulation for the Thoracolumbar Junction

The sitting position is ideal for mobilization of the thoracolumbar junction, which is important in pregnancy from both a physiological and an anatomical point of view.

The thoracolumbar junction is where postural curve changes occur in both the anteroposterior and lateral planes; it is the center of the sympathetic nervous system that relates to the pelvis and the pelvic organs; the blood supply to the pelvis relates to this junction with the bifurcation of the aorta at L1; and the psoas muscles will act as "rails" that the baby will ride on during the journey down into the pelvis and thus the outside world. The numerous lymph and venous blood channels returning blood to the heart are found at this junction, too. Ribs 10 and 11, which are attached to, and function with, the crura of the diaphragm, are to be found here; so too are the quadratus lumborum muscles as they attach to the lower ribs and aid in deep respiration.

All in all, this place plays a major role in normal well-balanced function during pregnancy. Unfortunately, as described in Chapter 3, Scheuermann's disease affects this junction very frequently, causing restriction of movement. Pregnancy and the softening action on the ligaments of the hormones once again give the osteopath an opportunity, not found outside pregnancy, to mobilize and restore function to this essential zone. You cannot change distorted bone shape, but you can stretch shortened ligaments and give back some segmental mobility in cases of chronic restriction.

There are a number of contraindications to this technique. As it can exaggerate a lumbar lordosis, the presence of a spondylolisthesis is an absolute contraindication. Bilateral leg pains, paresthesia, or increased knee jerk or ankle jerk reflexes, especially if they occur in both legs and are increased with respect to the upper extremities, and if accompanied by bladder or bowel signs or numbness in the "saddle" region, are rare signs in pregnancy, but if they are found in the case history or on examination, the patient should be referred to hospital as a matter of urgency for magnetic resonance imaging (MRI) to exclude spinal cord involvement. Any of these signs or symptoms is a contraindication to the sitting extension technique. If the patient is in the acute phase of symphysis pubis dysfunction, where the weight of the gravid uterus is falling on the pubic symphysis and causing it to separate, that again is a contraindication to use of this technique.

Position of the patient

The patient sits on a chair or on the treatment table, with her feet on the ground and with her arms crossed, so that her hands hold onto her biceps and her head rests on her forearms. She must keep hold of the biceps at all times.

Position of the osteopath

The osteopath stands in front of the patient, his hands passing through her linked arms to come to meet in the middle of her thoracic spine. His feet are placed parallel to each other. The height of the treatment table should be such that she has her feet on the floor. If need be, he will have to bend his knees to accommodate this.

Ambition of the technique

Apart from the effects mentioned above, the sitting technique opens the rib angles, increases the intercostal spaces, and articulates and stretches the thoracic, thoracolumbar and lumbar spines into extension, thus aiding the development of the lumbar lordosis and shifting the weight of the gravid uterus directly onto the pelvis, where it needs to be at the end of the third trimester.

Application of the technique

The technique is performed by movement of the osteopath forwards and backwards in a rhythmical manner, lifting the patient's arms up as he pulls back so that they describe an arc of movement, as in Figure 6.20. His fingers fix on the vertebrae in the mid-thoracic spine, thus transferring motion to the thoracolumbar junction and beyond, pulling them gently into extension (Fig 6.21). The patient can feel the stretch right down to the low lumbar spine and pelvis as the technique's traction effect pulls the vertebral segments apart.

By fixing the vertebra with his fingers and moving his body in a small circular motion, the osteopath takes the vertebra into a circumduction articulation which stretches the ligaments and capsules of each vertebral segment in turn. For this technique, the osteopath has his feet parallel to each other.

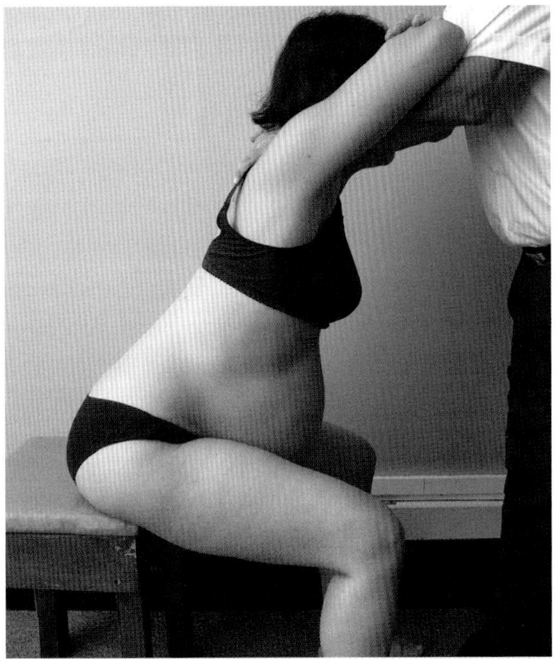

Fig 6.20
The patient moves into an arc of extension as she is pulled upwards through her arms.

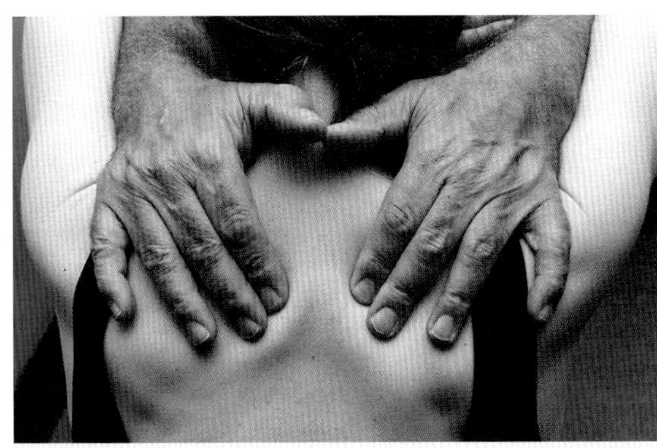

Fig 6.21
The osteopath's fingers on the transverse processes, fixing the vertebra concerned as it moves into extension.

High-velocity, Low-amplitude (High-velocity Thrust) Techniques and the Lumbar Spine in Pregnancy

Direct high-velocity, low-amplitude (HVLA) techniques, otherwise known as high-velocity thrust (HVT) techniques, are certainly indicated in pregnancy, as long as they are modified to be used with the most minimal lever that effectively achieves their ambition, and to avoid abdominal compression at all costs.

Modification of the Lumbar Roll Technique in Pregnancy

"Lumbar roll" techniques are indicated when there are facet joint restrictions in the lumbar spine. These can be of traumatic, postural, or visceral origin and may be acute, subacute, or chronic. They are painful, causing a local traumatic inflammatory response with accompanying muscle hypertonia and spasm, and are diagnosed by comparative palpation of neighboring apophyseal or facet joints.

The normal parameters and principles of HVLA/HVT techniques apply. This is a minimal leverage thrust. The minimum amount of leverage is used to "lock" the ligaments around the joint and focus the force through the facet joints concerned. These include flexion/extension, side-bending or lateral flexion to each side, rotation to each side, and then gliding in both planes, and an element of compression and distraction. Readers are referred to the texts of Professor Laurie Hartman for more on this subject (see Chapter 4).

The usual rotation of the patient towards the treatment table, as in a normal lumbar roll technique, is contraindicated. Instead, a side-bending or "body drop" technique is safer.

Position of the patient

The patient lies on her side in the three-sided square position, with the painful side upwards. This is a side-bending and not a rotation thrust. The thrust uses minimal leverage with a small element of lateral compression.

Position of the osteopath

The osteopath stands facing the patient.

Ambition of the technique

This is a very specific technique designed to open the facet joint affected.

Application of the technique

The osteopath asks the patient to straighten the lower leg, hyperextending the knee and resting the lower ankle at the corner of the table. He bends the upper knee and rests the foot on the bottom leg at mid-calf at the highest (Fig 6.22).

Reaching under the patient, he contacts her bottom shoulder and bends his knees (Fig 6.23). This is very important because, if he does not do it, he

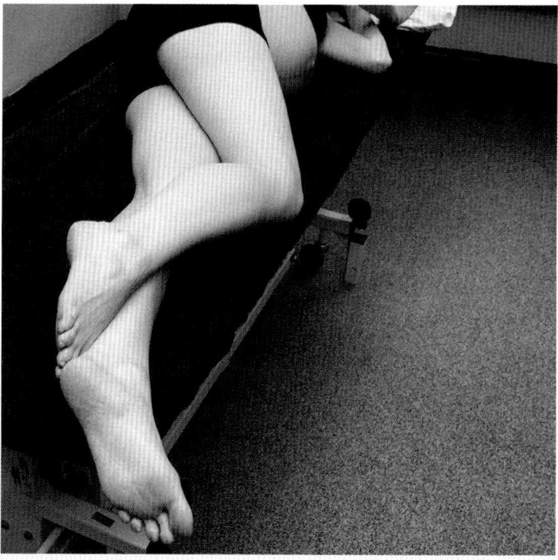

Fig 6.22
Modified lumbar roll: the position of the lower extremity.

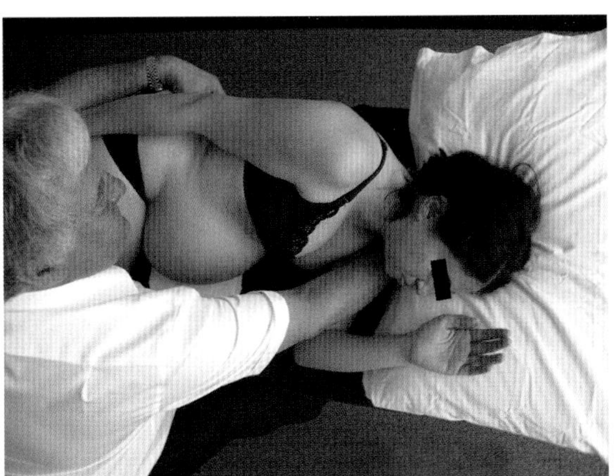

Fig 6.23
Reaching under the patient with one hand, the osteopath pulls the shoulder towards him, using more trunk flexion than rotation, until he feels the motion in the fingers of the other hand.

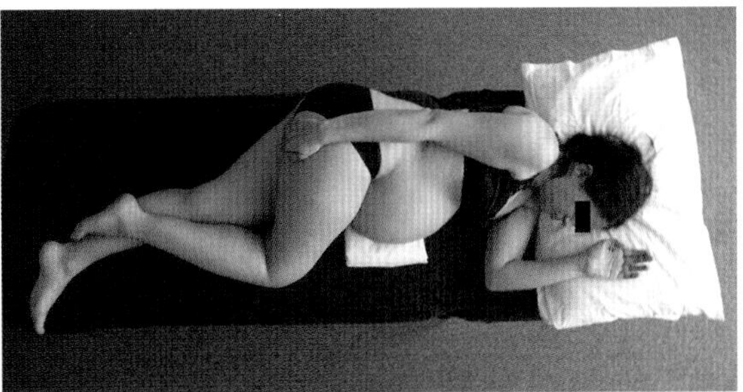

Fig 6.24
Note that the patient's top arm rests along the length of her body, so as to avoid the common fault of introducing rotation too early.

will apply the upper lever rotation too early. If he is tall, he may need to adjust the height of the table. He pulls the patient's bottom shoulder towards him, flexing her trunk until he feels the tension arrive at his bottom hand, which palpates the interspace between the two halves of the lesioned segment.

In order to stop her trunk from rotating, the osteopath places the elbow of her top arm in extension, in line with her body (Fig 6.24), and secures her top hand under his forearm as in Figure 6.25. The commonest fault with this technique is too much rotation from the top lever too soon. The fixing of the top hand in this way should limit early rotation.

When he feels the tension arrive, he asks the patient to grasp the forearm on the same side as her top hand with her bottom hand, and gently allows the top shoulder to fall back. This is all the rotation that is needed. The table height should be adjusted downwards if need be, so that the osteopath's weight can rest on the patient's pelvis. The caudad arm now introduces a minimal element of compression

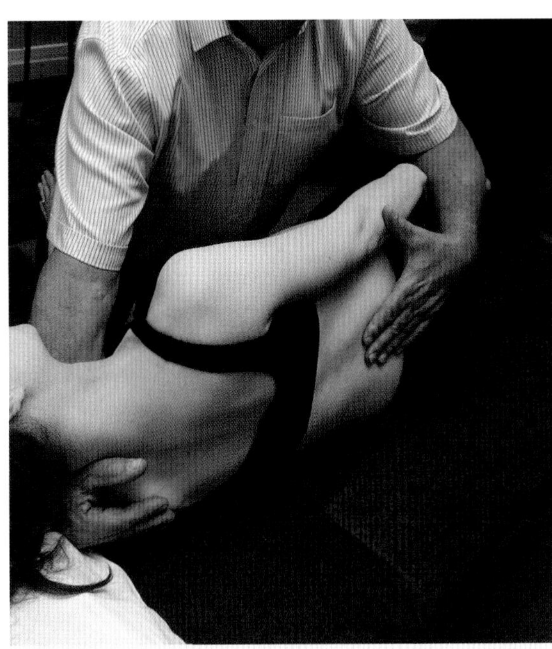

Fig 6.25
Flexion of the trunk down to the palpating hand at the level of the lesion.

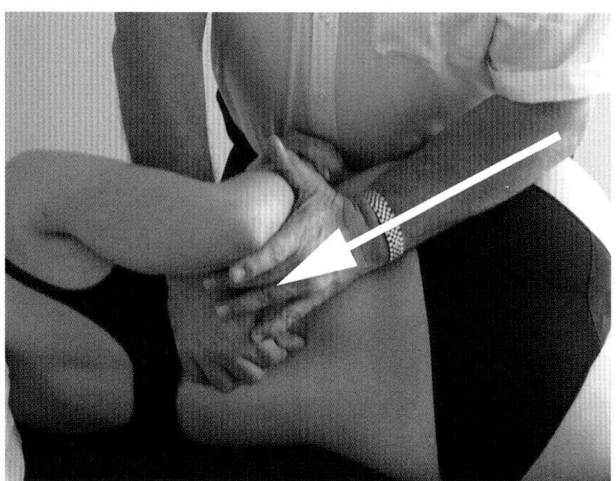

Fig 6.26
The direction of the thrust is into side-bending, with a very short and controlled "body drop" to open the top facet joints.

directly towards the table through her pelvis – *never the abdomen* of the patient – and the final "locking" is achieved with subtle movements of each of the parameters from the top lever. Once the top and bottom levers are such that the tension is where it is wanted, a short, sharp impulse from the caudad arm is directed towards the table to separate the facets. This is done with a very small, sharp "body drop," where the weight of the operator momentarily goes through the bottom lever arm onto his supporting leg (Fig 6.26). This creates a shock wave effect, opening the lesioned segment.

There has been considerable debate in the profession as to which facet should be uppermost: the lesioned facet or the normal facet of the segment concerned. Putting it another way, does the thrust open the top or the bottom facet? It is this author's opinion that it is the top facet that is affected because the levers are precisely set, and the impulse is of a very short amplitude and is limited by the bulk of the vertebral body. Provided the levers are minimal and there is a clear intention not to compress her abdomen, this is a safe technique because it avoids the use of rotation.

Reverse Thrust Technique for the Thoracolumbar Junction

The thoracolumbar junction can be a difficult area to manipulate for the reasons already stated, yet it is commonly affected by facet joint restriction, which can be a cause of acute pain, or may be responsible for disturbed function in the ribs, diaphragm, associated sympathetic nervous system, and structures attached to the ribs and diaphragm in this area. It is also a place where secondary restrictions caused by lesions in the lower lumbar spine occur because of disturbances that are caused in the antero-posterior and lateral plane curves of the spine. Once again, as she changes her posture, this part of the spine is an important place for movement, and so this technique is commonly used and can be invaluable in your treatment of the pregnant patient.

Position of the patient

The patient lies on her side, with the painful or restricted side upwards.

Position of the osteopath

The osteopath faces her, in the same position that he would adopt for a simple lumbar roll technique.

Ambition of the technique

This is a manipulation to release facet locking at the thoracolumbar junction. It is a reverse technique, compared to the classical version, to avoid excess rotation of the lower lever, which might cause abdominal compression.

Application of the technique

The patient is placed into the same position as before for a minimal leverage technique. The osteopath focuses the upper and lower levers using the same parameters, so that all of the focus is at the lesioned segment concerned. This is a manipulation for the top facet.

The first part of this reverse thrust for the thoracolumbar junction is as for the set-up for the lumbar roll technique. The focus is T12/L1.

It is important for the osteopath's feet to face towards the head of the patient and for his leading arm to be in contact with her axilla because the impulse is directed towards her chest, so that it does not go towards her abdomen (Fig 6.27).

His upper hand applies a small compression towards her chest and down into the treatment table. Once the osteopath is fixed in this position, he simply swivels on the balls of his feet so that he is facing towards the patient's pelvis (Fig 6.28). This simple maneuver changes the technique so that it becomes a reversal of the normal lumbar roll. By doing this, the force comes from above, not below.

Now any force will be directed safely to the upper part of the lesion, and a short, sharp impulse back and down towards the table will have the effect of separating the facets of the lesioned segment and restoring normal vertebral function (Fig 6.29).

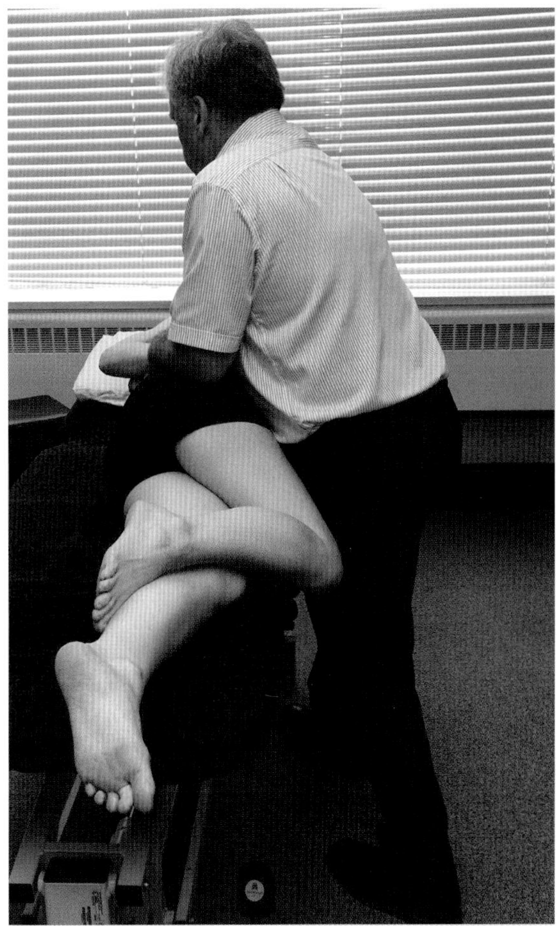

Fig 6.27
The position of the osteopath's feet at the start of the thoracolumbar reverse technique.

Visceral Techniques Below the Diaphragm

As mentioned in the previous chapter, the motility techniques of Barral[1] and others, which relate to specific findings of fascial and motility disturbances in certain organs, are going to be very difficult to apply because of altered fascial tensions. The movement of the organs below the diaphragm into new positions, caused by encroachment of the gravid uterus, means that the landmarks used to calculate the organ positions will change and the tensions on the supporting organs will be considerably different from normal.

This does not imply that visceral osteopathic techniques below the diaphragm are contraindicated; it simply means that the techniques are guided more by the bony anatomy and the attachments of the organs to the ribs and diaphragm.

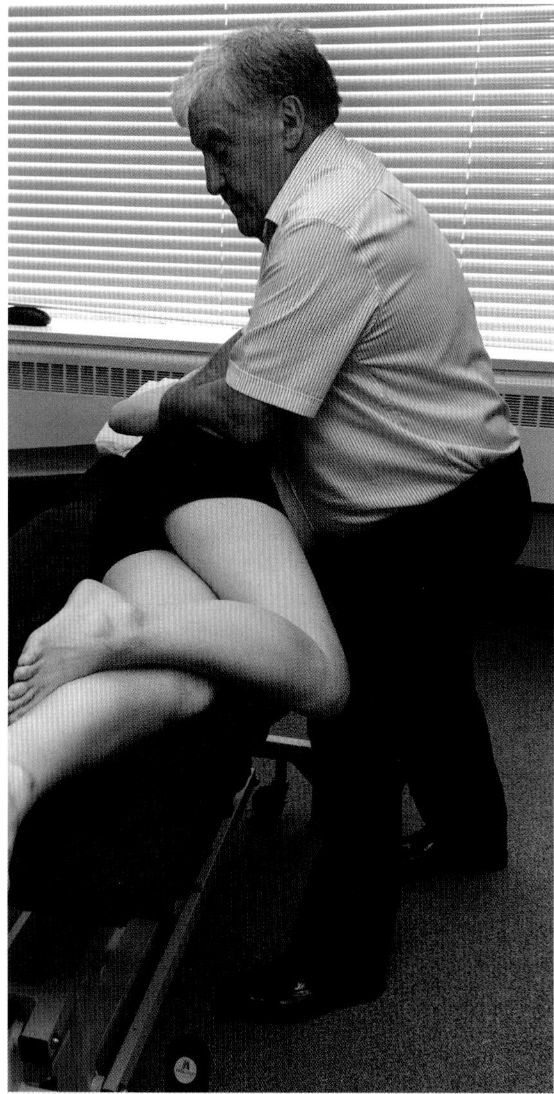

Fig 6.28
The osteopath is now facing down the table, towards the patient's feet.

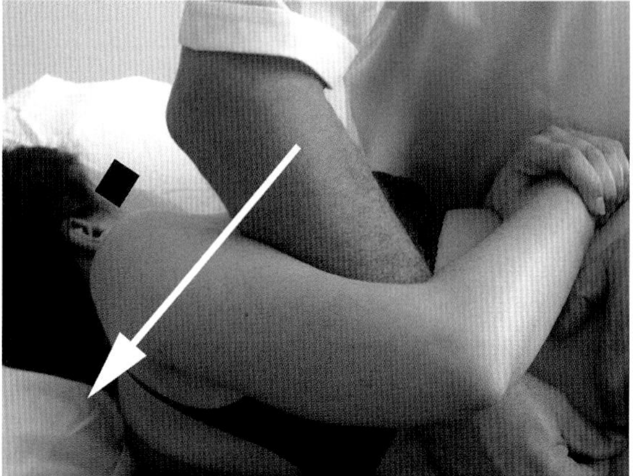

Fig 6.29
The technique takes the patient's shoulder away from the pelvis, avoiding any undue compression to the abdomen.

Certain specific syndromes of visceral dysfunction appear frequently in pregnancy, and some of these respond very well to osteopathic treatment approaches. What follows is not intended to be a set of recipes to be performed indiscriminately; instead, they should be thought of as treatment protocols.

Gastro-esophageal Reflux and Pregnancy

Gastro-esophageal reflux (GER, or GOR) is very common in pregnancy. It is caused by several factors, including relaxation of the lower esophageal sphincter by the pregnancy hormones, and the weight of the gravid uterus pushing the stomach contents up towards the chest and forcing them into the last part of the unprotected esophagus. The gradual change in the position of the stomach as it moves around the abdominal wall also means that the sphincter becomes looser. Lastly, reflux will be worse if the patient slumps in low armchairs after a meal, as this forces the stomach contents up into the esophagus.

The presence of gastric acid anywhere outside of the stomach will irritate the unprotected intestinal mucosa, either at the lower end of the esophagus or the upper end of the duodenum. The stomach has a rich, thick coating of mucus which acts to protect it against acid secretions and neutralizes the gastric acid. The longer that food remains in the stomach, the more chance it has to reflux and come back up; therefore, an important element in dietary advice for pregnancy is to think in terms of foods that pass quickly through the stomach and those that take time to digest.

Gastric acid outside the stomach leads to inflammation and spasm of the muscles of the esophageal wall at the gastro-esophageal junction and those of the diaphragm. The diaphragm spasm further irritates the esophageal wall, creating a vicious circle. This, in turn, leads to a viscero-somatic reflex, causing spasm and restrictions in the thoracic spine anywhere between T2 and T5. As the lower end of the esophagus and the upper end of the duodenum do not have a protective layer of mucus, as in the stomach, they can be prone to ulceration if they are exposed to irritation by reflux or reverse peristalsis.

In Figure 6.30, the attachment of the diaphragm to the esophagus by Bertelli's membrane is shown; spasm of the diaphragm will be seen to have the effect outlined above.

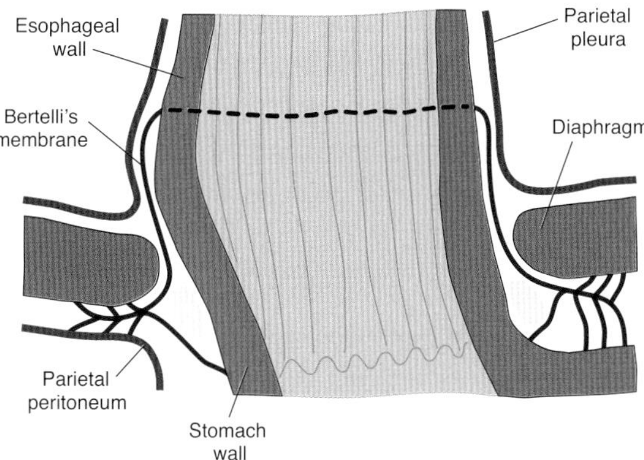

Fig 6.30
The attachments of the diaphragm and the esophagus.

Raw foods such as cucumber, especially if unpeeled, raw tomatoes, raw onion, and radishes are all slower to be digested. If the cucumber is peeled, the tomatoes poached and skinned, and the onions gently cooked before being eaten, reflux is less likely.

Meat and fish that are casseroled or poached, instead of fried or roasted, will also be digested more easily.

The pregnant patient should avoid all gassy drinks, including bottled water with gas, and should limit herself to a small glass of plain water with each meal. She should also steer clear of acid-containing fruit juices, if possible.

After a meal, she should be encouraged to sit on a dining chair, with a pillow behind her back, and to avoid low sofas or armchairs from mid-pregnancy onwards if this is practicable. In bed at night, if she suffers from reflux, she should sleep on her side, supported at 45 degrees with extra pillows. The flatter she lies, the more food will reflux. Towards the end of pregnancy, from around 30 weeks, patients are advised to eat the main meal of the day at lunchtime. In the evening, they can eat with the family but should miss out the main course and stick to soup, followed by something like ice cream. In this way, the stomach is almost empty by the time they go to bed and reflux is less likely to occur.

Diaphragm Lift Technique

Position of the patient

The patient sits on the treatment table with her feet over the edge and her hands on her hips, keeping them there at all times.

Position of the osteopath

The osteopath stands behind the patient, with one foot in front of the other.

Ambition of the technique

The technique is used to stretch the diaphragm laterally to break the spasm, and then allow the stomach and lower part of the esophagus to settle down into the abdominal cavity again. Lastly, the use of a gentle tension to the central tendon of the diaphragm "closes the door." It is an extension of the sitting technique applied to the lateral costal margin, seen earlier.

Application of the technique

The osteopath places the ulnar border of his hands along the costal margins, starting with his fingertips near to the xiphoid cartilage, as before.

He asks the patient to put her head back against the front of his shoulder. He takes a small step backwards, leaning back, and gently pulls the margins of the rib cage and diaphragm towards the sides (Fig 6.31). This has the effect of gently pulling at the esophageal hiatus in the diaphragm and opening it, allowing the trapped lower part of the esophagus to drop down into the abdominal cavity under the influence of gravity.

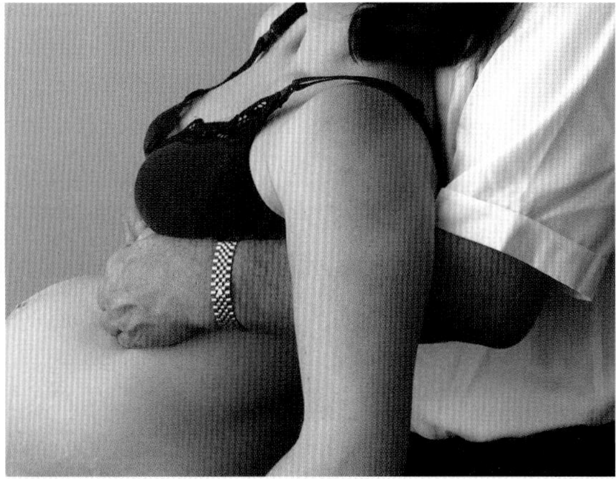

Fig 6.31
The patient's hands are on her hips and the osteopath leans back, taking her weight posteriorly.

 **Warning**

The osteopath's hands are very near to the breast tissue in this technique. Quite apart from being tender, this a sensitive area as far as ethics and patients' comfort are concerned. The osteopath must explain very clearly to the patient what he intends to do and why, in order to ensure that she is clearly informed as to the ambition of the technique and is in a position to give her informed oral consent. If English is not her native language, then use of a suitable adult interpreter must be considered. Once the explanation has been given and accepted, then the technique can proceed.

Using the tips of his fingers, he gathers the spare flesh under the rib margins, slowly moving from front foot to back foot as he does so. The finger pressure is very light, and in this way he can gather quite a lot of skin and superficial tissues under the ulnar borders of his hands (Fig 6.32). He takes care never to dig his fingers into the patient's flesh; instead, this is a light gathering process as his hands move deeper and deeper. The patient should be encouraged to tell him if he is unwittingly hurting her, as this should be a relatively painless technique.

When the osteopath has enough flesh gathered under his hands, he firstly moves his feet so that they are parallel, then, as he pushes with his chest at the same time as moving the patient forwards, she drops her head; he rolls his forearms, and his hands move into supination as his elbows move forwards against the patient's upper arms. He simultaneously lifts the patient up towards him as his hands "disappear"

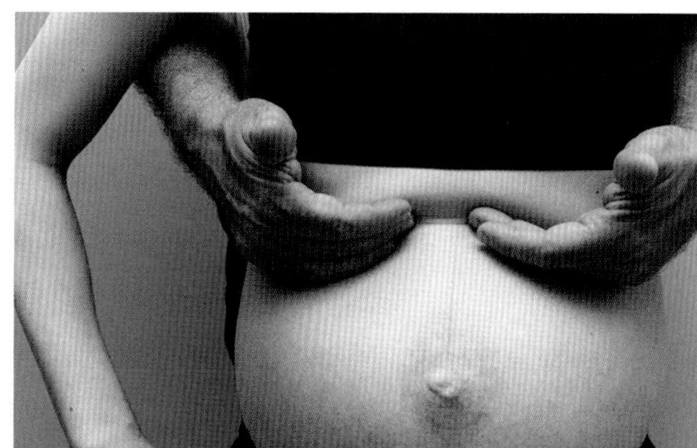

Fig 6.32
The ulnar border of the osteopath's hands are on the patient's costal margins.

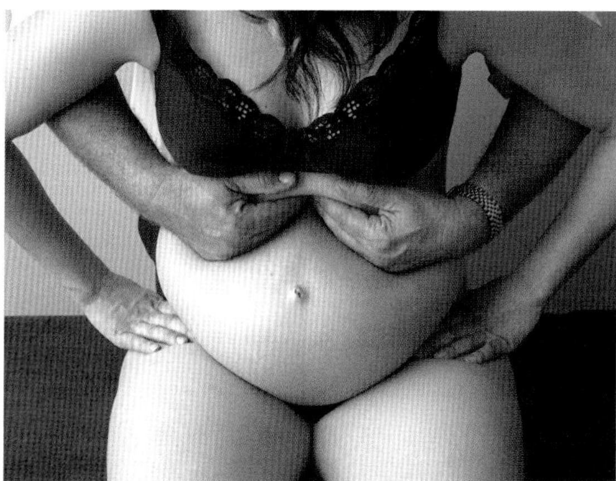

Fig 6.33
The patient rolls forwards and the osteopath pushes her arms forwards too as he supinates his wrists, allowing the ulnar border of his hands to move under the costal margins.

under the costal margins (Fig 6.33). He should not press with the fingertips.

If done carefully and slowly, and repeated until he has enough tissue under his fingers before the position is changed, the technique should – surprisingly – not cause discomfort.

With the hands and fingers in this position, the last movement of the fingers is behind the xiphoid, drawing the diaphragm slowly down. This has the effect of tightening the hole in the diaphragm after the stomach has gone back down into the abdominal cavity.

This is not an easy technique, as it requires timing and patient cooperation to ensure its success, but once mastered it will form a mainstay of your treatment of this condition.

The C2 to T2 Connection

There are very few findings in osteopathic practice that one can say with confidence exist in nearly every patient. A very common finding with GERD, however, is the lesion pattern of C2 and T2 on the left side of the spine at the level of the facet joints. This pattern exists, and again, there is a vicious circle of events serving to reinforce and maintain the chronicity of the problem.

As described earlier, the action of gastric irritation produces a viscero-somatic lesion at the level of the upper thoracic vertebrae. This is palpated as a muscular restriction or increased resistance to superficial and deep palpation locally, as well as motion restriction in all ranges, but notably flexion and extension.

The erector spinae muscles run parallel to the spine in the paravertebral gutter (Fig 6.34). The iliocostalis cervicis muscles arise from the angles of the 2nd, 3rd, 4th, 5th, and 6th ribs, and is inserted into the posterior tubercles of the transverse processes of the 2nd, 3rd, 4th, 5th, and 6th cervical vertebrae. Contraction and spasm of the fibers of this muscle will cause vertebral lesions at both the origin and the insertion of the muscle.

Irritation of the lower esophageal sphincter causes reflex contraction in the associated spinal muscles at T2 and T3, and between T4 and T5 on the left, because the stomach is on the left (Fig 6.35). These levels are

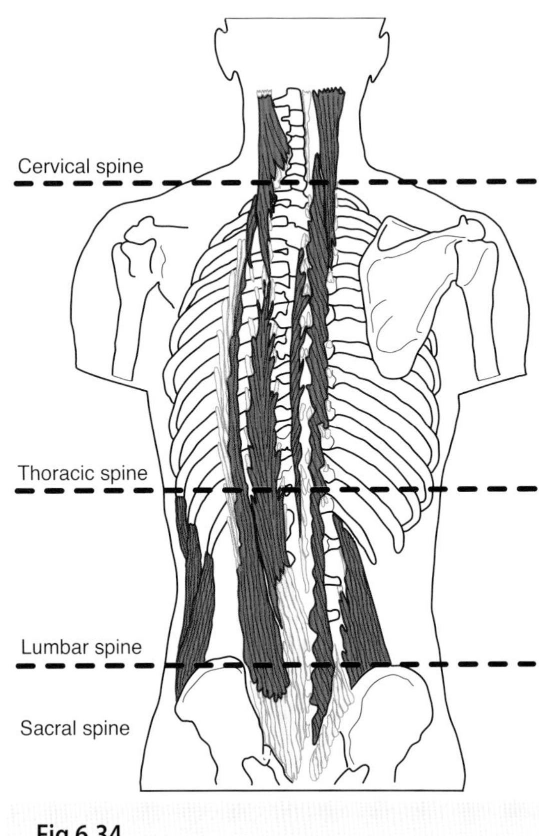

Fig 6.34
The erector spinae muscles.

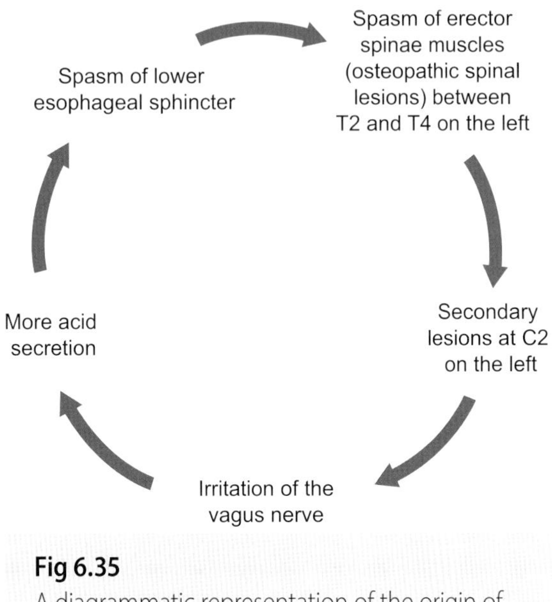

Fig 6.35
A diagrammatic representation of the origin of the C2–T2 lesion.

particularly affected because of the relevant viscerosomatic lesions at these levels at the foramen and the cord. This, in turn, causes a secondary lesion at C1/2 on the left. At this level, there is a small nerve running to the vagus nerve (Xth) which encourages secretomotor impulses to the gastric mucosa (Fig 6.36); therefore, excess acid, combined with a weak lower esophageal sphincter, can cause vagal stimulation, which brings about the vicious circle again.

Using a direct technique, such as an HVLA maneuver to the upper cervical spine to break facet fixation at C2 with the patient supine (Fig 6.37), followed by the "lift-off" technique to T2 described in Chapter 6 (Fig 6.38), will normalize the segmental motion, thus breaking the reflex pathways, allowing for less vagal irritation, and thus reducing esophageal irritation.

This works best with soft tissue relaxation techniques, functional techniques to the affected areas, and cranial techniques for the cranial base and the jugular foramen, through which the vagus nerve passes, as part of an overall treatment program. It is not just a recipe for manipulation by itself.

Treatment of Constipation During Pregnancy

Pregnant patients run the risk of chronic constipation during pregnancy. This can be due to a number of factors. The gravid uterus literally sits on the ascending and descending colons and blocks the movement of food residues. Food enters the ascending colon via the cecum, and the cecum has to contract with sufficient force to move a column of food residue with the consistency of wet sand towards the head against gravity. It has to pass the hepatic flexure to

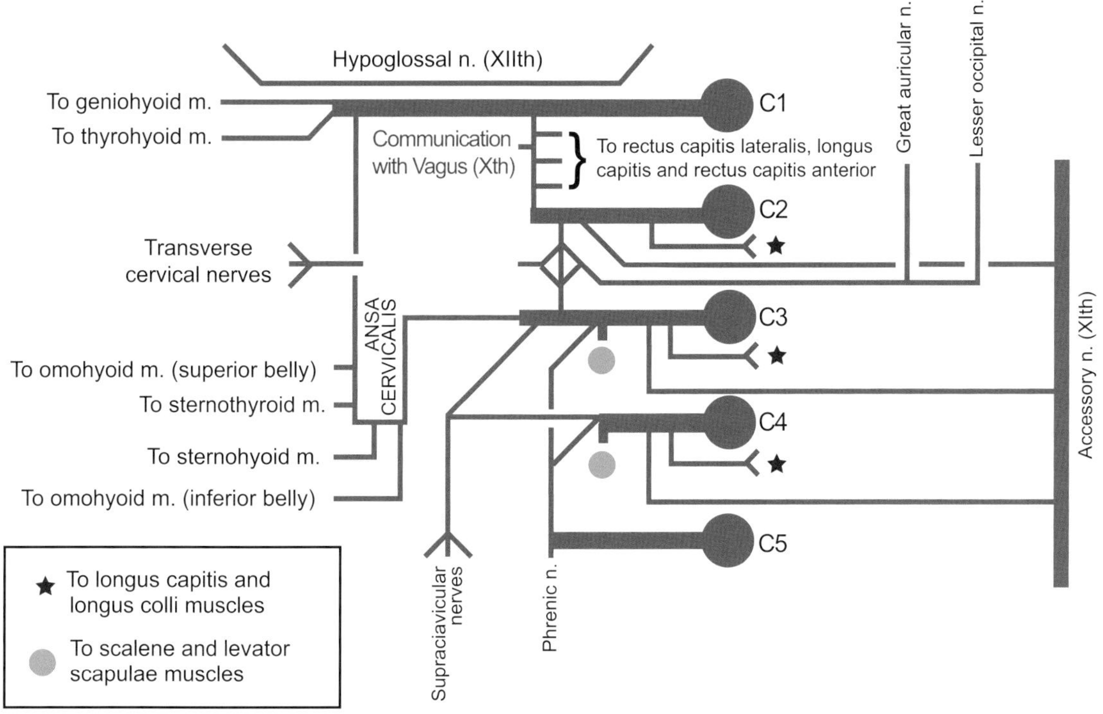

Fig 6.36
The superior cervical plexus showing the vagus nerve connection.

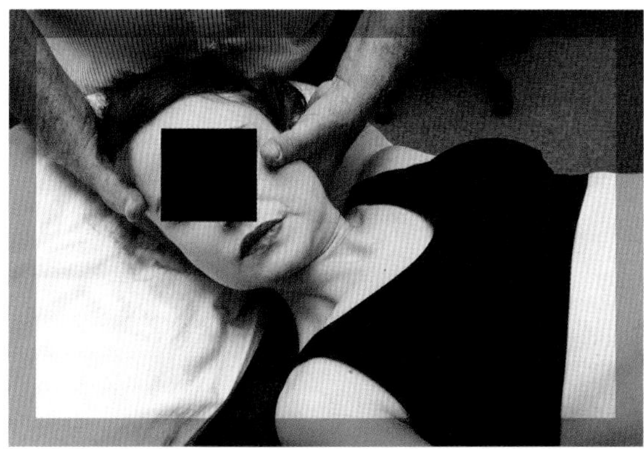

Fig 6.37
The "cradle hold "manipulation for C2 on the left.

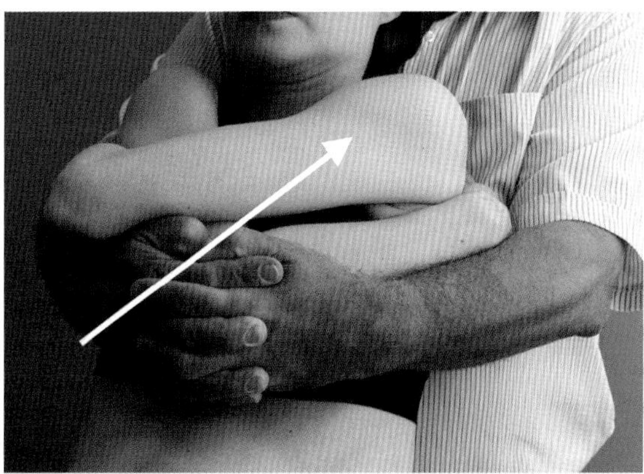

Fig 6.38
The "lift-off" technique for T2. Note the impulse is not a lift as such but a force directed towards the osteopath's chest.

enter the transverse colon. However, the angle will close if there is a ptosis of the transverse colon, making the passage of the food slow and heavy. It then has to rise up (the splenic flexure is higher than the hepatic flexure; Fig 6.39), again against gravity, and pass another potentially closed angle before it proceeds via the descending colon to the sigmoid and the rectum.

The longer the food residue stays in the gut, the drier it becomes, as there is increased time available for the absorption of water from the lumen of the

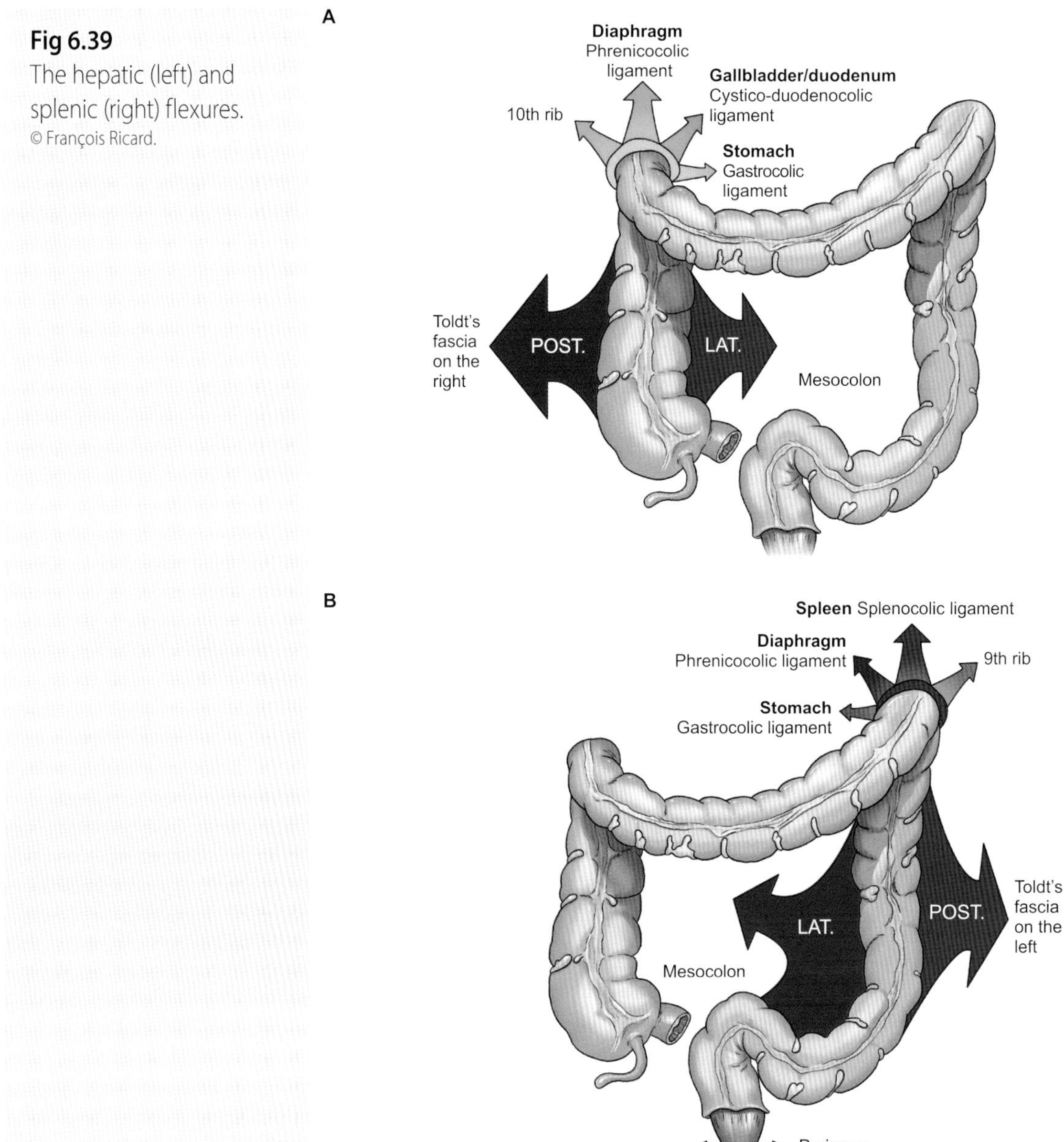

Fig 6.39
The hepatic (left) and splenic (right) flexures.
© François Ricard.

gut back into the bloodstream. The slower transit of food materials enhances the absorption of iron and calcium in the upper part of the intestine, and the action of the hormone calcitol adds to this, so that, 6 months into the pregnancy, calcium absorption is twice that of non-pregnant women. These two factors alone mean that the patient runs the risk of chronic constipation. Apart from making her feel heavy, bloated, and uncomfortable, if she strains at stool this can predispose to hemorrhoids, and tensions within the pelvis and anal canal.

As described in Chapter 5, there is considerable variation in the position of the abdominal organs as they are compressed and moved by the weight of the gravid uterus. If the cecum is heavy, it will descend into the pelvis, as will the sigmoid on the opposite side under the weight of the heavy, dry contents.

Normally, the movement of food in the gut is aided by peristalsis and the massaging action of the diaphragm. Towards the end of the pregnancy in particular, the descent of the diaphragm will be much less as the ribs flare and the fundus rises. This, again, predisposes to constipation, and also to visceral adhesions between the walls of the cecum and sigmoid and the walls of the pelvis. There is usually a sliding movement of the abdominal organs against each other, enhanced by the secretion of peritoneal fluid. If the organs come to lie in the pelvic bowl due to ptosis, they can form adhesions or dry areas between the two surfaces, which further restricts organ mobility (Fig 6.40).

Gentle "visceral thrust" techniques, designed to separate these two adherent surfaces, are well tolerated by the patient and effective at encouraging flow of peritoneal fluid and organ motion.

Visceral "Thrust" Techniques

The following is not an HVLA technique. The object is to create a shock wave that is transmitted between the two adherent layers to separate them and to allow the peritoneal fluid to flow and lubricate both surfaces.

Position of the patient

The patient lays supine and propped up at 45 degrees, with pillows under her knees.

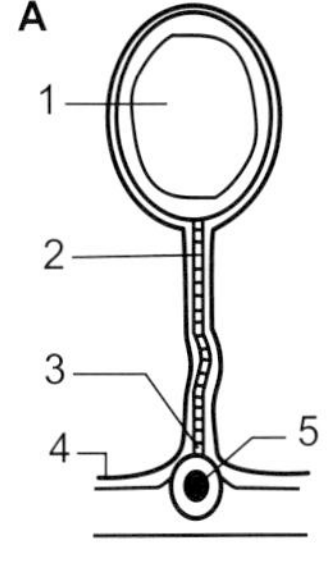

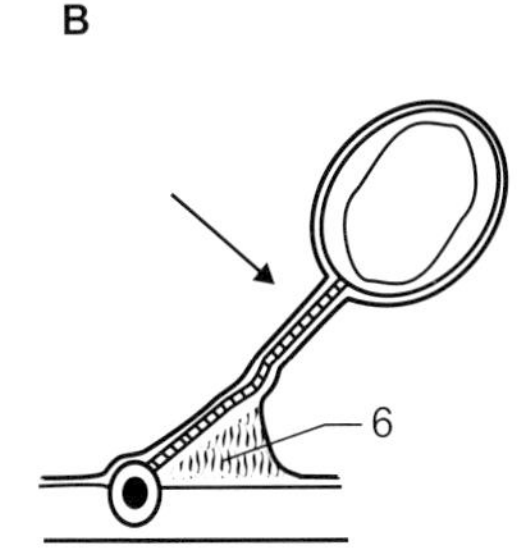

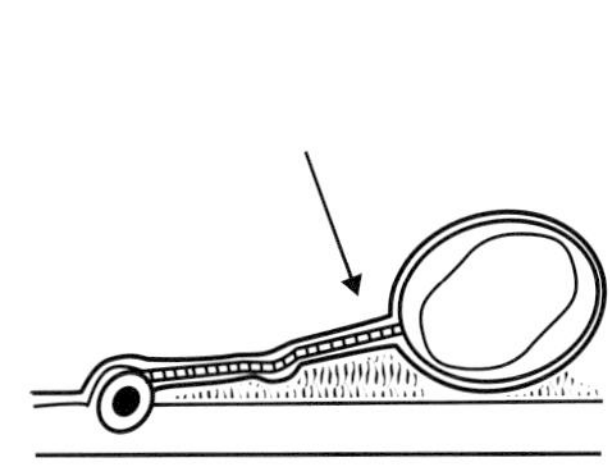

Fig 6.40
Formation of a visceral adhesion. (A) The viscera is mobile with no adhesions. (B) The adhesions builds. (C) A fully bound-down organ. Key: (1) Gastrointestinal tract; (2) Mesentery; (3) Root of the mesentery; (4) Posterior parietal peritoneum; (5) Retroperitoneal vessels; (6) Beginning of an adhesion.
© François Ricard.

Position of the osteopath

The osteopath stands on the right side of the patient, at the level of the pelvis and facing inwards.

Ambition of the technique

The technique is used to mobilize adhesions between the cecum and the wall of the pelvis on one side, and the sigmoid colon and the wall of the pelvis on the other.

Application of the technique

Using the length of his little finger, the osteopath attempts to slide it down the wall of the pelvis, very gently separating the cecum away from the bone. His right hand supports the left and ensures that he is not pushing down, but rather gently sweeping or "dissecting" the space between his hand and the wall of the pelvis (Fig 6.41). If he feels an adhesion, he takes a deep breath and, while exhaling, shudders through the border of the little finger, creating the shock wave. He never pushes at the tissues or there will be a reactive spasm within the abdominal wall; instead, he uses the lightest possible force to separate the tissues. This is a difficult technique to learn, but in time, with the application of minimal force and repeated attempts to create the shock wave, the osteopath can achieve very good degrees of relaxation and thus restore mobility of the cecum within the pelvic bowl.

For the sigmoid colon, the technique is applied from the other side.

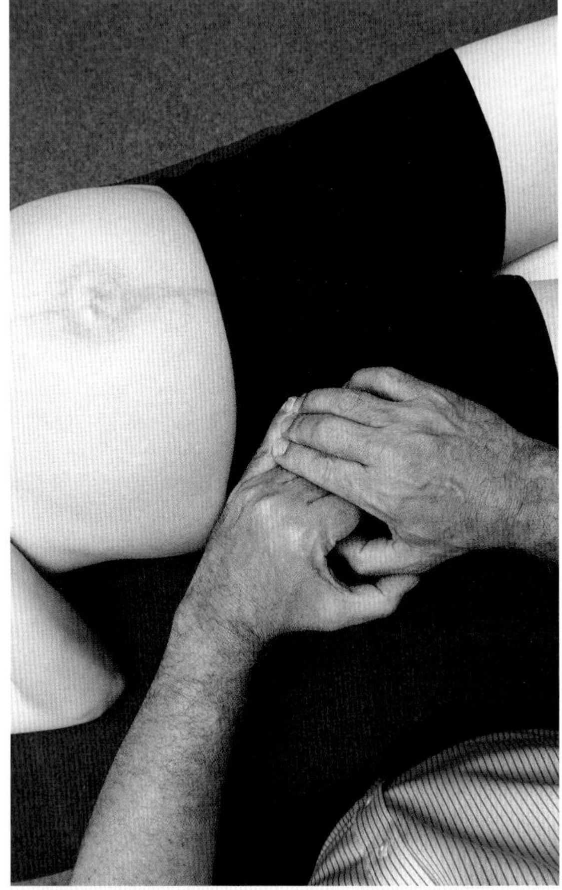

Fig 6.41
The "visceral thrust" technique.

Functional Techniques and the Colon during Pregnancy

Functional techniques applied to the cecum are perfectly possible in the early and middle stages of pregnancy before the patient puts on much weight. Towards the end of the pregnancy, the gravid uterus rests too heavily on the posterior abdominal wall and blocks out any sensations that are possible with these very subtle techniques.

Position of the patient

The patient lies in the supine position, with her neck and shoulders supported by a pillow. She should not be in this position for more than

10 minutes because of the weight of the gravid uterus falling on the inferior vena cava. She may prefer a pillow under her knees.

Position of the osteopath

The osteopath sits at the patient's pelvis, on her right side and facing towards her head.

Ambition of the technique

The objective is, once again, to free the cecum from any visceral adhesions, and to allow it to contract and to move the intestinal contents up and round the colon.

Application of the technique

The osteopath uses the usual parameters of flexion/extension/rotation left and right, and side-bending left and right. In addition, he will add the parameters of translation of anterior–posterior motion, and laterally motion, and a final parameter of cephalad motion (towards her head) and caudad motion (towards her sacrum).

Once again, he is going to look for ease and bind in each parameter, holding the ease and rejecting the bind, until he feels the minimum of tension under his palpating hand, and then, with exhalation, he follows passively until the motion comes to rest at a balance point (Fig 6.42). This will mean that all the tissues acting on the cecum are relaxed and the mobility of the organ is restored or "normalized." The technique should be repeated two or three times until the cecum is felt to move freely.

Normalization of the Kidneys

As outlined in Chapter 5, the kidneys have a lot of extra work to do during pregnancy.

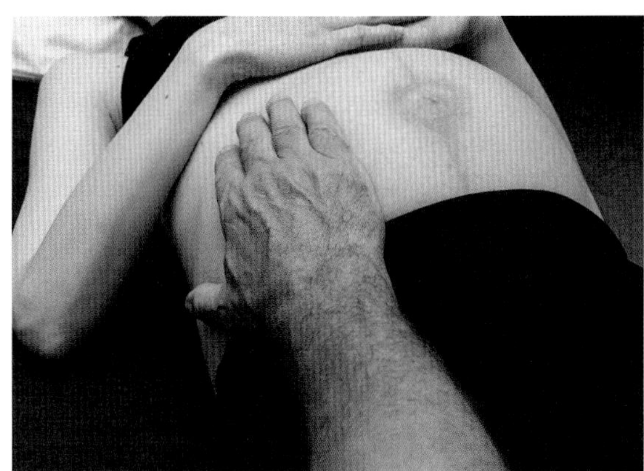

Fig 6.42
Functional technique to the cecum during pregnancy.

Normal motion of the kidneys should remain unchanged, as they are retroperitoneal and their position is not greatly affected by the rise of the gravid uterus. They slide superiorly and inferiorly around the rib cage with each breath taken, very much as before (Fig 6.43). However, it is always worth checking the mobility of the kidneys and the prerenal fascia, as restrictions can occur and should be dealt with using a myofascial release technique.

Position of the patient

The patient sits on a stool or with her legs over the end of the treatment table.

Position of the osteopath

The osteopath sits by her side, facing her. His hands are applied around the lower border of the 12th rib. He gently rests the whole of his palmar surfaces against the skin, assessing the volume of the tissues under his palpating hands. This is a volumetric technique.

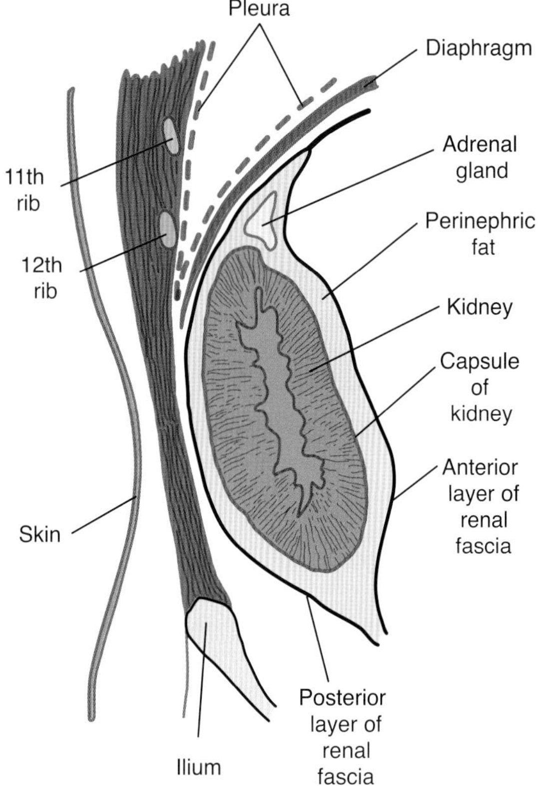

Fig 6.43
The fascia around the kidney.

Ambition of the technique

The aim is to normalize fascial tensions and kidney motion as it rises and falls with inspiration and expiration. Normal motion should then relate to normal function.

Application of the technique

The same parameters of flexion, extension, rotation, and side-bending as used before will apply. However, the change here is to the feeling of the volume of the tissues under the hands, rather than the tissues themselves. The kidney is not a hollow viscus and so it will feel different to, say, a cecum or a lung mass. The patient is treated sitting, which allows the kidneys to fall under the effects of gravity, and so caudal motion is easier felt here. The volume is palpated towards the ease of each parameter, stacking them to achieve the minimal possible tension (Fig 6.44). Then the position is held for up to 20 seconds until a global release is felt. This, again, is followed passively until the motion stops. The biggest difference between this myofascial release and any other functional technique release is the depth of relaxation gained by waiting for longer.

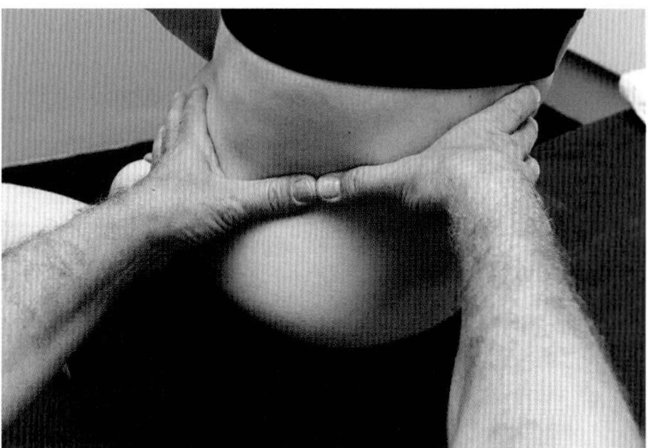

Fig 6.44
"Normalization" of the kidneys, releasing any fascial adhesions.

For a more detailed explanation of the differences between these positional release techniques, the reader is directed towards Leon Chaitow's excellent book, *Positional Release Techniques*, published by Churchill Livingstone.[2]

References

1. Barral JP, Mercier P. *Visceral Manipulations.* Eastland Press, 1988.
2. Chaitow L. *Positional Release Techniques.* Churchill Livingstone, 2016.

The Pelvis: Changes in Anatomy and Physiology During Pregnancy 7

The Anatomy of the Lumbopelvic Spine

The joints of the lumbopelvic complex that are important from an obstetric point of view include:

- the L5/S1 facet joints
- the two sacroiliac joints
- the pubic symphysis
- the sacrococcygeal joints.

Anatomy of the L5/S1 Joint and its Significance in Pregnancy

The complex of joints that exists between the last lumbar vertebra and the sacrum consists of the intervertebral disc, the facet joints between the inferior surface of L4 and the superior surface of L5, and the facet joints between the inferior part of L5 and the sacrum at the first sacral segment. These are all synovial joints with a joint capsule rich in nociceptive fibers.[1] The whole spine is reinforced by the anterior and posterior longitudinal ligaments (Fig 7.1). Where the ligaments meet the intervertebral discs, they blend with the fibers of the annulus fibrosus. The discs themselves consist of a jelly-like nucleus pulposus and the rings of the fibrocartilaginous annulus.

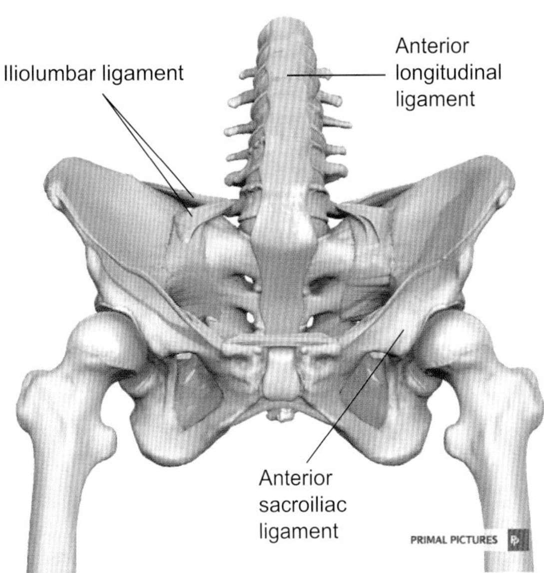

Fig 7.1
The iliolumbar ligaments and the anterior sacroiliac ligaments.

We know that the posterior third of the annulus, where it blends with the posterior longitudinal ligament, also contains many pain-sensitive fibers, especially where there is degeneration of the disc.[1]

Lumbosacral transitional vertebrae are common congenital anomalies of the human spine (Fig 7.2).[2] Either the fifth lumbar vertebra may show assimilation to the sacrum (sacralization), or the first sacral vertebra may show transition to a lumbar configuration (lumbarization). Although the condition has an incidence of over 12% in the general population, knowledge of the exact clinical implications is poor.

The association between lumbosacral transitional vertebrae and low back pain has been debated since it was first described by Bertolotti almost a century ago. Furthermore, several conflicting studies have been published regarding the association of the finding with other spinal pathology.

There seems to be a relation with early disc degeneration above the transitional vertebra in young patients. However, these differences fade with age as they are masked by other degenerative

Fig 7.2
Anomalies between the last lumbar and the first sacral segment.

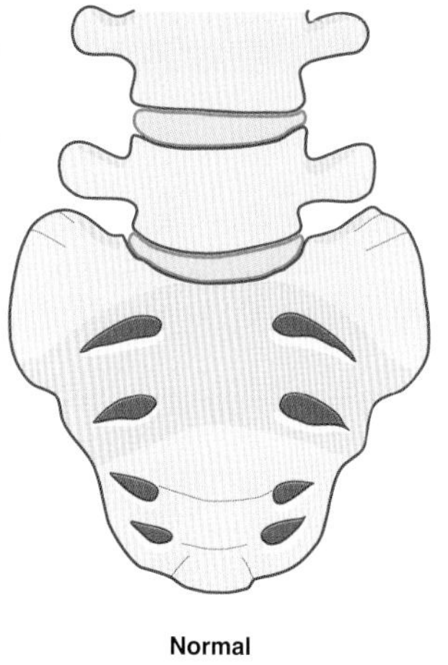

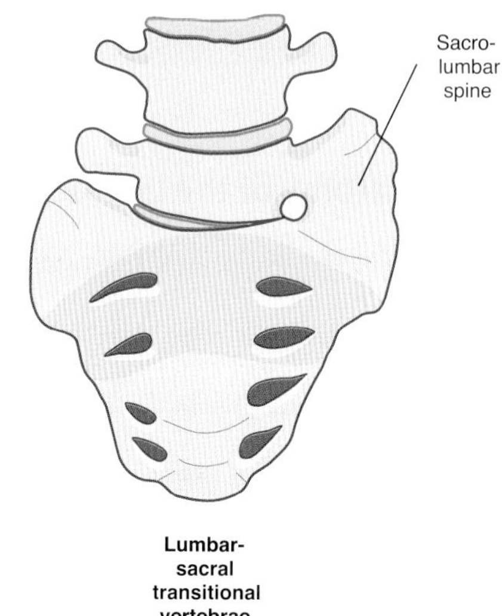

changes of the spine. From a pregnancy point of view, the development of a deep lordosis at the end of the pregnancy involves a hyperextension that takes place at these facet joints. The joints are not normally weight-bearing structures, but if they do become weight-bearing and are also anomalous in their development, then inflammation, pain, and muscle spasm can occur. Once again, there will be a predisposition to all of this because of the ligamentous laxity of pregnancy, which allows more free play between the joints and thus potential facet locking or imbrications. It will also have implications for the way that structural manipulative techniques are carried out during pregnancy.

The Pelvic Ligaments

These can be subdivided into two different groups, according to function. Firstly, there are the true pelvic ligaments connecting bone to bone, and secondly, there are the gynecological ligaments, which will be discussed later in this chapter. In the latter stages of pregnancy, both sets of ligaments will be softened by the hormone relaxin, thus allowing a small amount of bone separation and facilitating the descent and passage of the presenting part, usually the fetal head and shoulders.

The True Pelvic Ligaments

The Sacroiliac Ligaments

The sacroiliac joint is classified as a synovial joint. The sacral surface is covered with hyaline cartilage, while the iliac surface is covered with more of a fibrocartilage. This allows for a degree of compressibility within the joint.[3] The joint capsule is composed of two layers: an external fibrous layer, which contains abundant fibroblasts, blood vessels, and collagen fibers, and an inner synovial layer. Anteriorly, the capsule is clearly separated from the overlying ventral sacroiliac ligament; posteriorly, the fibers of the capsule and the deep interosseous ligament are intimately blended. Inferiorly, the capsule blends with the periosteum of the contiguous sacrum and innominate bones.

Like other synovial joints, the sacroiliac capsule is supported by its overlying ligaments, some of which are the strongest in the body. The ventral or anterior sacroiliac ligaments are quite weak and little more than a thickening of the capsule anteriorly and inferiorly. Clinically, according to Lee,[4] when the sacroiliac joint is hypermobile, these ligaments are often a source of pain.

The interosseous sacroiliac ligament is the strongest of the group and completely fills the space between the lateral sacral crest and the iliac tuberosity (Fig 7.3). The fibers are multidirectional and can be divided into a deep and a superficial group. Again, according to Lee, this structure is the primary barrier to direct palpation of the sacroiliac joint in its superior part.

The dorsal or posterior sacroiliac ligament attaches medially to the entire length of both the intermediate and the lateral sacral crests, and laterally to the posterior superior iliac spine and the inner lip of the iliac crest. It contains fibers which run transversely, obliquely, and vertically, connecting the joint with the sacrotuberous ligament and thus the extensor mechanism of the hip joint, and with the thoracolumbar fascia.

The Iliolumbar Ligaments

The iliolumbar ligament is comprised of two bands arising from the tip of the transverse process of the 5th lumbar vertebra. The anterior band inserts onto the anterior margin of the iliac crest, while the posterior band inserts onto the posterior margin of the iliac crest. The quadratus lumborum muscle arises from and between these two bands (Fig 7.4).

Clinically, when testing for movement in the sacroiliac joint with the patient supine, a force is driven down the shaft of the femur; the sulcus at

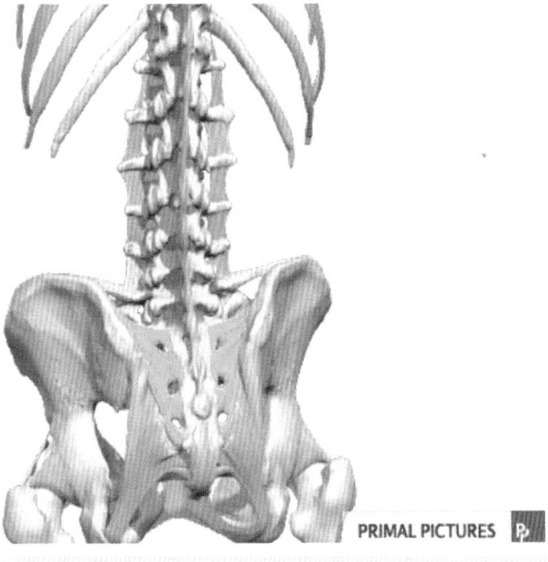

Fig 7.3
The interosseous and posterior sacroiliac ligaments.

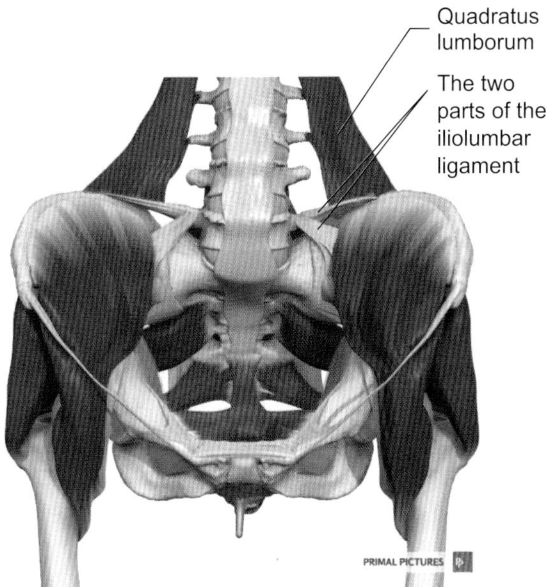

Fig 7.4
Quadratus lumborum and the iliolumbar ligaments.

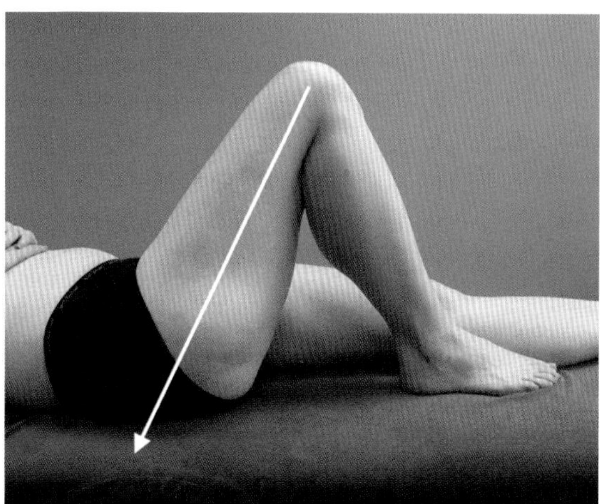

Fig 7.5
The sacroiliac joint shearing with the foot on the table.

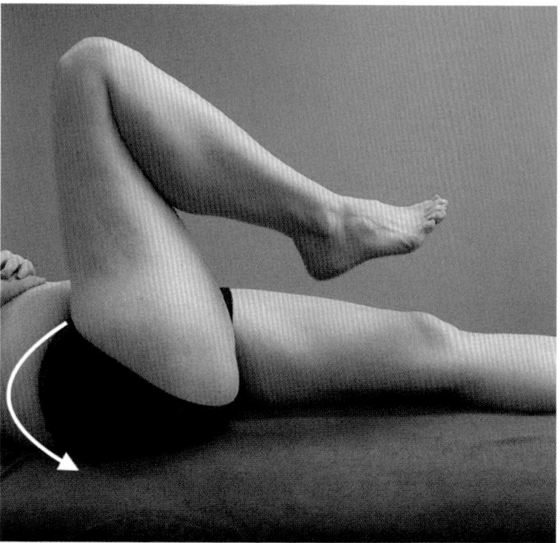

Fig 7.6
Taking the foot off the table stresses the iliolumbar ligaments, which negates the accuracy of the maneuver as a differential diagnostic test between the sacroiliac joint and the iliolumbar ligament.

the posterior superior iliac spine is palpated as the joint opens and closes, and the ilium is driven away from the sacrum. It is very important to keep the patient's foot on the table (Fig 7.5): lifting the leg rotates the whole pelvis and so any pain that is reproduced can stem from either the sacroiliac joint or the iliolumbar ligament, which contains many nociceptive fibers. If the foot is lifted from the table, this is not an accurate differential diagnostic test (Fig 7.6).

The Sacrotuberous and Sacrospinous Ligaments

The sacrotuberous ligament attaches medially to the posterior superior iliac spine, to the transverse tubercles of S2–4, and to the lateral margins of the lower sacrum and coccyx (Fig 7.7). Its fibers run in an inferior lateral and anterior direction, to converge as a thick band attaching to the medial part of the ischial tuberosity.

The sacrospinous ligament attaches medially to the lower lateral aspect of the sacrum and the coccyx. Laterally, the apex of this triangular ligament attaches to the ischial spine. It is closely connected to the coccygeus muscle and thus may be a source of coccygeal pain post partum, especially if the second stage of labor has been prolonged, or sometimes if the patient has been in the lithotomy position in stirrups without support for the lumbar spine.

The Sacrococcygeal Ligaments

These ligaments are in three bands: anterior, lateral, and posterior. The anterior band is the continuation of the anterior longitudinal ligament, and the posterior band a continuation of the posterior longitudinal ligament attaching the coccyx to the last sacral segment. The lateral ligaments connect the sacrum and coccyx laterally.

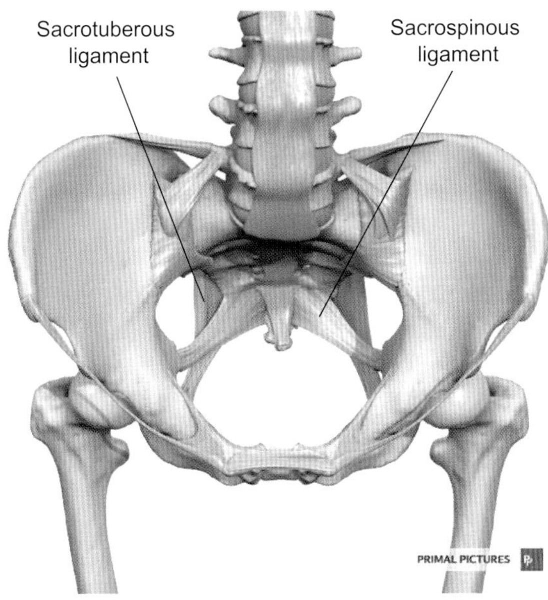

Fig 7.7
The sacrotuberous and sacrospinous ligaments.

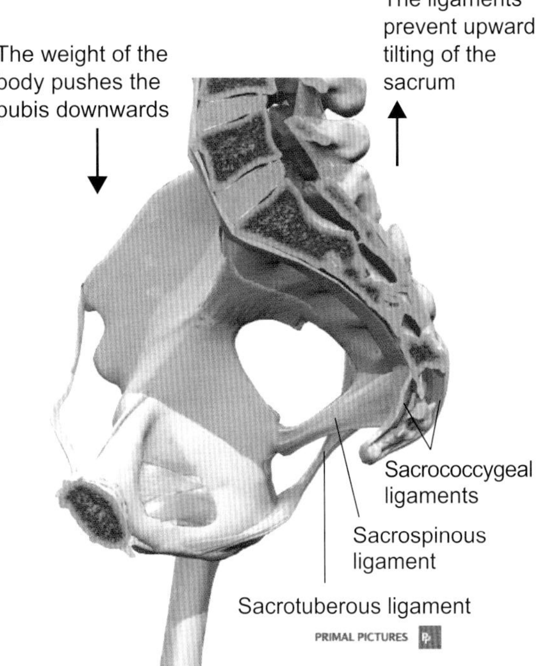

Fig 7.8
Pelvic ligaments preventing upward tilting of the sacrum.

Clinically, these are important for the reasons already described (Fig 7.8); postpartum coccygeal pain is not uncommon, and is often the consequence of a rapid or uncontrolled second stage. Patients report not being able to sit on their coccyx for feeding or even to sit up in bed. The pain can persist for many months after labor, but coccygeal pain post partum is treatable by manipulation per rectum and should be considered in patients who have this sort of history.

Ligaments of the Pubic Symphysis

The pubic symphysis is a unique joint consisting of a fibrocartilaginous disc, sandwiched between the articular surfaces of the pubic bones. It resists tensile, shearing, and compressive forces, and is capable of a small amount of movement under physiological conditions in most adults (up to 2 mm shift (0.08 inches) and 1 degree of rotation). During pregnancy, circulating hormones such as relaxin induce resorption of the symphyseal margins and structural changes in the fibrocartilaginous disc, increasing symphyseal width and mobility.

The pubic symphysis is a true symphysis and is not a synovial joint as such. There is a thick fibrocartilaginous disc between the two pubic bones. The bony surfaces are covered by a thin layer of hyaline cartilage. There are many ligaments supporting the joint from above, anteriorly, and posteriorly (Fig 7.9).

The superior pubic ligament is a thick, fibrous band connecting the bones above; the arcuate ligament performs the same function from below.

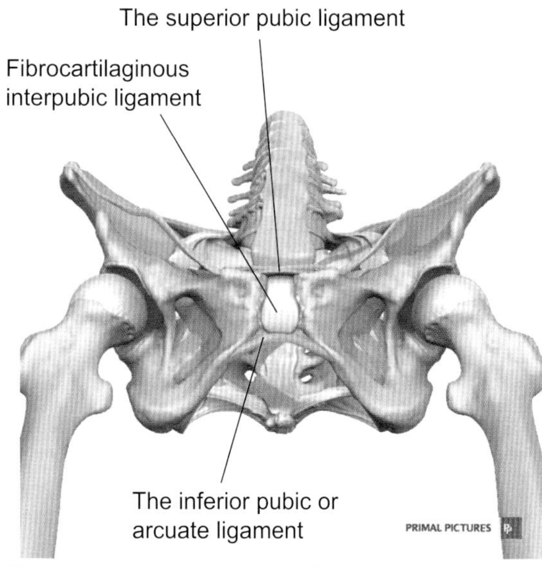

Fig 7.9
Pelvic ligaments of the pubic symphysis.

Both ligaments blend with the fibrocartilaginous disc. The posterior ligament is thin and blends with the periosteum; the anterior ligament is very thick, containing both transverse and oblique fibers. It is reinforced by fibers from the aponeurosis of the rectus sheath and by fibers from adductor magnus.

From an obstetric point of view, the pubic symphysis must be able to "separate" during the labor process to allow for passage of the fetal head. The reinforcement anteriorly and superiorly allows for a widening inferiorly and posteriorly. If there is dysfunction in one of the sacroiliac articulations, it can lead to torsion through the pelvis, known as the pubic ring syndrome (see later in this chapter). This can produce pain radiating from the pubis (pubalgia), as well as pain in the opposite compensating sacroiliac joint. It is commonly seen during the mid and latter months of pregnancy.

Low Back Pain and Pregnancy

The commonest presenting symptom among our pregnant patients will be back pain in one form or another. The evidence and theories relating to low back and pelvic pain in pregnancy are explored in detail in Chapter 5.

Review of Gynecological Anatomy

The Hard–Bony Passages

The bony pelvis is divided obstetrically into the false pelvis and the true pelvis by the pelvic brim, which is bounded by the pubic crest, the iliopectineal line on the innominate bone, and the anterior border, ala, and promontory of the sacrum (Fig 7.10). The shape and structure of the true pelvis are of great obstetric

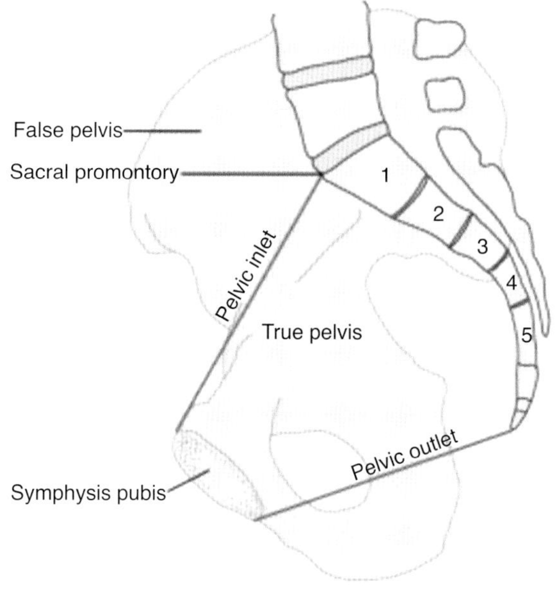

Fig 7.10
The funnel shape of the pelvis, showing a wide inlet and a narrow outlet.

importance. The shape and structure of the false pelvis have little significance.

The outlet of the pelvis is bounded by the arcuate ligament (which forms the inferior part of the pubic symphysis), the ischial tuberosities, and the sacrotuberous ligaments laterally, and by the sacrum and coccyx posteriorly.

Zones of the pelvis

The contour of the birth canal varies at different levels. For descriptive purposes, it is defined by three zones: the pelvic brim, the pelvic cavity, and the pelvic outlet. These are important because they will define the amount of room available for the passage of the fetus.

Brim or pelvic inlet. This zone is bounded by the upper border of the pubis in front, the iliopectineal line laterally, and the sacral promontory posteriorly.

Pelvic cavity. This extends from the brim above to the pelvic outlet below. The anterior wall is formed by the pubic bones and the symphysis pubis, and the posterior wall is formed by the curve of the sacrum. The lateral walls are formed mainly by the obturator internus muscle. The cavity is circular in shape, and while it is not possible to measure the diameters exactly, they are generally considered to be 12 cm (4.7 inches).

Pelvic outlet. In most obstetric textbooks, two outlets are described: the anatomical and the obstetric. The anatomical outlet is formed by the lower borders of each of the bones, together with the sacrotuberous ligament. The obstetric outlet is of greater practical significance because it includes the narrowest part of the pelvis, through which the presenting part of the fetus must pass. This narrow part lies between the sacrococcygeal joint, the two ischial spines, and the lower border of the symphysis pubis.

Midwives and obstetricians measure these structures with their fingers vaginally when examining and assessing the patient and evaluating the potential for vaginal delivery. If the space is deemed too narrow for the size of the baby, the patient is said to have cephalopelvic disproportion (CPD) and will be offered an elective cesarean section. Obstetrically, it is better practice to have an elective section than an emergency section if the passages are found to be too narrow once labor has started.

From an osteopathic point of view, in the UK, although we are legally restricted from helping at the birth itself unless we are specifically invited to do so by the midwife or the doctor, we are ideally situated to assist in preparation for labor. Maximum mobility between the pelvic bones is essential if they are to separate during delivery and allow passage of the fetal head. This is particularly important in the case of the sacroiliac joints and the joints of the coccyx and pubic symphysis. Relaxin will soften and unwind the collagenous ligaments holding the bones together, and so ligament-stretching techniques, aimed at giving maximum mobility to the joints, will result in a shorter and better controlled labor. One would not expect a marathon runner to perform without expert training and physical fitness before the race.

Obstetrically, the analogy is the same. We should prepare the pregnant patient for the hardest physical day's work of her life by stretching the joints controlling the bony passages. Turning the baby is considered by the authorities as an obstetric procedure and thus is not the work of the osteopath, but myofascial and gentle stretching techniques for the abdominal muscles and fascia will give the developing child as much space as it needs to present itself to the pelvis in the easiest way for it to pass down into and through the birth canal.

The pelvic floor

The pelvic floor is made up of the soft tissues which form the outlet of the pelvis. The most important of these is the strong pelvic diaphragm, slung like a hammock from the walls of the pelvis. Through it pass the urethra, the vagina, and the anal canal. The pelvic floor supports the weight of the abdominal and pelvic organs, and its muscles are responsible for the voluntary control of micturition, defecation, parturition, and particularly relaxation to allow baby to be born. There are superficial and deep muscle layers.

The superficial muscles contain four main structures. The external anal sphincter surrounds the anus and is attached by a few fibers to the coccyx. The transverse perineal muscles pass from the ischial tuberosities to the center of the perineum, which is called the perineal body (Fig 7.11). The bulbospongiosus muscle passes from the perineal body forwards around the vagina to the pubic arch. The ischiocavernosus muscles pass from the ischial tuberosities along the arch to the substance of the clitoris.

Deep transverse perineal muscles
Piriformis
Levator ani
Perineal body
Urethral sphincter
Obturator fascia
Puborectalis
PRIMAL PICTURES

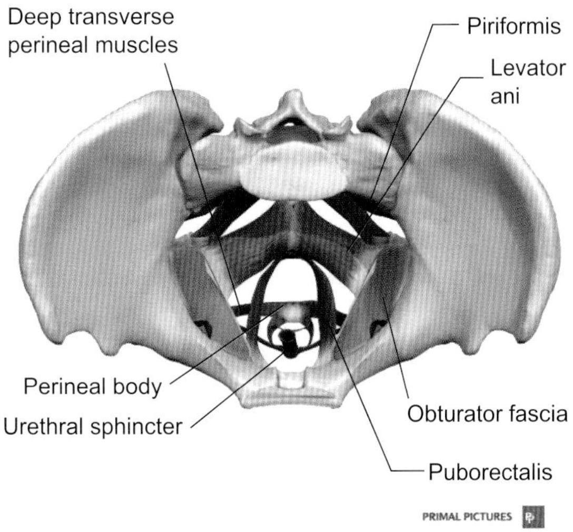

Fig 7.11
The perineal body and its muscular attachments.
© Informa UK Ltd (trading as Primal Pictures), 2020.

The deep layer is composed of three pairs of muscles, which together are known as the levator ani muscles (Fig. 7.12). Each levator muscle has three parts which attach various pelvic structures to the coccyx.

The pubococcygeus muscle passes from the pubis to the coccyx, with a few fibers crossing over the perineal body to form its deepest part. The iliococcygeus muscle passes from the fascia covering obturator internus to the coccyx. The ischiococcygeus muscle passes from the ischial spine of the pelvic wall to the coccyx.

Between the muscle layers, and also above and below them, are the layers of the pelvic fascia; this forms part of the transverse layer of the pelvic floor which is continuous with the vertical chains of fascia described by Paoletti (see Chapter 3).

The piriformis muscle

This is a pyramid-shaped muscle in the gluteal region. It originates at the anterior sacrum, the lowest

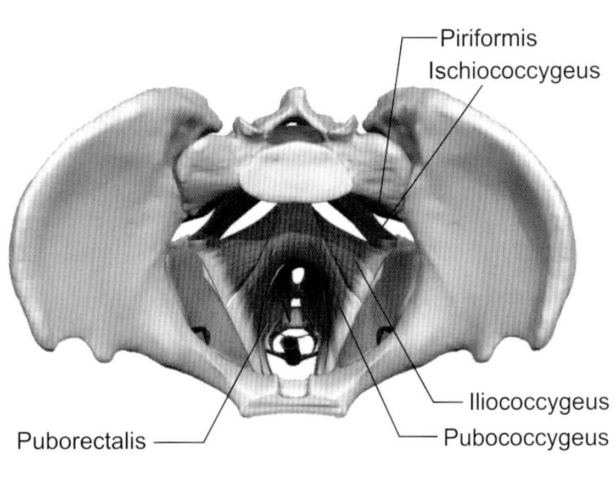

Fig 7.12
The levator ani muscles.
© Informa UK Ltd (trading as Primal Pictures), 2020.

portion of the spine, and the superior margin of the greater sciatic notch, extends through the greater sciatic foramen of the pelvis, and attaches to the greater trochanter of the femur (Figs 7.13 and 7.14). The piriformis muscle lies parallel to and beneath gluteus maximus.

The common peroneal nerve often runs through the piriformis muscle, and in about 15% of the population so does the sciatic nerve. In most people, the sciatic nerve runs underneath the piriformis muscle. In either case, piriformis can sometimes exert pressure on the sciatic nerve, which, at this point, can be as thick as the human thumb. It causes the piriformis syndrome, a condition that is more common in those whose sciatic nerve runs through the muscle.

Piriformis runs down, out, and back, to be inserted into the greater trochanter of the femur. The function of piriformis is to externally rotate and abduct the thigh.

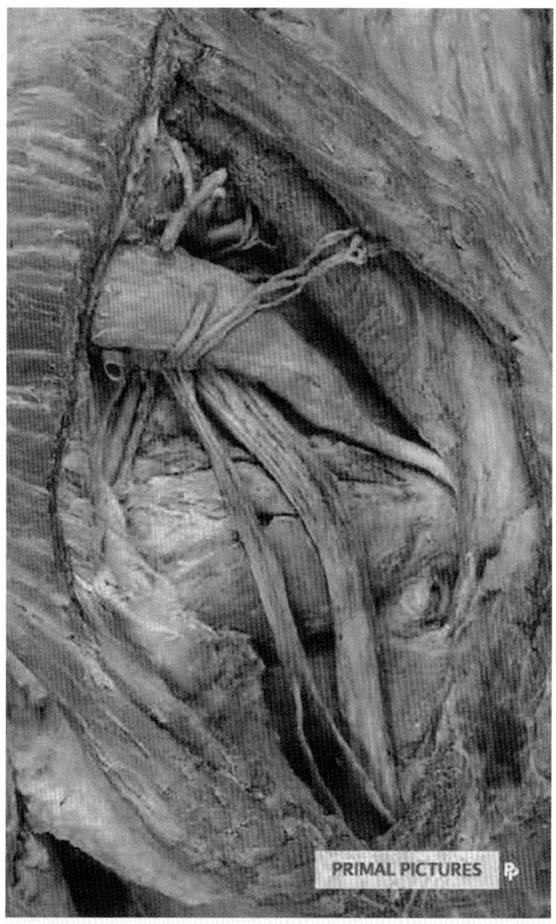

Fig 7.14
The piriformis muscle.

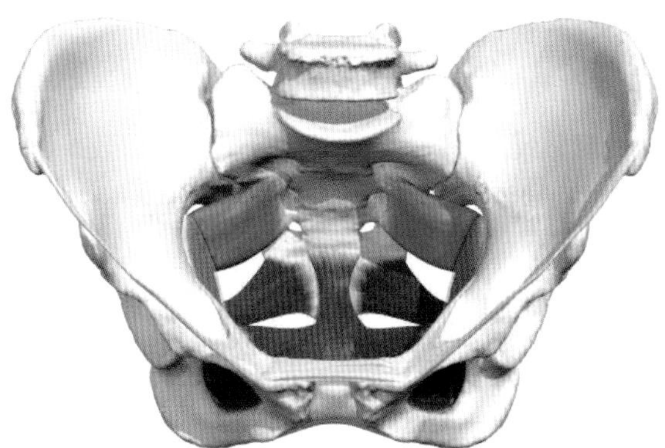

Fig 7.13
The piriformis muscle.

The obturator internus muscle

This muscle arises from the inner surface of the antero-lateral wall of the pelvis, where it surrounds the greater part of the obturator foramen. It is attached to the ramus of the pubis, the ischium, and the inner surface of the pelvic wall below and behind the pelvic brim, reaching from the upper part of the greater sciatic foramen above and behind to the obturator foramen below and in front (Fig 7.15).

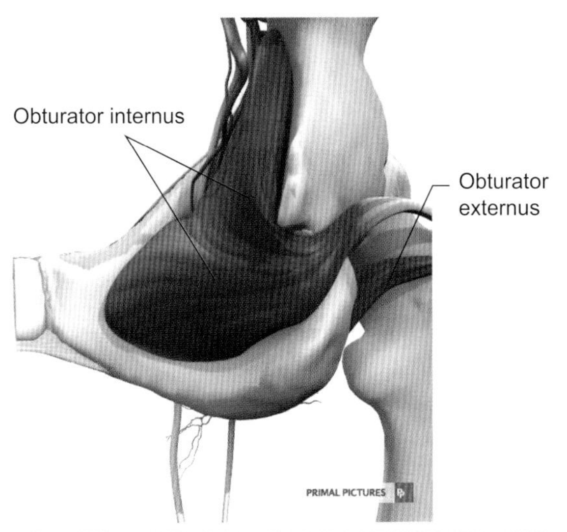

Fig 7.15
The obturator muscles.
© Informa UK Ltd (trading as Primal Pictures), 2020.

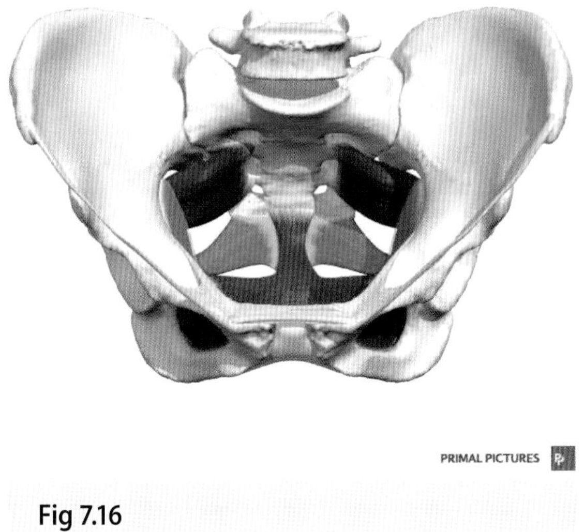

Fig 7.16
The coccygeus muscle.
© Informa UK Ltd (trading as Primal Pictures), 2020.

It also arises from the pelvic surface of the obturator membrane, except in the posterior part; from the tendinous arch which completes the canal for the passage of the obturator vessels and nerve; and, to a slight extent, from the obturator fascia, which covers the muscle.

The fibers converge rapidly toward the lesser sciatic foramen, and end in four or five tendinous bands, which are found on the deep surface of the muscle. These bands are reflected at a right angle over the grooved surface of the ischium between its spine and tuberosity.

The coccygeus muscle

This is a muscle of the pelvic wall, located posterior to levator ani and anterior to the sacrospinous ligament (Fig 7.16). It is a triangular plane of muscular and tendinous fibers, arising by its apex from the spine of the ischium and sacrospinous ligament, and inserted by its base onto the margin of the coccyx and onto the side of the lowest piece of the sacrum. In combination with levator ani, it forms the pelvic diaphragm. It assists levator ani and piriformis in closing in the back part of the outlet of the pelvis.

From these broad origins, the sides of the pelvic floor slope downwards and forwards, forming a sling or gutter-shaped structure through which the urethra, vagina, and rectum must pass (Fig 7.17).

The structures related to the upper concave surface of the pelvic floor are:

- the bladder anteriorly, resting on the pubococcygeus portion of levator ani
- the uterus and vagina behind the bladder, the vagina passing through the gap between the two levator muscles
- the broad ligaments and the pelvic connective tissue containing the uterine venous plexuses
- the ureters, which lie on the pelvic floor beneath the broad ligaments, and pass forwards to the bladder

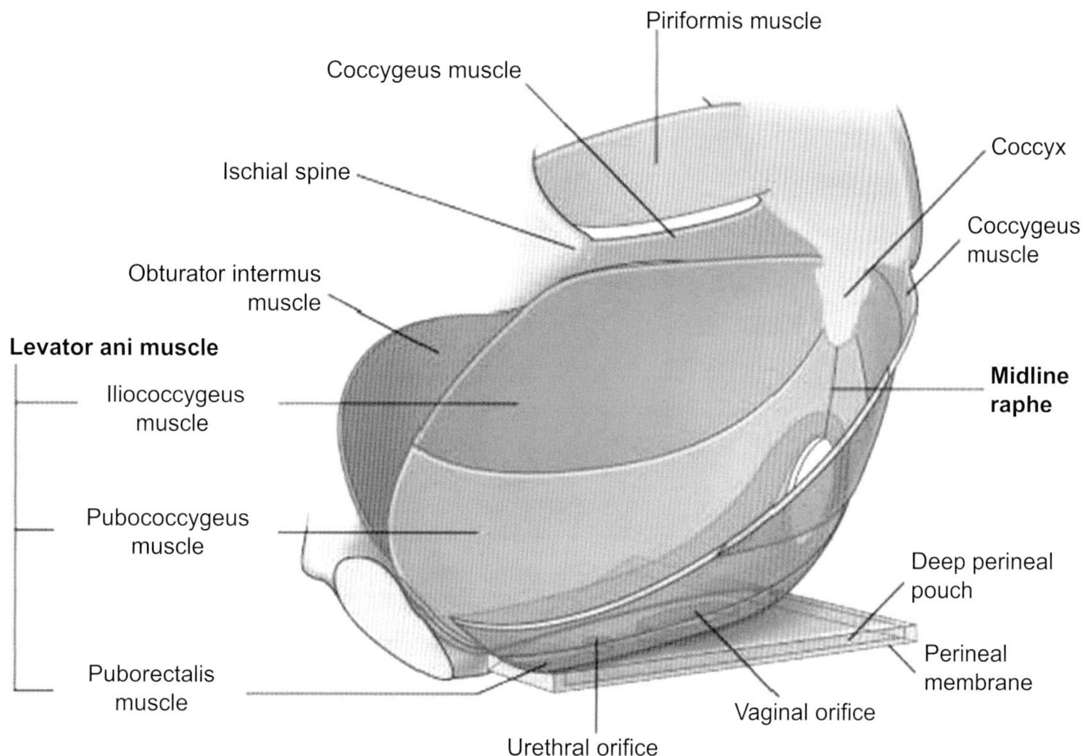

Fig 7.17
The gutter or sling-shaped pelvic floor.
From Gray's Anatomy for Students, 4th edn, Richard Drake, A. Wayne Vogl, Adam Mitchell. Copyright Elsevier, 2019. Reproduced by kind permission of the publishers.

- the uterine and vaginal arteries above and below the ureters
- the rectum behind the uterus and vagina, passing through the gap between the two levator muscles.

Between the levator muscles and penetrated by the urethra and the vagina is the superior layer of condensed connective tissue known as the urogenital diaphragm.

The Gynecological Ligaments

As mentioned before, there are two sets of ligaments in the pelvis: the true pelvic ligaments and the gynecological ligaments. The gynecological ligaments are subdivided into the ligaments of the uterus and the ligaments of the cervix.

The Uterine Ligaments

The first and most important ligament of the uterus is the broad ligament (Fig 7.18).

The broad ligaments are formed from folds of peritoneum at the base of the abdominal cavity, which are draped over the fallopian tubes. They hang down like a curtain and spread from the sides of the uterus to the side wall of the pelvis. The distal ends of the

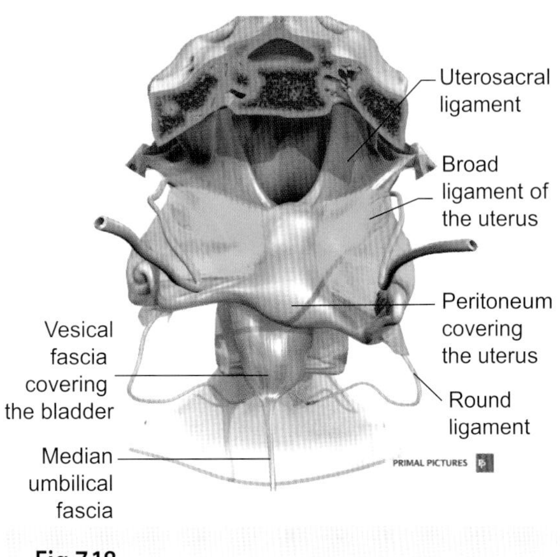

Fig 7.18
The ligaments and fascia covering the uterus.
© Informa UK Ltd (trading as Primal Pictures), 2020.

fallopian tubes protrude from the folds of the broad ligament posteriorly and lie free.

Between the two layers are the uterine arteries and veins, the round ligament, and the ligaments of the ovary and the lymphatics. The ovary is partly covered by a separate posterior fold of the broad ligament called the mesovarium, but the surface of the ovary is devoid of peritoneum to allow for exit of the eggs.

The fallopian tubes lie in the upper edge of the broad ligament, which is termed the mesosalpinx. The ureters pass through the base of the broad ligament in close relation to the uterine artery.

Together with the uterus, the broad ligament forms a septum across the female pelvis, dividing that cavity into two compartments. In the anterior part is the bladder and in the posterior part is the rectum. The broad ligament is believed to hold the uterus in its normal position within the pelvis and maintains the relationship of the fallopian tubes to the ovaries and the uterus, a role that might be important in reproduction. However, the broad ligament plays a minimal role, if any, in pelvic support. The principal support of the uterus is provided by the pelvic floor.

Problems with the broad ligament are most likely to arise during pregnancy, which can cause tension in the ligament, leading to hip or pelvic pain. Rarely, an ectopic pregnancy can occur on the broad ligament. All ectopic pregnancies are potentially dangerous. Also, an unusual complication that may appear during delivery or after delivery is a broad ligament hematoma, which is basically a large bruise.[5]

The round ligaments

These have little value as a support mechanism for the uterus but tend to help maintain an anteverted uterine position. They arise from the corners of the fundus of the uterus in front of and below each insertion of the fallopian tube, and pass between the folds of the broad ligament through the inguinal canal, to be inserted in the folds of the labium majus (Fig 7.19).

The retroverted or retroflexed uterus

Unfortunately, the retroverted uterus (tilted or tipped uterus) is a syndrome that has been diagnosed and treated, in some cases surgically, for as long as women have been going to see gynecologists. There is no evidence that it is anything other than normal; certainly, it is not symptomatic in any way in the absence of pathology.

A retroverted uterus is tilted backwards instead of forwards. This contrasts with the slightly "anteverted" uterus that most women have, which is tipped forwards toward the bladder, with the anterior end slightly concave. A retroflexed uterus is very similar, in that the fundus is thought to lie towards the spine.

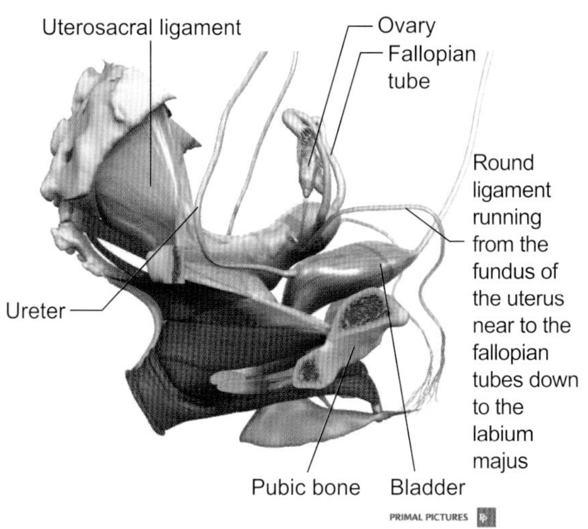

Fig 7.19
The round ligaments.

Between 1 in 3 and 1 in 5 patients are thought to have a uterus that sits in the pelvis in this way.[6] In most cases, a retroverted uterus is genetic and is perfectly normal, but there are other factors that can cause the uterus to be retroverted. Some cases are caused by pelvic surgery, pelvic adhesions, endometriosis, fibroids, or pelvic inflammatory disease, or may be found post partum. The condition usually does not pose any medical problems, though it can be associated with dyspareunia (pain during sexual intercourse) and dysmenorrhea (pain during menstruation). Uterine position has no effect on fertility.

A tipped uterus will usually right itself during the 10th to 12th week of pregnancy. From an osteopathic point of view, as long as the uterus is normally mobile and exhibits a normal motility pattern, it should be left alone. Attempts to change the position with visceral manipulation techniques will serve no purpose unless the patient has symptoms, but for fertility issues there is no evidence that the position of the uterus in the pelvis has any effect at all.

The Ligaments of the Cervix

The uterus is supported by the pelvic floor and maintained in position by several ligaments. The ones at the cervix are the most important.

The transverse cervical ligaments, or the cardinal ligaments, fan out from the sides of the cervix to the walls of the bony pelvis (Fig 7.20).

The uterosacral ligaments pass backwards from the cervix to the sacrum. These structures are often invaded by deposits in endometriosis and can cause dragging back pain if overstretched during a long labor. The differential diagnosis is annulus fibrosus or disc pain, and should be part of the evaluation of

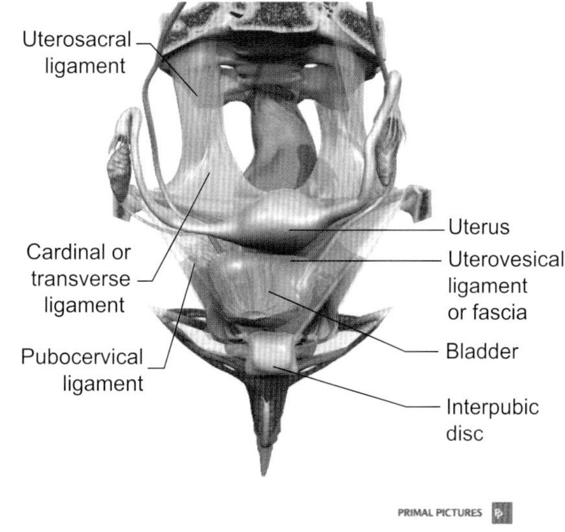

Fig 7.20
The ligaments of the cervix and the uterine fascias.

the pregnant patient and postpartum questioning in osteopathic practice.

The pubocervical ligaments pass forwards from the cervix under the bladder to the pubic bones. If they are overstretched during labor, patients can present with postpartum pubalgia.

Changes to the Uterus in Pregnancy

The most obvious and important changes take place within the uterus.

The uterus has three layers. The outer serous layer forms ligaments that hold it to the pelvic walls. The middle muscular layer has three muscle layers, used in labor. The inner layer is the lining of the uterus, or the endometrium (known as the decidua in pregnancy).

The decidua becomes thicker and very heavily vascular under the influence of progesterone and estrogen, produced by the corpus luteum of pregnancy. This is particularly important at the fundus and the upper body of the uterus because this is where the placenta ideally is going to implant. The decidua is thinner and less vascular in the lower pole of the uterus. It provides a glycogen-rich environment for the blastocyst until the trophoblast cells begin to form the placenta. Once the placenta is formed, it produces its own hormones and the corpus luteum is no longer maintained by human chorionic gonadotrophin (HCG). The corpus luteum then atrophies and becomes the corpus albicans.

Estrogen is responsible for the growth of the uterine muscle layers. There is an increase in size (hypertrophy) and an increase in number (hyperplasia) of muscle fibers in the uterine wall. The uterus grows in this way for the first 20 weeks of pregnancy, after which it simply stretches.

The uterus increases in weight from 60 g in the non-pregnant woman to 900 g (0.1 to 2 pounds) at term, and in size from 7.5 × 5 × 2.5 cm (3 × 2 × 1 inch) to 30 × 23 × 20 cm (12 × 9 × 8 inches).

The uterus is able to stretch in this way because progesterone encourages relaxation of the smooth muscle layers.[7] These muscle layers are divided into an outer longitudinal layer, a middle oblique layer, and an inner circular layer (Fig 7.21). During pregnancy, each layer becomes more differentiated and organized to be able to play its part in expelling the fetus at term.

The circular layer has a role in stretching the lower segment and cervix during labor. The middle or oblique layer is involved in the contractions necessary to expel the fetus at the end of pregnancy, but more importantly, this action is needed to entrap and enmesh bleeding vessels and stop bleeding once the placenta is delivered, as the uterus shrinks back to a near-normal size. This is essential to prevent postpartum hemorrhage. The longitudinal outer layer of muscles contracts and retracts during labor, causing the upper segment of the uterus to thicken. The thickened upper layer acts as a piston to drive the fetus into the receptive lower segment of the uterus. The uterus contracts from above downwards, in spirals of contraction, to squeeze the fetus towards the uterine exit. A better example of the structure–function principle is hard to find!

Changes in the Uterine Blood Supply

The blood supply to the uterus increases to keep pace with growth and also to meet the needs of the functioning placenta. Estrogen causes new blood vessels to develop. Initially, they form a coiled network throughout the uterine walls, but as the uterus grows and stretches, they become straightened until after the birth, when the uterus involutes and shrinks; at this point, they become tortuous again (Fig 7.22).

Changes in Uterine Shape

Healthy growth of the fetus requires adequate space. After conception, the embedded blastocyst requires

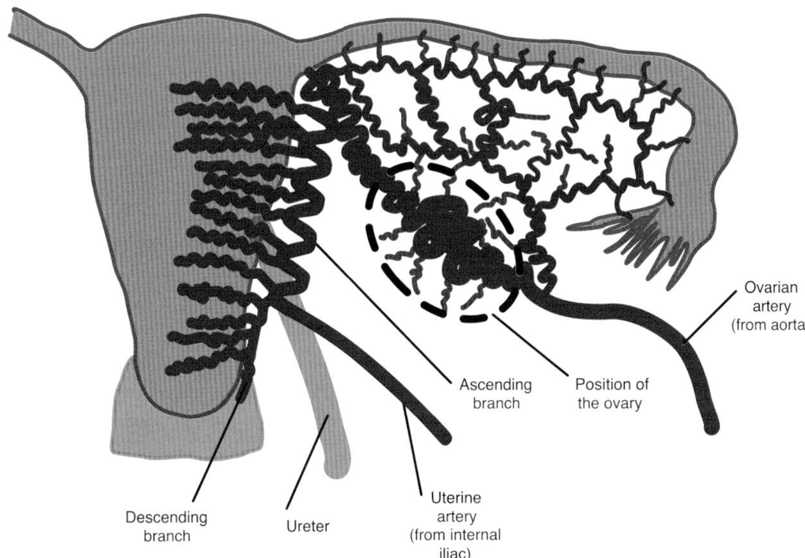

Fig 7.21
Coiling of the uterine blood supply.

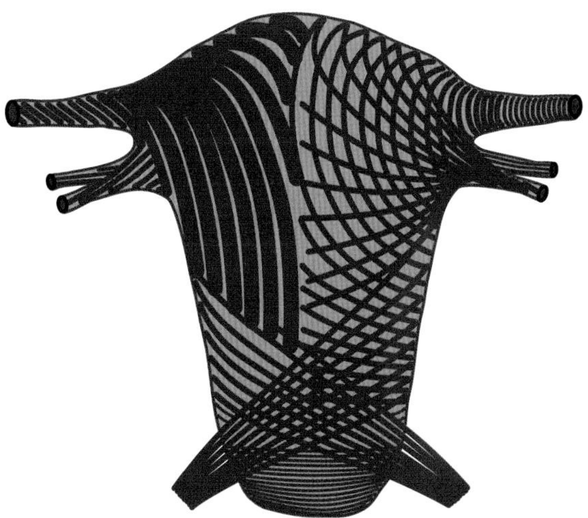

Fig 7.22
The direction of the muscle fibers in the uterus.
(After Llewellyn Jones.) © Faber & Faber.

a minimal change in shape and size, but the upper part of the uterus begins to enlarge due to the effects of estrogen. In early pregnancy, the uterus adopts a globular or teardrop shape to anticipate fetal growth and to accommodate increasing amounts of amniotic fluid and placental tissue (Fig 7.23).

By the 12th week, the uterus is no longer anteverted and anteflexed. It has risen out of the pelvis and is upright, often rotating to the right because pressure from the left sigmoid colon pushes it away. This is known as dextrorotation.

At 12 weeks, the fundus may be palpated abdominally above the pubic symphysis.

By the 20th week, the uterus is pear-shaped and now has a thicker and more rounded fundus. The fallopian tubes, being restricted by attachment to the broad ligaments, become progressively more vertical.

By the 30th week, the lower uterine segment can be identified. It lies above the internal os, and this is where the midwife will try to palpate the head of the baby (ballottement).

By the 36th week, the uterus will reach the level of the xiphisternum. Softening of the tissues of the pelvic floor, together with the good tone of the uterus,

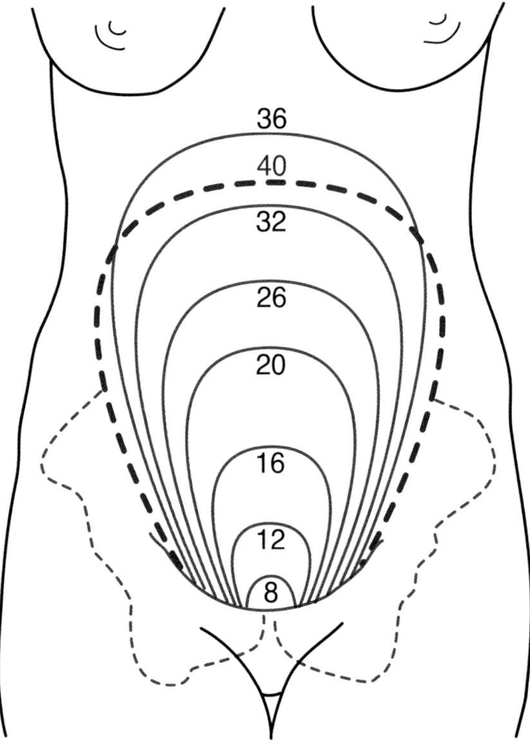

Fig 7.23
Changes in uterine shape and the height of the fundus during the weeks of pregnancy.

encourages the fetus to sink into the lower pole of the pelvis.

The head "engages" in primiparous mothers but often does not in multigravid women. This means that, around the 36th week, the head descends into the pelvis and rests on the bladder, causing urinary frequency and some deep pelvic discomfort.

References

1. Edgar MA. The nerve supply of the lumbar intervertebral disc. J Bone Joint Surg Br 2007 Sep;89-B(9):1135–9.
2. Bron JL, van Royen BJ, Wuisman PIJ. The clinical significance of lumbosacral transitional anomalies. Acta Orthop Belg. 2007 Dec;73(6):687–95.
3. Walker JM. Age related differences in the human sacroiliac joint; a histological study; implications for therapy. J Orthop and Sports Ther. 1986;7(6):325–34.
4. Lee D. *The Pelvic Girdle*. Churchill Livingstone, 1989.
5. Saleem N, Ali HS, Irfan A, Afzal B. Broad ligament haematoma following a vaginal delivery in primigravida. Pak J Med Sci. 2009 Jul–Sep;25(4):683–5.
6. O'Grady JP. Malposition of the Uterus; http://emedicine.medscape.com/article/272497-overview.
7. Kofinas AD, Rose JC, Koritnik DR, Meis PJ. Progesterone and estradiol concentrations in nonpregnant and pregnant human myometrium. Effect of progesterone and estradiol on cyclic adenosine monophosphate-phosphodiesterase activity. J Reprod Med. 1990 Nov;35(11):1045–50.

Treatment Techniques for the Pelvis During Pregnancy 8

Treatment techniques for the lumbar spine were dealt with in Chapter 6. This chapter will concentrate on treatment approaches for the pelvis.

Palpation of the Pelvic Floor Externally

 **Warning**

This technique requires palpation of tissues very close to the genital area. Therefore the verbal and, if need be, written consent of the patient must be obtained before the examination can proceed. A chaperone should also be offered.

Position of the patient

The patient is supine, with her head propped up on pillows, her knees flexed, and her feet flat on the treatment table.

Position of the osteopath

The osteopath is at the side of the treatment table, facing the patient.

Ambition of the technique

The technique is used to evaluate any difference in tone between the patient's right side and left side, and the posterior pelvic triangles. Is a difference in tone to be expected when the findings are compared to her standing posture? Does she have a short or long leg on one side? If so, a change in tension might be normal for her as her body tries to bring about a sacral base plane. Has she previously had children or surgery to the pelvic floor, resulting in scar tissue: for example, an episiotomy during a previous childbirth?

All of these questions and observations are very important when examining the pelvic floor because any tensions that are palpated might be physiological and not pathological. If that is the case, a decision has to be made as to whether to leave them alone or to treat them.

Application of the technique

To palpate the patient's right side, the osteopath stands on the same side of the table, with the patient supine.

Using his right hand, he asks the patient to lift her buttocks and sit on his fingers, leaving the thumb free to palpate the ischial tuberosity (Figs 8.1 and 8.2).

Then, rolling his wrist inwards into supination, he palpates the response to light pressure on the tissues immediately medial to the tuberosity. The direction of his force is towards the table for the posterior triangle of the pelvic floor.

It is essential for the osteopath never to lose contact with the ischial tuberosity, so that at all times this is maintained as an external technique. With this technique, only the posterior pelvic floor is assessed, as the thumb never goes forward of the line connecting the two ischial tuberosities.

The osteopath can also use an indirect technique. Comparing hip rotation both internally and externally on each side, with the patient supine, will also show an imbalance in the tissues of the pelvic floor because the piriformis and obturator externus muscles are rotators of the hip. Here, as before when testing the muscular response, the osteopath feels for the quality of end stop in hip joint rotation.

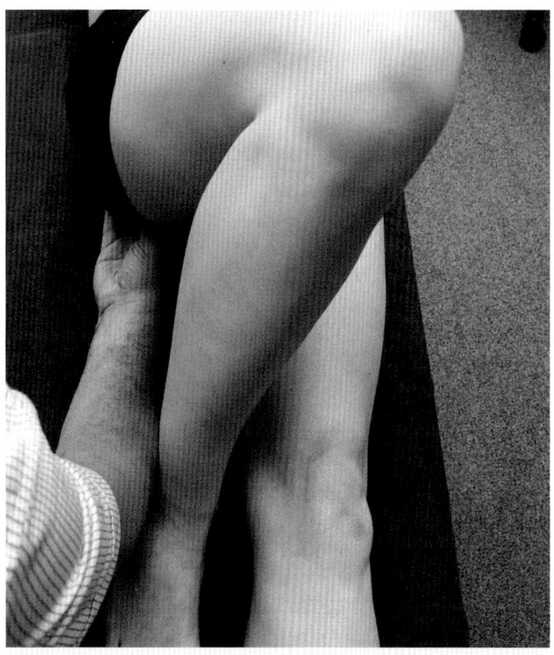

Fig 8.1
Palpation of the pelvic floor via the ischial tuberosity.

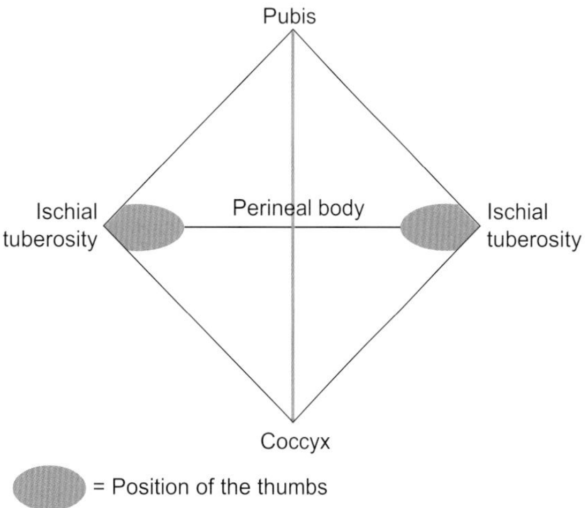

Fig 8.2
Diagrammatic representation of the thumb position in relation to the perineal body.

Muscle Energy Technique (MET) to Reduce the Tone of the Piriformis Muscle

As described in Chapter 7, piriformis is a very important muscle in obstetrics. Not only does it maintain tension in the pelvic floor, but it is frequently involved in cases of sciatica or sacroiliac joint strain because the origin of the muscle is the inferior pole of the sacroiliac joint. If there is tension in the muscle, or even muscle spasm, the following technique can bring a rapid reduction in pain.

Position of the patient

This technique is traditionally performed with the patient prone; however, in pregnancy, it is always better to do this technique with her side-lying.

Position of the osteopath

He stands facing the patient. The technique can, however, be carried out from behind the patient, if preferred.

Ambition of the technique

The aim is to release tension in the muscles of the buttock, including piriformis and the gluteal muscles. It is very useful for treating increased tension in the piriformis muscle, the obturator muscles, and all of the other hip rotators which go to form the posterior part of the pelvic floor, and which, all too often, are seen to be tense in cases of pelvic ring syndrome.

Application of the technique

The technique is performed using isometric contraction. The patient's knee is flexed to 90 degrees and the osteopath places the palm of his hand against the external malleolus of her ankle (Fig 8.3). Starting with the knees together, the patient is asked to push

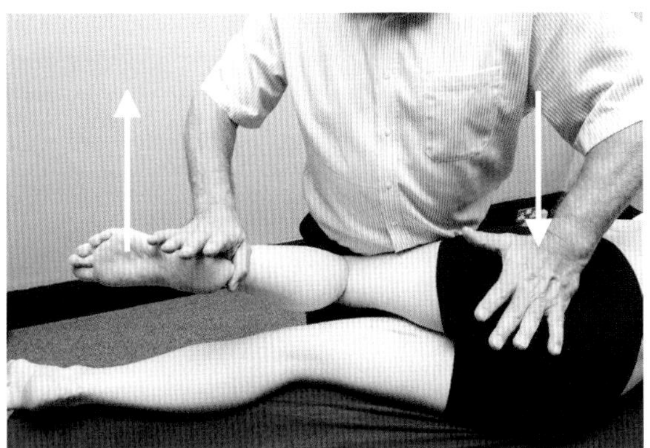

Fig 8.3
Muscle energy technique used to balance tone in the piriformis muscle.

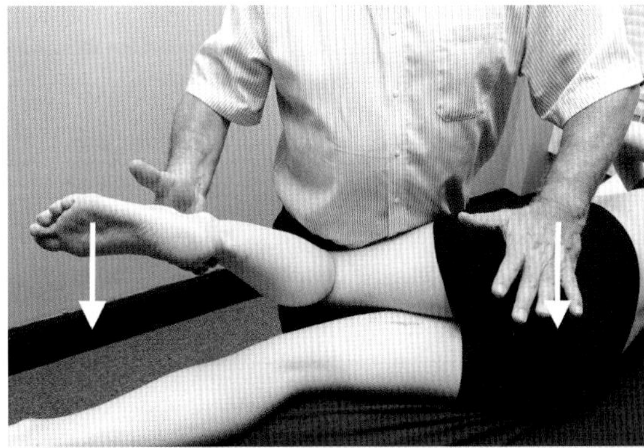

Fig 8.4
The patient pushes her ankle downwards and the resistance is as before.

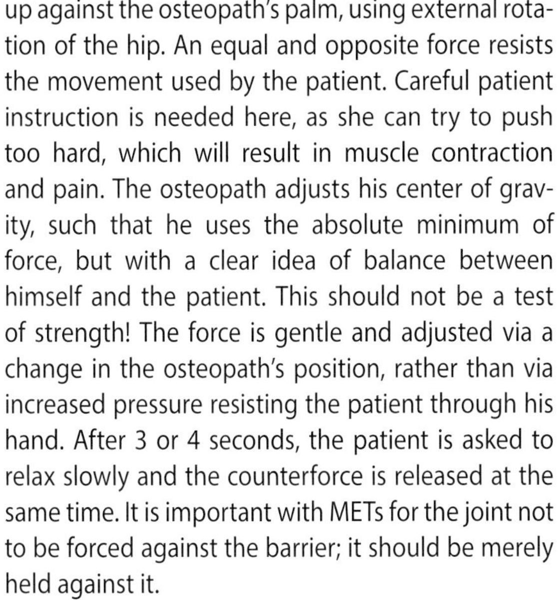

up against the osteopath's palm, using external rotation of the hip. An equal and opposite force resists the movement used by the patient. Careful patient instruction is needed here, as she can try to push too hard, which will result in muscle contraction and pain. The osteopath adjusts his center of gravity, such that he uses the absolute minimum of force, but with a clear idea of balance between himself and the patient. This should not be a test of strength! The force is gentle and adjusted via a change in the osteopath's position, rather than via increased pressure resisting the patient through his hand. After 3 or 4 seconds, the patient is asked to relax slowly and the counterforce is released at the same time. It is important with METs for the joint not to be forced against the barrier; it should be merely held against it.

The patient is given control of the force, which further increases the safety aspects. The technique is repeated three or four times, with increasing degrees of external rotation each time.

The patient's ankle pushes upwards, and the resistance is through the buttock, aimed at the tight piriformis muscle down towards the table: an inhibition force.

Finally, the osteopath transfers his hand to hold the medial malleolus and the patient pulls down against his resistance, using internal rotation of the hip (Fig 8.4). This again is repeated three or four times, with increasing degrees of rotation, and in this way the forces producing external and internal rotation are balanced and the pelvic floor relaxes.

Articulation or Ligamentous Stretch Technique for the Sacroiliac Joint with the Patient Supine

Position of the patient

These techniques can be performed with the patient supine or side-lying, but not prone. She flexes the hip of the side to be treated, and if the technique is designed also to stretch the fibers of the iliolumbar ligament, the foot can come off the table.

In the supine position, this is an extension of the diagnostic technique.

Position of the osteopath

The osteopath stands at the level of the patient's hips and facing the head of the treatment table.

Alternatively, he can sit on the edge of the table, facing her.

Ambition of the technique

The aim is to stretch and mobilize shortened sacroiliac or iliolumbar ligaments.

Application of the technique

With one hand palpating the superior pole of the sacroiliac joint, at the level of the posterior superior iliac spine, the osteopath applies a firm pressure down the shaft of the femur (Fig 8.5). The response in the sacroiliac ligaments and joint capsule is felt, and the joint is stretched and mobilized with small movements of adduction, abduction, and circumduction, with more or less flexion as required. The maneuver is repeated rhythmically.

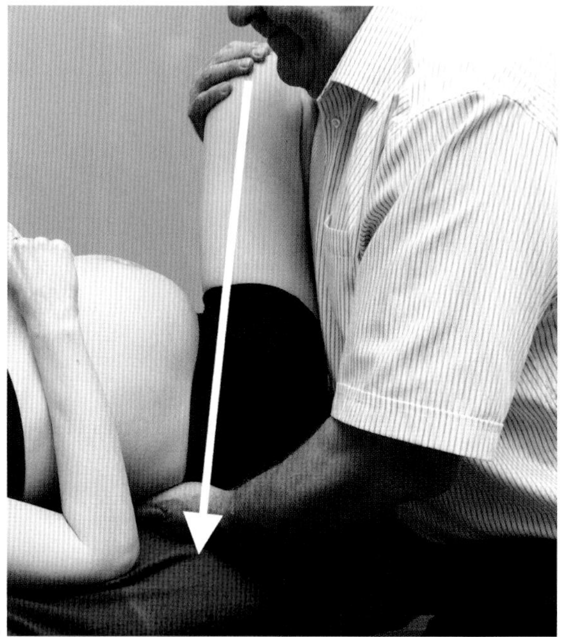

Fig 8.5
Posterior sacroiliac ligament stretching, with the patient supine.

Articulation or Ligamentous Stretch Technique for the Sacroiliac Joint with the Patient Side-lying

Position of the patient

The patient lies on her side in the form of a three-sided square, as seen in Chapter 5, with the painful side uppermost.

Position of the osteopath

The osteopath stands facing the patient at the level of her hips.

Ambition of the technique

The aim is to stretch and mobilise painful articular ligaments and capsular structures.

Application of the technique

The fingers of both of the osteopath's hands are used to palpate the joint line. Using his chest, he gently compresses her ilium, rocking his weight forwards and backwards, and stretches the posterior and internal ligaments of the joint, as well as the joint capsule (Fig 8.6). If limitation of movement is felt more at the superior or the inferior part of the joint, the technique should focus on these restrictions.

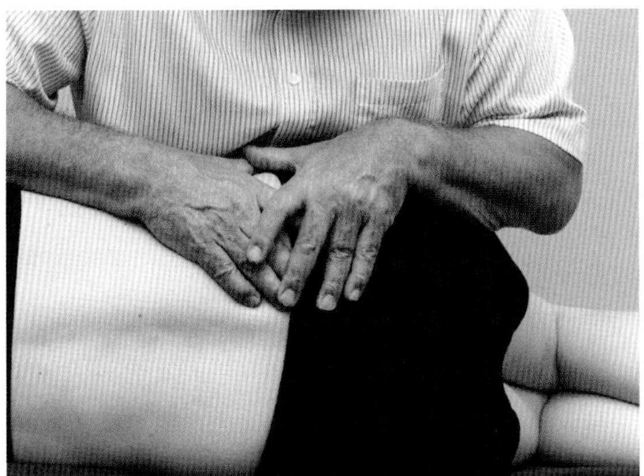

Fig 8.6
Ligamentous stretch technique for the sacroiliac ligaments.

Another very useful addition is the figure of eight articulation technique, seen in Chapter 5 at the lumbar spine. With the patient in the same position and the osteopath gently leaning on the ilium as before, he applies force in a figure of eight in the horizontal plane. The force is directed from the osteopath's shoulder girdle. The focus of the force is at the center of the eight, which can be at the posterior superior or posterior inferior iliac spine, specifically for the poles of the sacroiliac joint. This is repeated in the vertical plane. The result is a gentle but global mobilization and stretch of the painful sacroiliac ligaments and joint concerned.

Sacroiliac Joint Lesions: Theories and Techniques

The technique textbooks present many ways of manipulating and mobilizing the sacroiliac joint. Classic technique describes lesions in terms of bone position: for example, the innominate anterior or the sacrum posterior. Also, "upslip," "inflare," or "outflare" lesions are seen in the diagnosis of lesion production and direction of force for manipulation.

The difficulty with these theories of joint lesion production is that the anatomy is at variance with the theory. The sacroiliac is not a plane joint; it is corrugated, with hills and valleys on corresponding ilial and sacral surfaces. Also, the toughest and hardest ligaments in the body secure and fix the joint anteriorly, posteriorly, and internally, thus preventing any upslip or flaring of the innominate bone on the sacrum of more than a millimeter or so. It is the same with so-called anterior and posterior innominate lesions. The ilium simply cannot rotate on the sacrum in this way. The reader is referred to I A Kapandji's *The Physiology of the Joints, Volume 3* for more detailed information about these ligaments and about sacroiliac joint movement.[1]

Notwithstanding the above, the sacroiliac joint, being a synovial joint, can suffer from facet locking or imbrications at the superior and inferior poles in the same way that spinal apophyseal joints lock or block. This will produce restriction and pain at the superior and inferior parts of the joint on palpation, as described. It also means that high-velocity, low-amplitude techniques can be used to open the superior or inferior pole, as required.

To treat these restrictions, modifications of the standard techniques are used to avoid compression of the patient's abdomen.

Reverse Manipulation for a Super Pole Lesion at the Sacroiliac Joint

Position of the patient

The patient is on her side, with the painful side uppermost, lying in the form of a three-sided square.

Position of the osteopath

The osteopath stands in front of her.

Ambition of the technique

To avoid any abdominal compression in pregnancy, this technique was developed by the author to release a restriction at the superior pole of the sacroiliac joint.

Application of the technique

She is placed in the minimal leverage position, with her bottom leg hyperextended at the knee and the bottom ankle resting near to the corner of the treatment table (Fig 8.7).

A common error with this technique is to introduce rotation of the top lever too early, thus overlocking the joint. To avoid this, the osteopath places the patient's top arm in line with her body (Fig 8.8), holding it with his forearm.

He uses his caudal hand to palpate the L5/S1 interspace, which allows ligamentous locking of the spine down to the pelvis and not beyond.

With his cranial hand, he introduces flexion from the shoulders down to the L5/S1, as a pure lever alone and not in combination with any other levers (Fig 8.9). Then he asks the patient to clasp her top forearm at the elbow and he gently introduces the minimum amount of rotation needed to locate the tension.

All the while, he is stabilizing the bottom lever with his thigh.

With the levers of flexion, and a small degree of reverse rotation at the shoulders, the patient is stable on the treatment table.

The osteopath now uses his cranial hand to stabilize the shoulders as he walks around the head of the treatment table and comes to stand behind the patient.

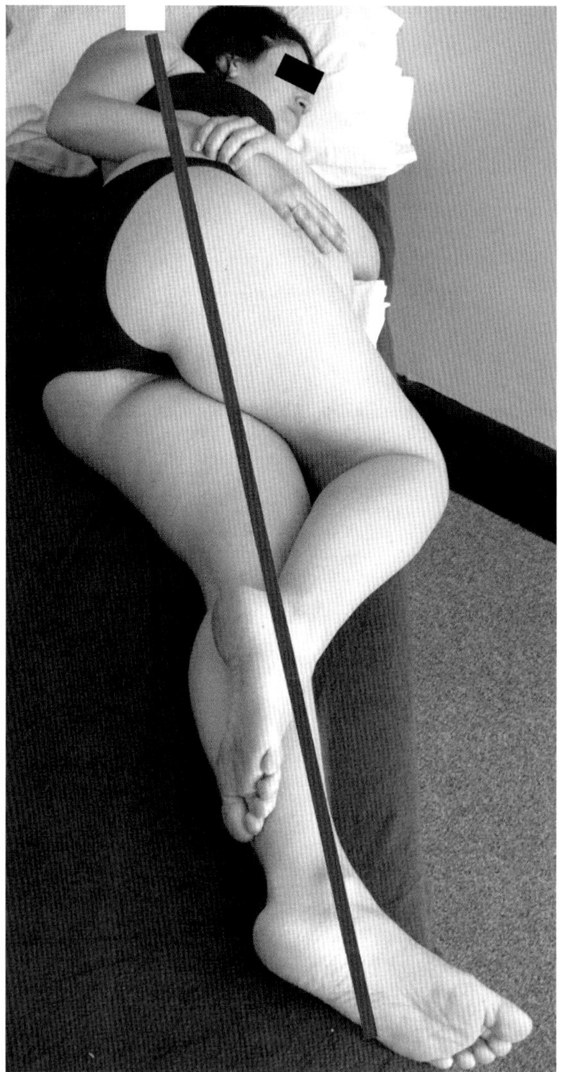

Fig 8.7
The "minimal leverage line" passing from the shoulder via the hip and the hyperextended knee to the ankle.

He introduces his cranial arm between the patient's crossed arms and her trunk, externally rotating his

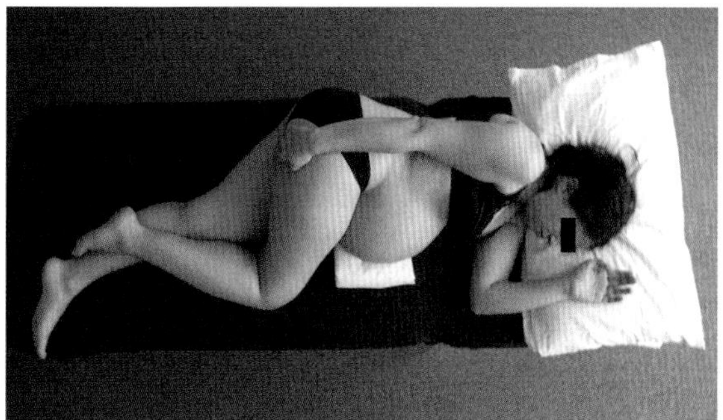

Fig 8.8
The top arm is held alongside the body when applying the top lever, to avoid over-rotation of the shoulder.

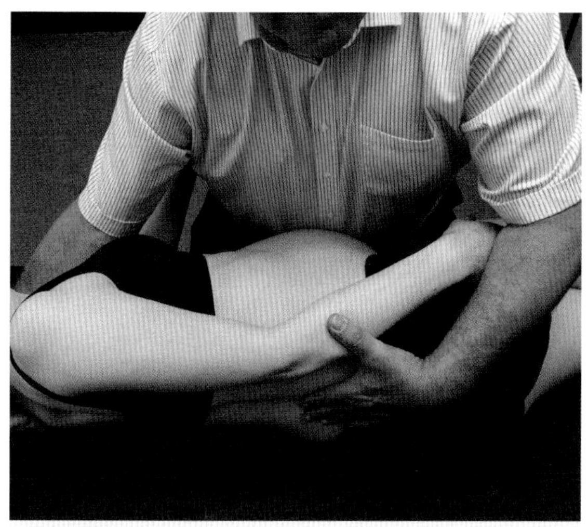

Fig 8.9
Introducing flexion of the whole lumbar spine right down to the L5/S1 interspace, so as to localize force to the sacroiliac joints.

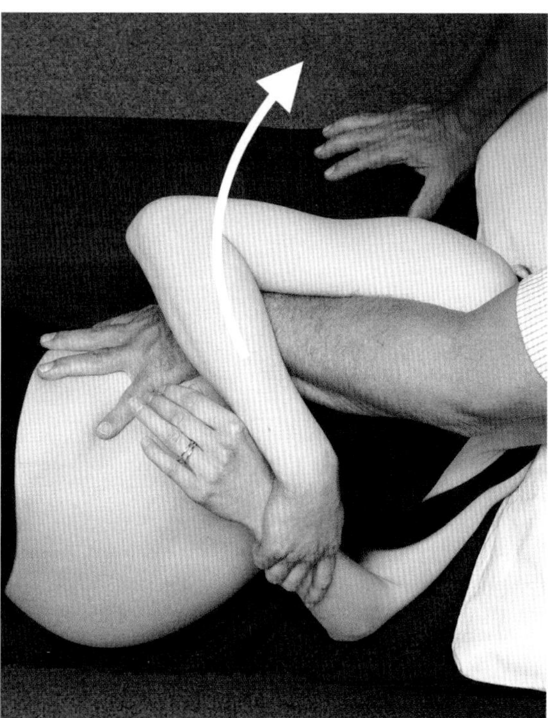

Fig 8.10
The cranial hand and forearm are employed to hold the patient's shoulders back.

arm and widening his hand so as to palpate the low lumbar spine again (Figs 8.10 and 8.11).

He asks the patient to clench his arm against her body. This isometric contraction further stabilizes the upper lever. By small adjustments of his body, the osteopath focuses the tension towards his palpating hand.

One of his hands is placed on the patient's iliac crest, so that his arm is externally rotated and the elbow is hyperextended. This will direct all the force from his arm directly towards her ilium, focused on the posterior superior iliac spine and thus directing the action down the shaft of the femur (Fig 8.12). This is achieved with the osteopath's elbow in full extension, which assists in contracting the pectoral muscles and directing the force.

The impulse is transmitted with a gentle momentum as the osteopath contracts his pectoral muscles,

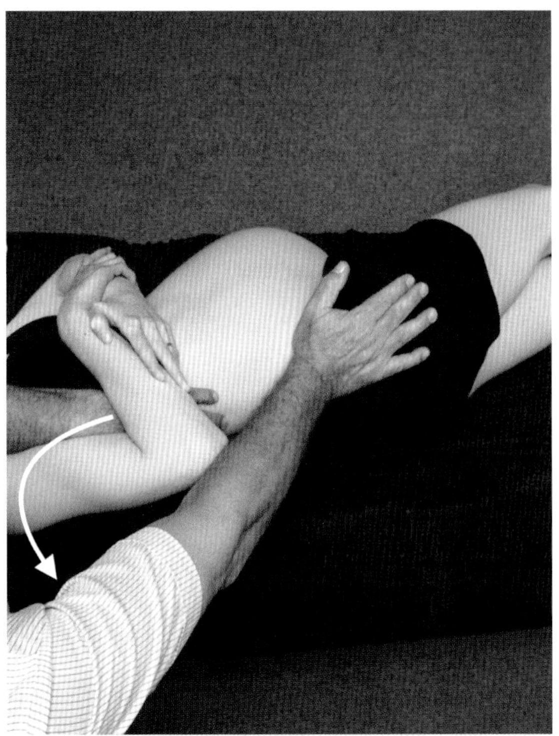

Fig 8.11
The arrow shows the cranial hand being used to rotate the shoulder backwards, while the fingers of the same hand are employed to palpate the low lumbar spine to maintain the focus of the levers.

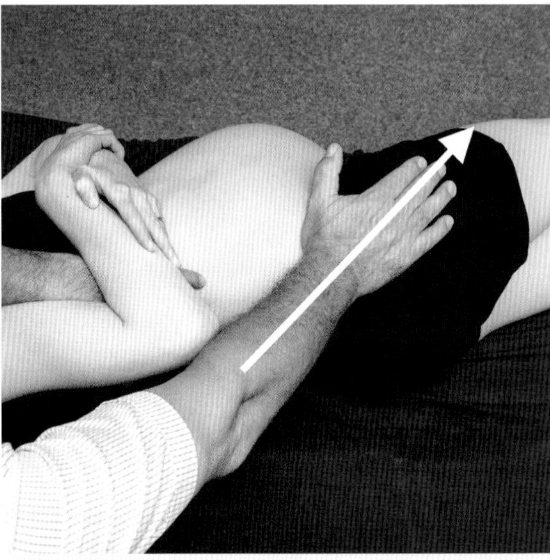

Fig 8.12
The impulse is directed towards the shaft of the femur.

accompanied by a short, sharp exhalation. The thrust moves the innominate in a direction away from the sacrum, breaking fixation at the superior pole.

"Leg Tug" Manipulation

This is not a tug as such, merely a shock wave sent along the leg from the ankle to the hip, which breaks facet fixation at either the superior or the inferior pole, whichever evaluation dictates. The leg should never be pulled sharply with any degree of force. This is a gentle technique, done with momentum.

Position of the patient

The patient is supine, with pillows supporting her head and her lumbar spine.

Position of the osteopath

The osteopath stands at the foot of the treatment table and a little to one side, facing the patient.

Ambition of the technique

The aim is to break facet fixation at either the superior or the inferior pole of the sacroiliac joint.

Application of the technique

The osteopath grasps the leg above the ankle, using the hand hold shown in Figure 8.13. This means that the impulse does not come from the ankle or the foot.

For the superior pole, he adducts the limb, holding it with flexion and internal rotation (Fig 8.14). For the inferior pole, he abducts the limb with extension and external rotation.

He makes a circle of his two arms and hands, adjusting his position by raising and lowering the limb, and applying tension along the limb by leaning backwards. It is important for the patient's knee to be kept in hyperextension. When he feels the tension arrive at the joint, he gently oscillates the limb, producing a wave of motion along the body (Fig 8.15). After a few moments, he applies a very gentle impulse via his pectoral muscles along the limb, producing a small shock wave which opens the affected locked joint.

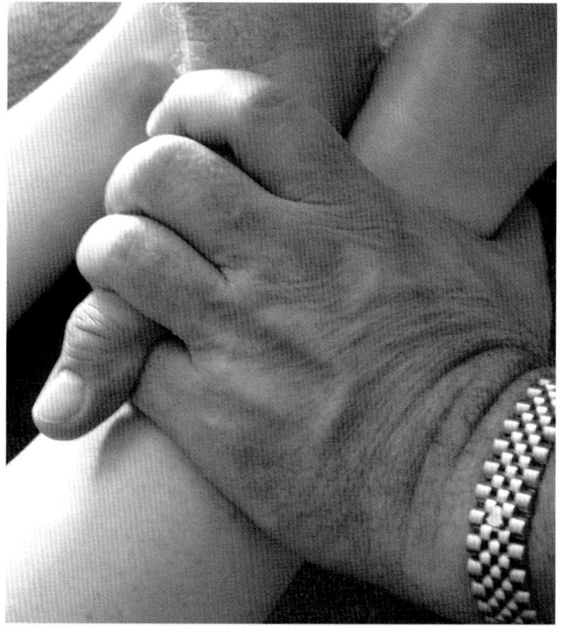

Fig 8.13
The hand hold for the leg tug technique.

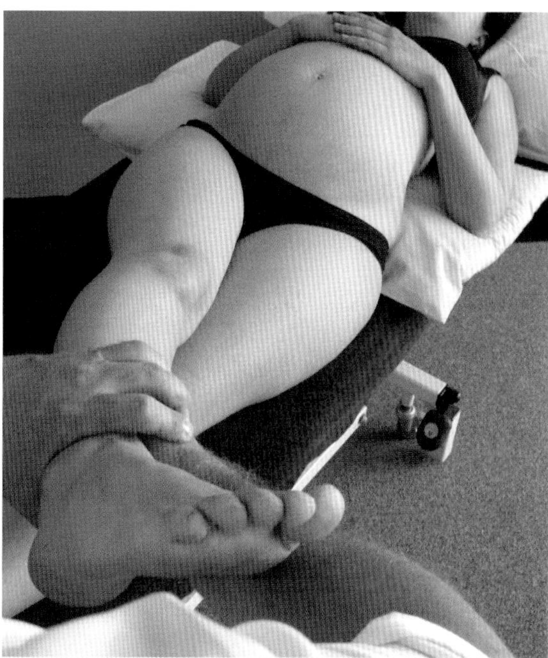

Fig 8.14
The leg tug for the superior pole of the sacroiliac joint.

High-velocity, Low-amplitude (HVLA) Technique for the Superior Pole of the Sacroiliac Joint (Superior Pole Lesion) with the Patient Sitting

Position of the patient

She sits at the end of the treatment table, either astride and facing along the length of the table, or astride a chair with her arms crossed over her

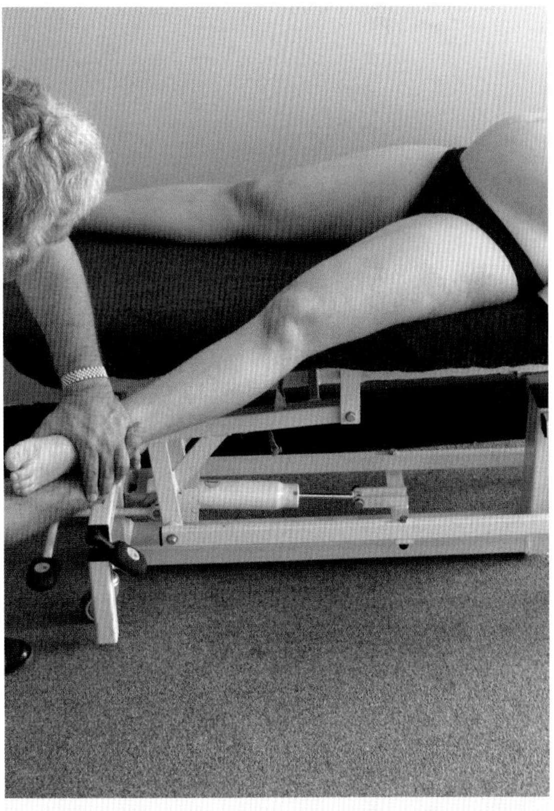

Fig 8.15
The leg tug technique for the inferior pole lesion of the SIJ.

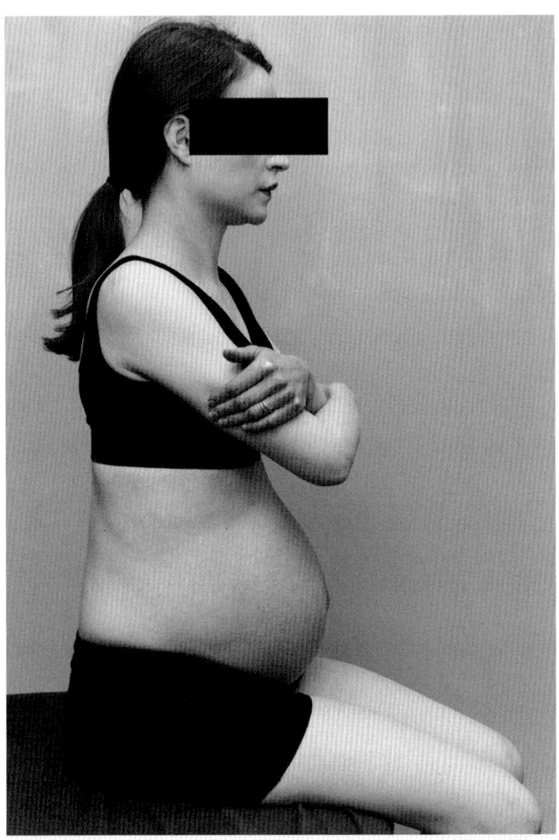

Fig 8.16
The patient sitting for an HVLA technique for a superior pole lesion of the sacroiliac joint.

chest. In late pregnancy, where there is a risk of overstrain to the pubic symphysis with the legs hyperabducted, the technique should be performed with the patient sitting with her legs over the side of the table. The patient crosses her arms firmly (Fig 8.16).

The position of the osteopath

The osteopath stands behind the patient if she is at the end of the table astride, or on the opposite side of the lesion if her legs are over the side of the table.

Ambition of the technique

Some patients find it difficult to be on their backs in the later stages of pregnancy, so this technique was developed to allow for manipulation of the superior pole of the sacroiliac joint with the patient sitting.

Application of the technique

For a left-sided lesion, the osteopath's right arm comes around the patient's body and grasps her left shoulder, so as to control movement through it.

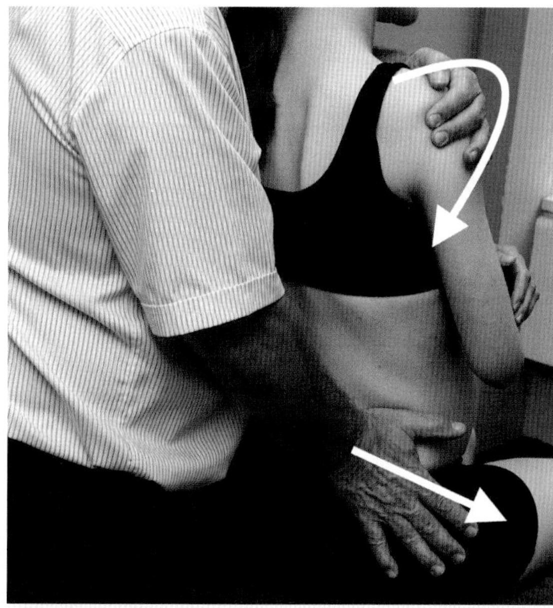

Fig 8.17
Position of the osteopath for the sitting sacroiliac joint thrust technique.

The osteopath's right elbow is applied firmly to his right side, while the base of the hand is externally rotated and applied to the patient's posterior superior iliac spine.

His left arm introduces lumbar flexion, left side-bending, and right counter-rotation, while the base of his right hand fixes tension to the right sacroiliac joint (Fig 8.17). With a small movement of his body weight forwards and into the lesion, he applies a short-amplitude, high-velocity thrust to the posterior superior iliac spine. The movement of the body, with left side-bending and right reverse rotation, ensures accurate ligamentous locking to focus the forces.

Pubalgia and the Pelvic Ring Syndrome

Symphysis pubis dysfunction (SPD) and pubalgia of pregnancy are both descriptions of the same thing: pubic pain in pregnancy.

In an article from 1992, Ostergaard et al.[2] describe the condition as being a pelvic insufficiency during pregnancy: a condition with pain at the pubic symphysis and/or the sacroiliac joint developing in connection with pregnancy or delivery. No unambiguous criteria for the diagnosis of pelvic girdle relaxation exist, but Ostergaard maintains that the following findings commonly occur:

- direct tenderness at the pubic symphysis and/or sacroiliac joint
- waddling gait
- pain on change of position, especially turning in bed at night
- a positive Trendelenburg's sign
- pain on iliac compression test
- pain on iliac gapping test
- pain on sacral pressure test.

The problem can be a common one, with figures of 7.6–18.5 per 1,000 deliveries reported. The incidence is increased in multiparous patients and women with occupations which strain the back. Recurrence is seen in 41–77%.[2] The condition usually appears for the first time in the 5th to 8th months of pregnancy, but can occur earlier in hypermobile women.

The standard medical approaches to treatment vary, according to the resources available. Physiotherapists who have a special interest in women's health have patients referred to them both privately and under public healthcare systems such as the National Health Service in the UK. The problem is that it would be rare to find a physiotherapist who has double postgraduate training in both women's health and musculoskeletal care. Physiotherapists can give their patients a pelvic support garment to wear, such as a belt or Tubigrip bandage, and crutches if walking is difficult. Patients may also be given gentle exercises to help strengthen the muscles supporting the joint, along with general advice about posture and activities to avoid. Delivery options and positions can also be discussed. If necessary, patients can be referred to an occupational therapist for other aids to make their daily life easier.

Patients with this problem need to have the whole pelvic ring evaluated, not just the pubic symphysis alone.

If one sacroiliac joint is locked, it can create a torsion effect throughout the pelvis. This can exaggerate hypermobility on the other side and pain at the pubis, as the fibers of the fibrocartilaginous disc soften with the effects of relaxin and other hormones, and thus become tensioned or twisted.

Assessment of the pelvis is done by performing the standing, side-lying, and supine tests referred to in Chapter 2.

The pubic symphysis is also evaluated.

Warning

Once again, this is regarded by the registration authorities as a sensitive area; practitioners must be familiar with the codes of practice, and use consent forms and offer chaperones in each case.

Evaluation of the Pubic Symphysis

Position of the patient

The patient is supine, with her legs flat on the treatment table.

Position of the osteopath

The osteopath stands at the side of the treatment table, facing the patient.

Ambition of the technique

The aim is to evaluate the pubic symphysis and see if there is a problem that is causing pubalgia.

Application of the technique

The steps are illustrated in Figures 8.18 to 8.24.

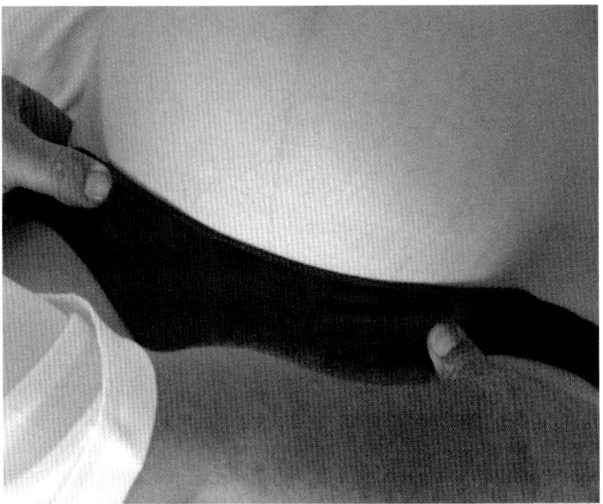

Fig 8.18
Step one: The osteopath uses his thumbs to palpate the anterior superior iliac spine.

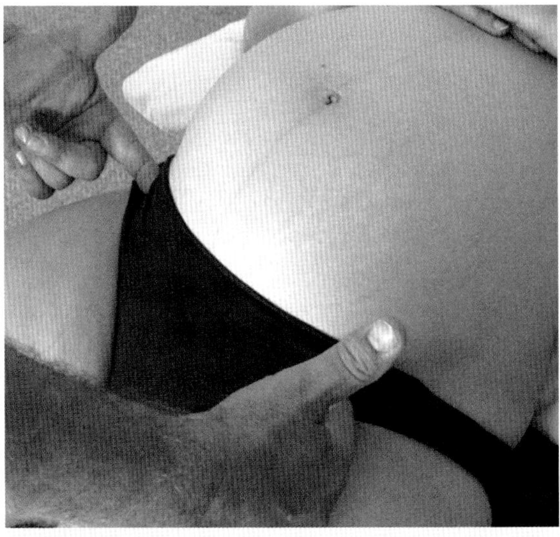

Fig 8.19
Step two: Change the thumbs for the index fingers.

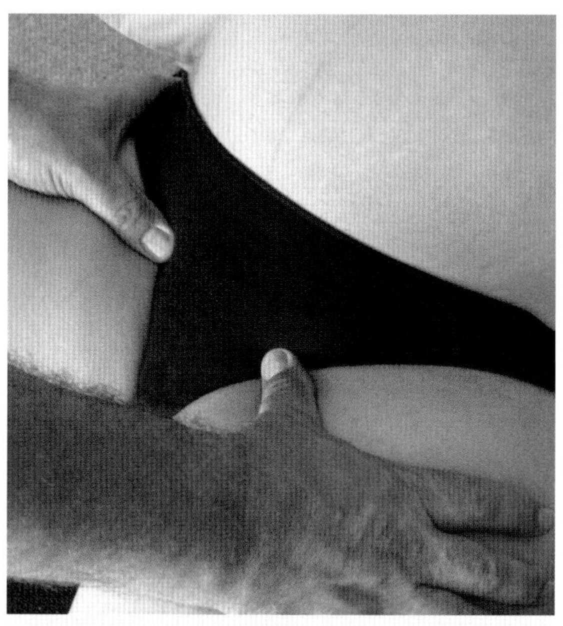

Fig 8.20
Step three: Use the thumbs to palpate the ramus of the pubis lateral to the symphysis.

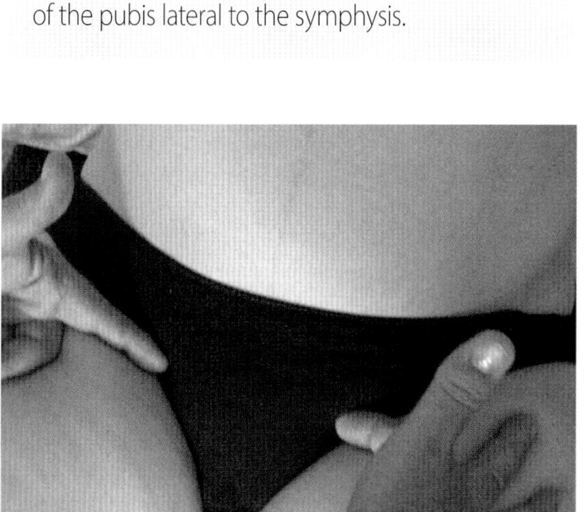

Fig 8.21
Step four: Change the thumbs for the index fingers, as before.

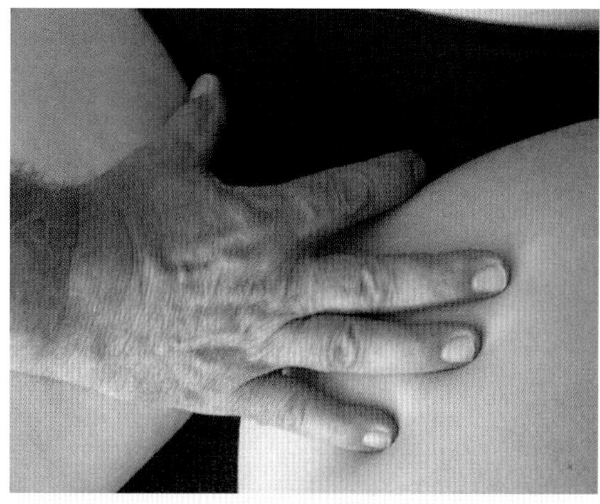

Fig 8.22
Step five: The osteopath now moves alongside the patient, producing a line formed by the index finger at one ramus and the thumb at the other.

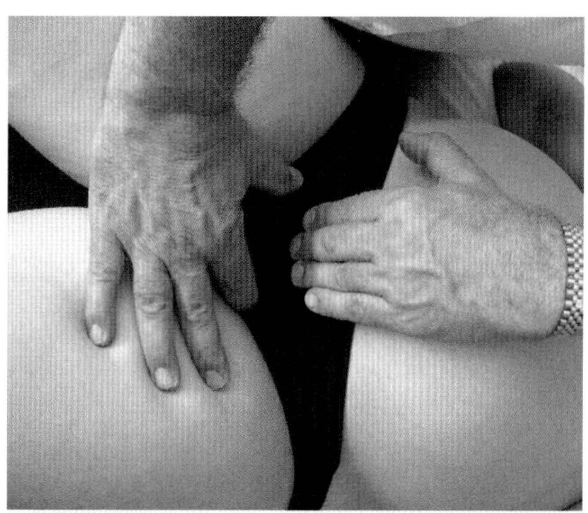

Fig 8.23
Step six: Using the fingernails of the free hand, a line is palpated marking the superior border of the symphysis.

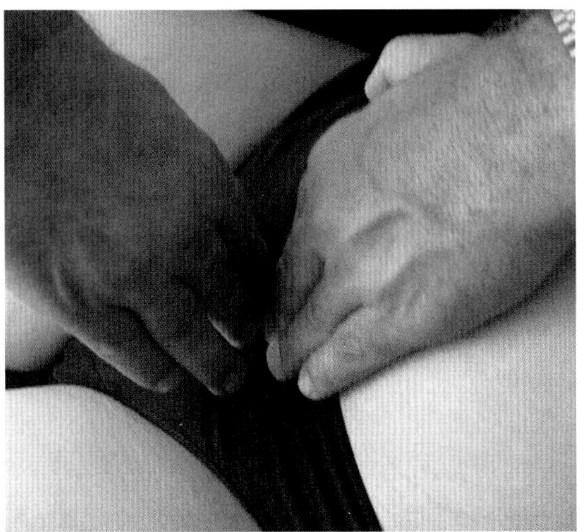

Fig 8.24
Step seven: At this line, the fingernails of the two hands come together. This is the superior border of the pubis, the center of which is the pubic symphysis.

Using this method, the joint can be palpated in an ethical manner with accuracy and precision. The joint cannot be evaluated inferiorly or posteriorly without a vaginal technique, which is rarely indicated in pregnancy

Common findings include gaps in the joint; a step, suggesting pelvic torsion or any other positional variation from the norm; and tenderness and sometimes even edema over the joint line. Pain at the joint line is a common finding. It is rare to have a separation of the surfaces superiorly because of the reinforcement to the joint provided by the aponeurosis of the abdominal muscles. A step could indicate a shearing of the joint on walking.

Once the diagnosis of pelvic ring syndrome is proved, the restricted sacroiliac joint should be manipulated, using the techniques above, and then a gentle MET is employed for the pubis itself. This is sometimes referred to as the "shotgun" technique for reasons that have disappeared into the mists of time, and it should be noted this is not an HVLA technique because the pubic symphysis is not a synovial joint.

MET or "Shotgun" Technique for the Pubic Symphysis

Position of the patient

The patient lies supine on the treatment table, with her head supported by pillows as before.

Position of the osteopath

The osteopath stands alongside her, facing towards the side of the treatment table with his hands resting gently on the inner surfaces of both of her knees (Fig 8.25).

Ambition of the technique

The aim is to use a muscle energy technique involving bilateral contraction of the patient's adductor muscles, so as to correct any lesion that exists at the pubic symphysis.

 **Warning**

The key to this technique is careful instruction of the patient, including a warning that she might hear a click and there might be a momentary twinge of pain at the pubis. If patients are forewarned as to the possibility of a twinge of pain, then they are not taken by surprise and they willingly give consent for the procedure.

Application of the technique

The osteopath gently shakes the knees, encouraging the patient to relax, then, at the count of three, she

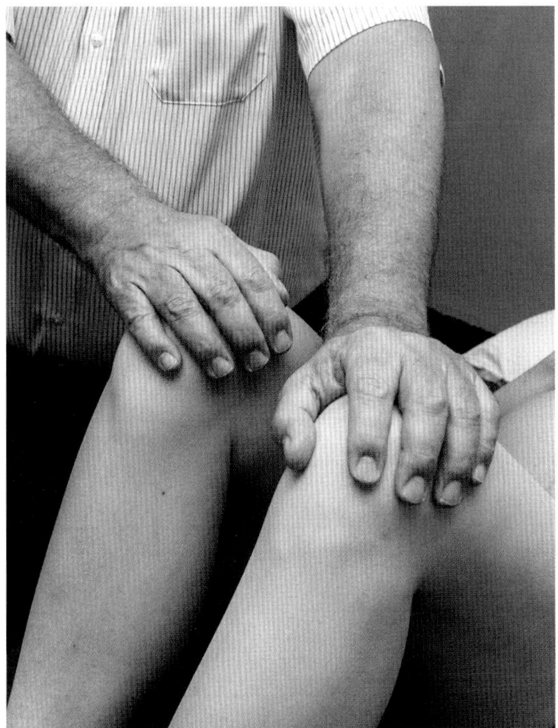

Fig 8.25
The MET "shotgun" technique for the pubic symphysis.

very rapidly "claps" her knees and the osteopath contracts his pectoral muscles, resisting the adduction maneuver. He never pulls the knees apart. This causes the adductor muscles to contract, pulling down on the pubic ramus and thus "correcting" the lesion. The origin of the pop or snap is a mystery because the joint is not a synovial joint.

Self-help for Patients with Pelvic Ring Syndrome

Exercises

The exercises described in Box 8.1 can be prescribed for pregnant patients who have pelvic ring syndrome.

BOX 8.1

Self-help exercises for pubalgia

These exercises should be performed three times each day.

If an exercise causes pain it should be discontinued.

Abdominal stabilization

- Sitting with your feet resting on the floor, gently pull in your lower abdominal muscles, as if you are hugging your baby. Hold for 5 seconds. Repeat 5 times. Continue to breathe normally throughout.

Pelvic floor

- Sitting tall, squeeze to close around the vaginal and rectal openings. Lift and hold for 5 seconds. Repeat 5 times. Breathe normally throughout.

Gluteal muscles

- Sitting or standing, squeeze the buttocks together. Hold for 5 seconds. Repeat 5 times.

Latissimus dorsi muscle

- Sit on a chair in front of a treatment table or closed door. Grasp the door handle or table with both hands and pull towards you. Hold for 5 seconds. Repeat 5 times.

Hip adductor muscles

- Sitting down, put your fist or a rolled towel between your knees. Squeeze your knees together. Use no more than 40% of your maximal force. Hold for 5 seconds. Repeat 5 times.

Self-help and management tips

Some hints on management are listed in Box 8.2.

BOX 8.2

Self-help and management tips for pubalgia

Getting into and out of bed

- Sit on the edge of the bed, keeping your knees close together, and then lie down on your side, lifting both of your legs up sideways.
- Reverse this to get out of bed.
- Do not attempt to pull yourself up from lying on your back.

Rolling over in bed

- Keep your knees together.
- Do not roll with your knees apart.

Getting up from a chair

- Keep your knees close together, put your hands on your knees, and lean your nose over your toes to stand up.

Sitting down

- Do the reverse to sit down.
- Ensure that you feel the chair at the back of your legs first.

Getting into a car

- Sit down first and then swing your legs in, keeping your knees together.

The use of sacroiliac binders and belts remains contentious. Some belts work for some patients and some are better for others. Belts should be worn low down under the anterior superior iliac spine and should never compress the abdomen. They are generally better tolerated outside of the patient's clothing. Other belts just go around the pelvis.

The Coccyx

The sacrococcygeal junction is a frequent source of pain during the latter stages of pregnancy and also post partum.[2,3,4] In the non-pregnant patient, magnetic resonance imaging (MRI) or a plain lateral view X-ray is part of the routine examination process. Neither of these options is immediately available during pregnancy.[5] The diagnosis and treatment of coccyx pain are the subject of debate in the medical journals, and opinion on treatment is often inconclusive.[6,7]

The pain is local to the coccyx, and the differential diagnosis is between local ligament pain, fracture, or referred pain.

Differential Diagnosis of Coccyx Pain

If the pain to the coccyx is referred, the commonest site of the problem is the last lumbar disc.

A history of direct trauma obtained from the case history is an important finding. A direct fall onto the bottom, or repeated trauma such as horse riding or driving over speed bumps, is not uncommon. The last lumbar disc is designed to accept these minor traumas but the coccyx is not.

A history of pain on standing, rather than sitting or walking, is unlikely to be a coccyx injury. Sitting in flexion – that is, slumped in an easy chair – will aggravate a disc lesion but will be easier with a coccyx injury than sitting upright with the spine in extension, as the latter will cause real pain as the weight comes to rest directly on the coccyx itself. A soft chair is better tolerated than a hard chair for coccyx patients, while the reverse is true for a disc lesion.

Pain coming from the coccyx can be felt on defecation; if it were a disc lesion, the pain would be associated with straining at stool, rather than the passage of a hard stool as it passes the sensitive coccyx. Care is needed here because codeine is often prescribed in one form or another for acute musculoskeletal pain and will constipate a patient, encouraging her to strain at stool.

If the pain is referred, it could also be coming from the sacroiliac joints, especially after a long or protracted labor with postpartum pain. Questions relating to unilateral weight-bearing are going to be useful in this case.

Lastly, in the history of postpartum pain it is essential to establish whether there has been damage or surgical trauma to the pelvic floor during the delivery.

Episiotomy

An episiotomy is a common surgical procedure during childbirth. The term describes a surgical incision made in the perineum, the area between the vagina and anus (Fig 8.26). Episiotomies are done during the second stage of labor to expand the opening of the vagina and prevent tearing of the area during delivery of the baby.

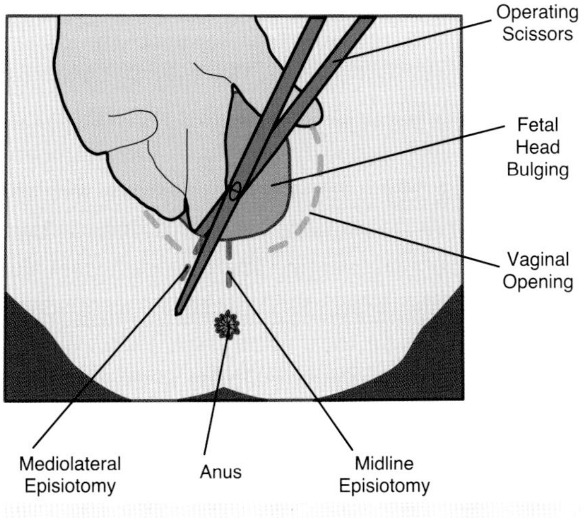

Fig 8.26
A medio-lateral episiotomy.

They are done for several reasons, the most important of which is evidence of maternal or fetal distress. They may also be carried out if the baby is premature or in breech position, and its head could be damaged by a tight perineum; if the baby is too large to be delivered without causing extensive tearing; if the delivery is being assisted by forceps; or if the mother is too tired or unable to push.

The arguments for and against an episiotomy versus a natural tear and the effects on healing are still current in the obstetric profession, but if the scar is extensive or poorly healed, it can lead to postpartum tension in the pelvic floor and pain if the coccyx is deviated from the midline or pulled forwards.

Examination for Coccyx Pain

On standing examination, all active movements, such as flexion with or without lateral flexion, will cause pain in disc cases but no pain in coccyx cases. Extension may be painful in either case.

Sitting tests will provoke pain in extension for coccyx cases and flexion for disc cases. There is a direct provocation test for the coccyx, which should remove any doubt about the origin of the pain: it is a sitting provocation test. With the patient sitting slumped and the osteopath standing behind her, the osteopath introduces his finger into the sacrococcygeal junction. Then he brings the patient back into a hyperflexed position while introducing pressure locally with his finger. A positive test will reproduce a sharp pain locally and is an indication for rectal manipulation.

With the patient supine, internal and external rotation of the hips should be tested. This often reveals a tension in one buttock or the other. The coccyx is normally supported by the posterior pelvic floor muscles, but if there has been a direct trauma to the region, it is often pushed forwards. A buttock with greater tone will tend to side-bend the coccyx towards it, creating a coccygeal torsion.

Pregnant patients are best examined side-lying. Direct pressure over the sacrococcygeal junction will invariably provoke pain in coccyx cases, while pain and restriction of motion at the last lumbar disc interspace will produce either local pain or referred pain to the coccyx. Direct palpation at the coccyx will not produce pain at the last lumbar disc.

A Per Rectum Technique for Coccygeal Manipulation

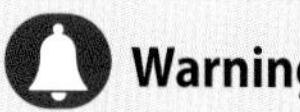

Warning

As this is a sensitive area, the osteopath should always consider the use of a consent form and a chaperone, and must discuss the technique with the patient before starting treatment. She should be sitting, not lying down, as this is more appropriate for warning her beforehand of something she might be anxious or apprehensive about. If the patient refuses the technique, or if she wants time to think about it or bring her own chaperone, the consultation ends there and she comes back for the treatment at the following visit.

Before this technique is performed, the patient should be asked to sign a consent form and be questioned about latex sensitivity. She should also be offered the services of a chaperone at this time. The chaperone can be a woman from your own practice or the patient can bring a female relation or a friend.

If she considers a chaperone unnecessary, the treatment may be undertaken on the same day. The use of a plastic model to show exactly what the internal and external fingers are trying to achieve is considered best practice.

Position of the patient

The patient lies on her side in the form of a three-sided square, with the tense or dominant buttock uppermost. She is covered with a sheet or a blanket, and her underwear is lowered to the knees. It is not necessary for her to remove her underwear completely for this technique.

Position of the osteopath

The osteopath stands behind the patient, facing towards the head end of the couch. Both hands are covered with latex gloves or hypoallergenic plastic gloves.

Ambition of the technique

The aim is to reduce the position of a flexed coccyx. This may also serve as a direct ligamentous or muscular inhibition technique for the pericoccygeal tissues.

Application of the technique

With one hand, the osteopath separates the cheeks of the buttocks and inspects the anus for skin tags and hemorrhoids or fissures because these should be carefully avoided during the technique. A small amount of lubricating jelly is introduced at the anus with the index finger of the opposite hand. This finger is then placed at the anal margin. The osteopath does not push against the anus as this only encourages tension; instead, he waits for the anus to relax. Then, with the other hand applying counter-tension to the perineum laterally, he gently puts a small amount of pressure on the anal margin with his fingernail. The anus will relax and allow the finger to enter the anal canal.

The rest of the fingers of the manipulating hand are clenched tight into a fist, so that the back of the carpal bones pushes against the perineum. This pressure is necessary because the internal finger should go right up past the coccyx to the sacrum. This is not a direct path but a curved route around the coccyx, which is probably flexed. Once the sacrococcygeal joint is located internally, the other thumb of the external hand is brought to the sacrococcygeal junction, thus grasping the coccyx between the two hands.

A functional technique is used to bring tensions around the coccyx to a neutral point. It is important to stress that the osteopath does not move the coccyx in the directions of the different vectors, but rather moves his own body into flexion, extension, and so on, perceiving the ease and bind responses at the coccyx.

If this technique fails, it is often because of poor technique. The coccyx is never pulled back but is allowed to assume its normal position itself. At the end of the maneuver, the osteopath can feel for tension in the lateral muscles and ligaments of the coccyx; if need be, he can use a gentle inhibition or massage technique to release tension in them.

Once the release of tensions is felt at the point of functional balance, the patient is asked to extend her legs and knees and gently roll towards the osteopath. It is this maneuver which will bring the coccyx back down to the supporting muscles of the pelvic floor again. Once the coccyx has descended, the osteopath grasps it between his internal and external fingers and the patient is asked to flex her knees as far as she can. The internal finger is removed, and the technique is complete.

Afterwards, the patient is asked to rock forwards and backwards on her buttocks; if they are free of pain, the technique has been successful. It can be repeated at the next visit if there is not a complete resolution of symptoms; if the pain is still there after the second treatment, it is likely that the ligaments around the sacrococcygeal junction are torn. If this is the case, she may need to see an orthopedic surgeon for an opinion regarding further treatment: for example, an epidural injection or a course of prolotherapy to sclerose the torn ligaments. In rare cases, she may need an opinion regarding amputation of the coccyx if she is post partum.[7,8]

Once again, it is important to stress that the examination and treatment of the coccyx are rarely done alone, but as part of a routine investigation of pain arising in the whole pelvic ring.

Techniques for Mobilization of the Pelvic Viscera During Pregnancy

As already described, the position of the uterus changes during pregnancy from being flexed forwards over the bladder and pubic symphysis to being vertical and upright. During the first part of the pregnancy, as the uterus rises out of the pelvis and the lumbar lordosis decreases, the broad ligament that encloses the uterus will also become more vertical. Joint mobility at the thoracolumbar and the lumbosacral junctions is of prime importance, to allow the verticality of the uterus to establish itself.

Specific visceral techniques directed to the uterus are possible at this time.

Normalization of Uterine Motion in Pregnancy

Position of the patient

The patient lies on her side.

Position of the osteopath

The osteopath stands behind her.

Ambition of the technique

The aim is to normalize uterine motion and allow for good mobility of the uterus within the pelvic and abdominal cavities.

Application of the technique

He lifts the bulk of the abdomen, allowing his hands to externally rotate at the wrists so as to come underneath the bump, lifting and supporting its weight (Fig 8.27). Starting down at the inguinal ligament, he feels for tensions in the abdominopelvic wall and releases them, using a myofascial or functional tension.

He continues to relax and release the uterus in this way right up to the diaphragm, before asking the patient to turn on to her opposite side so that he can perform the same technique there.

Uterine Lift Technique

Position of the patient

The patient sits on the treatment table, with her legs over the side.

Position of the osteopath

The osteopath stands behind her.

Ambition of the technique

The aim is to lift the uterus and bladder together to release any painful adhesions and to mobilize the body of the uterus in the vertical plane.

Application of the technique

The patient puts her hands on her hips and the osteopath places the ulnar border of his hands deep into the inguinal ligaments each side (Fig 8.28).

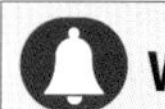
Warning

The notes regarding ethics and propriety apply as before.

The patient leans back against the osteopath, who leans back in turn, lifting the uterus towards him (Fig 8.29). Then, gently pushing the patient with his chest, he leans her forwards until his center of gravity is directly over his hands. He very gently lifts the uterus up towards him, and when he has taken the weight of the uterus, he mobilizes it with

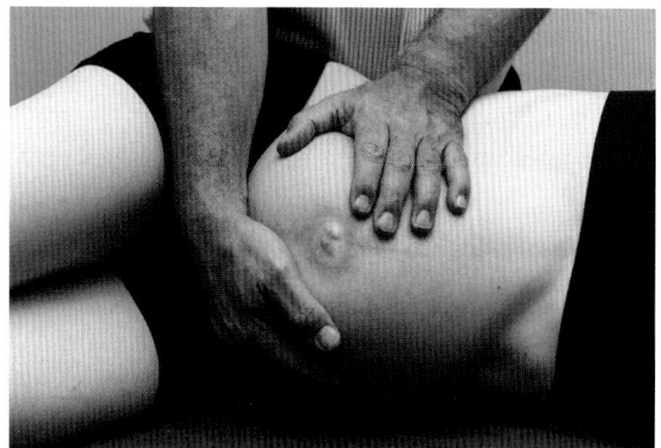

Fig 8.27
Normalization of uterine motion in pregnancy.

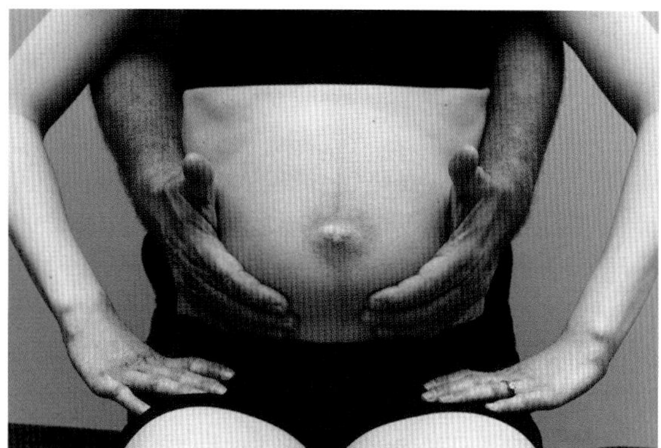

Fig 8.28
The uterine lift technique.

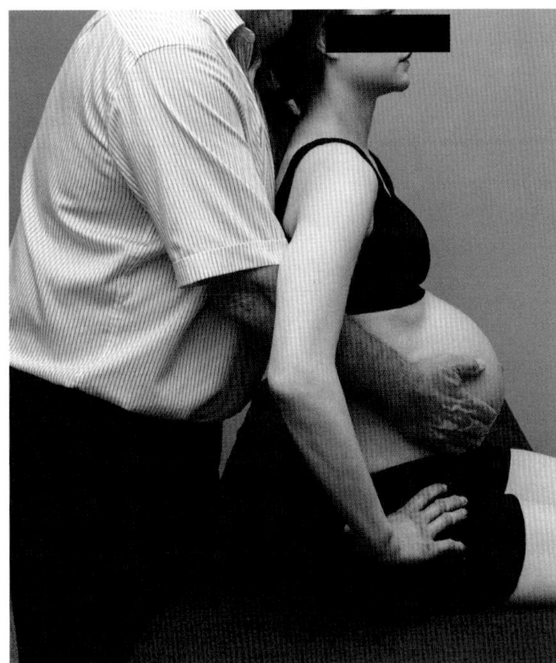

Fig 8.29
The osteopath leans back and lifts the uterus towards him, performing a functional technique to balance ligamentous tensions.

a functional technique. This will gently allow the uterus and the adnexa to release and relax.

Both of the above techniques are applicable at any stage after 20 weeks and are particularly helpful if the patient's abdominal muscles are tight and causing pain.

Patients can sometimes experience what are known as Braxton Hicks contractions. These are "practice" uterine contractions that can start as early as 18 weeks of pregnancy. They are described as a tightening of the uterine muscles, each tightening usually lasting for about half a minute. The patient may have this sensation once or twice an hour, or a few times a day.[9] Not every patient experiences these contractions. They take their name from John Braxton Hicks, the English doctor who first described them in 1872. Braxton Hicks contractions may just be a sign that the uterus is keeping its muscle fibers toned. It could be that these contractions maintain the uterus in good condition, ready for the rigors of labor.

Some experts think that the contractions also affect the cervix. In early labor, the cervix starts to become shorter and more pliable, ready to dilate and make way for the baby. It is possible that Braxton Hicks contractions give the cervix a rehearsal for the stretching stage.

Other experts think that Braxton Hicks contractions do not affect the cervix. They believe that the cervix does not change until the very last days of the pregnancy, or once the patient is in established labor.

Creating Space for the Baby Within the Pelvis

At the end of a pregnancy, unless the baby is in a breech or transverse position, the position of the head, and of the occiput in particular, is considered to be important to the way that the labor is going to progress. The "occiput anterior" position is ideal for birth; this means that the baby is lined up so as to fit through the pelvis as easily as possible. The baby is head down, facing the mother's spine. In this position, the baby's head is easily "flexed": that is, its chin is tucked into its chest, so that the smallest part of its head will be applied to the mother's cervix first. The diameter of the head, which has to fit through the pelvis, is approximately 9.5 cm (3.7 inches), and the circumference approximately 27.5 cm (10.8 inches). The position is usually "left occiput anterior" (LOA), though occasionally the baby may be "right occiput anterior" (ROA).

The swing of weight-bearing from posterior and onto the spine to anterior and onto the abdomen will help facilitate this change. Much has been written on the subject of optimal fetal positioning and how changing the mother's or baby's position during labor and before can allow the baby to turn and move into the ideal position, thus maximizing the potential for physiological descent in the birth canal.[10,11,12,13,14]

From an osteopathic point of view, techniques designed to open the pelvic outlet and to widen the ribs will also allow the fetus room to move if it can. These include craniosacral techniques designed to balance the sacrum between the two iliac bones, and to address tensions that might run through the long ligaments that connect the occipital bone at the back of the head to the sacrum in the pelvis.

The usual position to treat in this way is with the patient on her back or supine, but the weight of the gravid uterus on the blood vessels returning blood from the legs and pelvis to the heart means that she will be better treated on her left side during pregnancy (Figs 8.30 to 8.32).

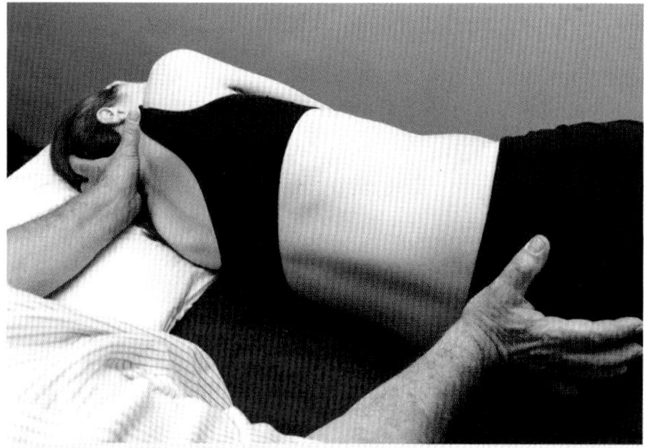

Fig 8.30
Craniosacral techniques during pregnancy are performed with the patient lying on her left side.

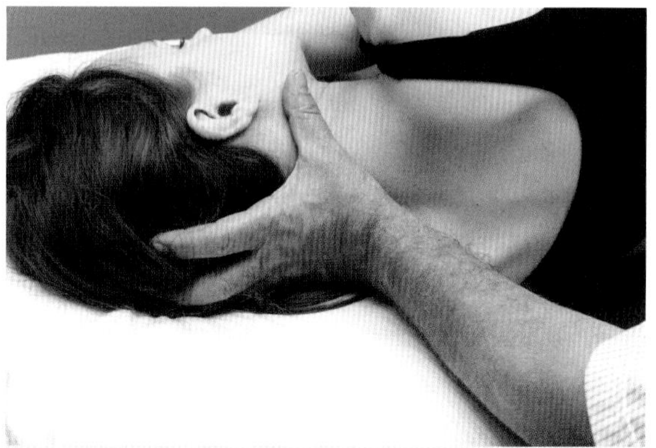

Fig 8.31
The position of the cranial hand with the patient lying on her left side.

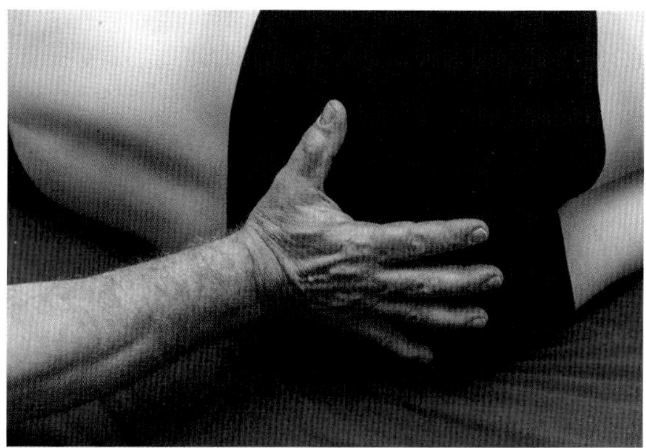

Fig 8.32
The position of the caudad hand with the patient lying on her left side.

Bimanual Contact for Treatment of Sacrum/Sacroiliac Joints Using an Involuntary/Craniosacral Approach

By Nicholas Woodhead, DO

During pregnancy, many women are unable to tolerate being treated supine with a midline sacral contact because this places an additional stretch on the already lax, and often sensitive, sacroiliac ligaments, particularly the anterior ligaments.

An alternative, more comfortable contact can be utilized by "cradling" the innominate bones and sacrum with both of the osteopath's hands, which provides good support for the potentially hypermobile sacroiliac joints, and good palpatory and therapeutic contact for the practitioner.

Position of the patient

The patient lies supine on the treatment table, with hips and knees flexed.

Position of the osteopath

The osteopath sits alongside the treatment table. The relative height of the table and the osteopath's chair is adjusted so that his forearm(s) and elbow(s) can rest comfortably on the table.

Ambition of the technique

The aim is to achieve balanced ligamentous tension in the sacroiliac ligaments.

Application of the technique

The osteopath's hands are placed under the patient's medial gluteal regions so that his fingers span the sacroiliac joints posteriorly; typically, the proximal or middle phalanges of the second to fifth fingers will extend across the joints, depending on the relative size of the patient and the osteopath's hands (Figs 8.33 to 8.35). The osteopath's arm nearest the treatment table will reach under the patient's flexed hips and knees, and his shoulder will be adjacent to, or even under, the patient's knee; his other lower

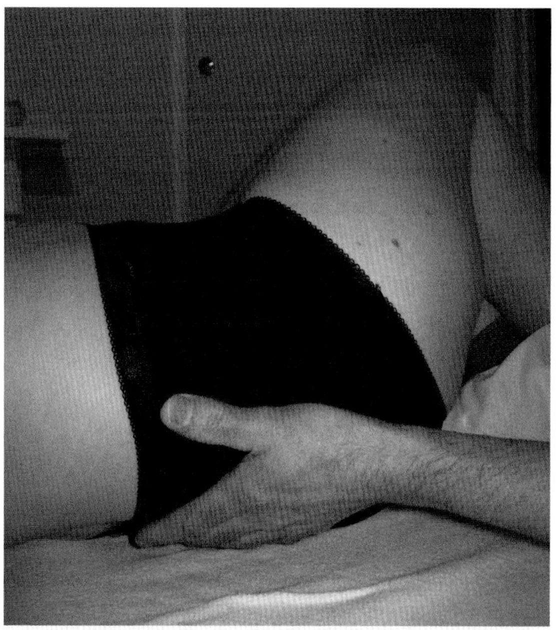

Fig 8.33
The hand hold showing the hand on one side.

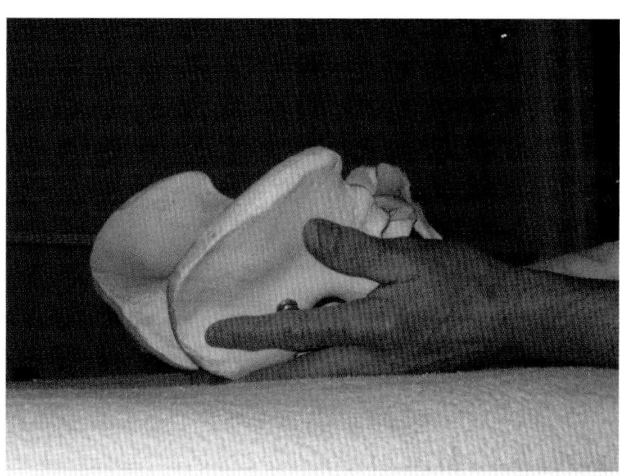

Fig 8.34
As in Figure 8.33, but using the skeleton to show where the hand is applied to the bone.

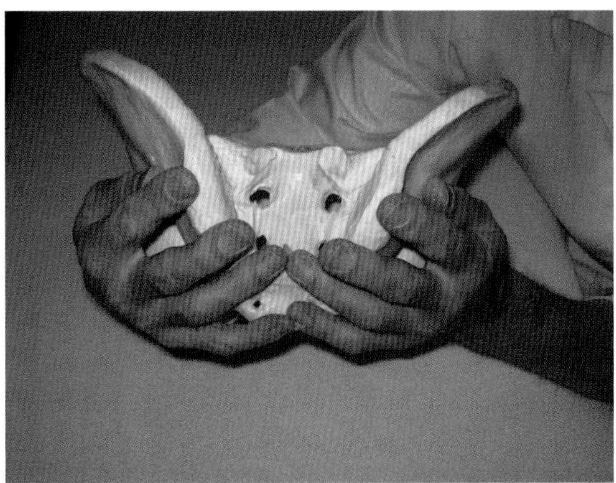

Fig 8.35
The bimanual hand hold.
© Nicholas Woodhead.

forearm is steadied on the edge of the table nearest to him.

With this contact the involuntary flexion and extension motion of the sacrum is less obvious than with a midline contact, but directional strains between the sacrum and innominate(s), and interosseous strains of these structures, are very readily palpated and a balanced tension approach to treatment easily employed to the sacroiliac and other pelvic ligamentous structures. With appropriate explanation and patient consent, the contact can be modified to place the fifth fingers under the coccyx to address involvement of the sacrococcygeal and sacrospinous ligaments.

External Cephalic Version

The procedure to turn the baby in the uterus is called external cephalic version (ECV). Many studies from around the world since the turn of the twenty-first century have shown that the number of babies remaining in the breech position at the end of pregnancy can be reduced by ECV. Many obstetricians base their practice on guidelines from the UK's National Institute for Health and Care Excellence (NICE),[10] which state that all women who have an uncomplicated singleton breech pregnancy at 36 weeks' gestation should be offered ECV. Exceptions include women in labor; those with a uterine scar or abnormality; fetal compromise; ruptured membranes; vaginal bleeding; and medical conditions. Where it is not possible to schedule an appointment for ECV at 37 weeks' gestation, it should be scheduled at 36 weeks.

If ECV is not possible or if it fails, the obstetrician will generally opt for an elective cesarean section. Therefore, a successful ECV would mean that the mother would have a chance at having a normal vaginal birth.

The success or failure of an ECV depends on a number of elements. In a paper published in 2011[15] that looked at the factors associated with success rates, a number of variables were examined that could potentially affect the outcome of the maneuver. It was found that ECV was successful in 52% of the 500 cases studied. The variables associated with better success were parity, placental location, amount of amniotic fluid, and type of breech.

On the day of the procedure, an ultrasound scan is performed to check the position of the baby. The baby's heart rate is checked for at least 20 minutes to confirm that it is healthy. In some hospitals, the procedure is done in the delivery suite; in others, it might take place in the usual room used for antenatal appointments.

It is standard practice to give an injection just under the skin of the arm to relax the uterine muscle during the procedure. The obstetrician will then try

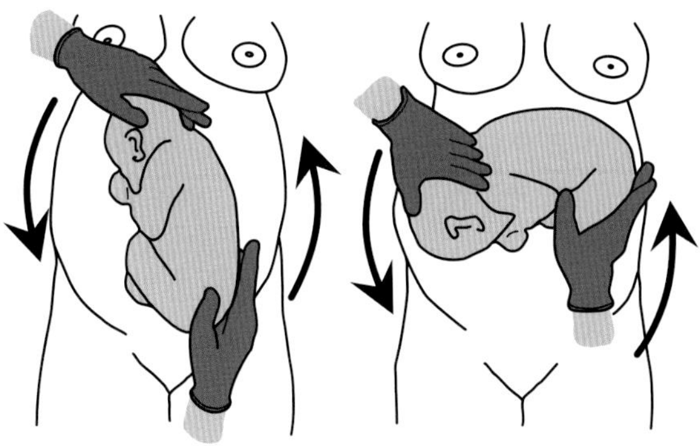

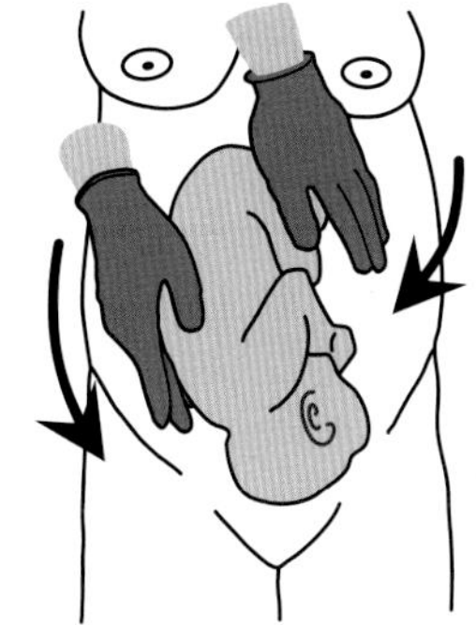

Fig 8.36
External cephalic version (ECV).

to bring the baby's bottom out of the pelvis and "massage" the baby around to a head-first position, by encouraging it to do a forward somersault (Fig 8.36). This may take up to 15 minutes. An ultrasound examination is usually performed afterwards to check the position of the baby and the placenta.

Not all EVC maneuvers work. Common reasons for babies reverting to their previous position include a short cord or a small child that just turns back for no known reason. However, if ECV is performed after 37 weeks, fewer than 5% of babies will turn back.[11]

Osteopaths should not attempt to perform an ECV because it is regarded as an obstetric maneuver and should be performed only by qualified personnel using ultrasound guidance before and afterwards.[15] However, there are a number of procedures that can be attempted before 37 weeks to attempt to give the baby more room so that, if it wishes, it will turn itself.

The first step is to encourage the mother to move into the all-fours kneeling position for 5–10 minutes four or five times each day. This allows the belly to hang down and gravity can stretch the abdominal muscles, allowing the uterus more room within the abdomen. If the abdominal muscles are looser, the pressure on the uterus is lower; decreased pressure within the uterus gives the baby more space to turn if it wishes to do so.

In the practice, a gentle myofascial or functional technique to the uterus, done in this position, can also release uterine tension.

Position of the patient

The patient is on all fours on the treatment table or resting on a pile of pillows.

Position of the osteopath

The osteopath stands at the side of the treatment table, level with her pelvis.

Ambition of the technique

The aim is to release abdominal muscle tone and allow space for the baby to turn.

Application of the technique

The osteopath reaches over the patient so that one hand is on either side of the abdominal mass. Using his own center of gravity as a reference point, he facilitates a still point or neutral point in the tissues, using a myofascial release into ease as before (Fig 8.37).

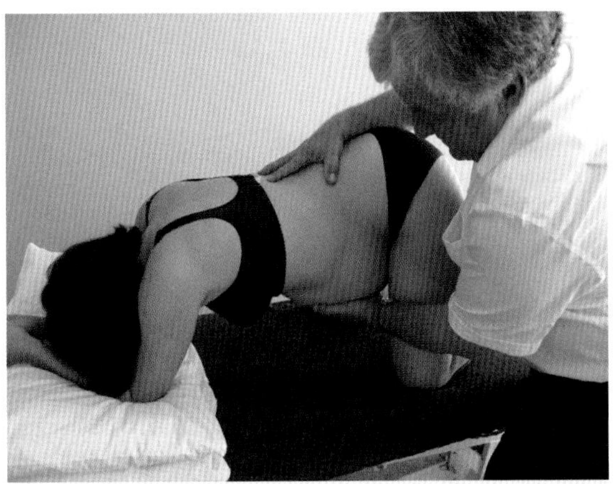

Fig 8.37
Creating space for the child to turn if it is capable, with the mother on all fours.

Use of Functional Techniques During Pregnancy

As already stated, functional techniques are excellent for use during pregnancy to unwind the ligaments controlling the position of the uterus as it grows and rises out of the pelvis. Similarly, myofascial unwinding techniques are very well tolerated by the mother, helping her to relax during treatment.

Functional techniques are also very helpful for sacroiliac strains when use of an HVLA technique is either contraindicated, or not wanted by the mother, or not possible.

Position of the patient

She lies on her side, with the top leg semiflexed and the bottom leg straight.

Position of the osteopath

The osteopath stands at the side of the treatment table, facing the patient.

Ambition of the technique

The aim is to release any intra-articular adhesions within the sacroiliac joint, or to release any muscular tensions in the tissues associated with the joints, such as piriformis, quadratus lumborum, or any of the ligaments connecting the ilium to the sacrum or the pelvis to the lumbar spine. It is thus a global technique.

Application of the technique

The osteopath takes her top leg and rests the shin across his abdomen (Fig 8.38). His hands fit around the ilium as if it were a cartwheel. Using his "belt buckle" as a focus for his center of gravity, he applies the usual parameters of flexion, extension, side-bending, translations, and rotations, palpating the movement of the ilium on the sacrum as he does so with his fingers at the posterior superior iliac spine. When he feels the first balance point, he asks the patient to breathe in, then hold the breath for a few moments until she relaxes; he follows the movement of the ilium totally passively until he reaches the final balance point of release.

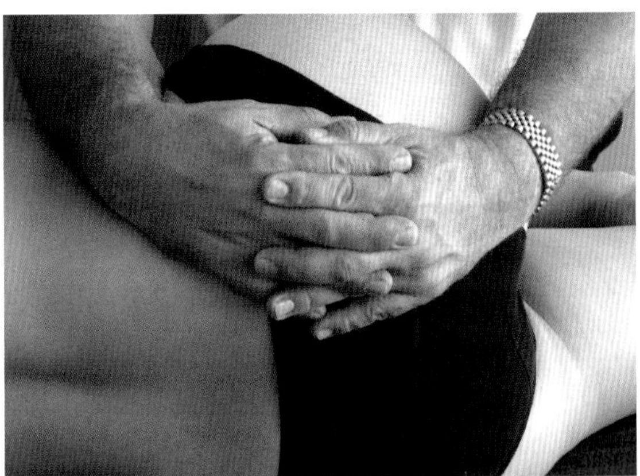

Fig 8.38
A global functional technique applied to the ilium.

References

1. Kapandji IA. The *Physiology of the Joints, Volume 3*. Blackwell, 2019.
2. Ostergaard M, Bonde B, Thomsen BS. Pelvic insufficiency during pregnancy. Is pelvic girdle relaxation an unambiguous concept? Ugeskr Laeger. 1992 Dec;154(50):3568–722.
3. Ryder I, Alexander J. Coccydynia: a woman's tail. Midwifery. 2000 Jun;16(2):155–60.
4. Jones ME, Shoaib A, Bircher MD. A case of coccygodynia due to coccygeal fracture secondary to parturition. Injury. 1997 Oct;28(8):549–50.
5. Nathan ST, Fisher BE, Roberts CS. Coccydynia: a review of pathoanatomy, aetiology, treatment and outcome. J Bone Joint Surg Br. 2010 Dec;92(12):1622–7.
6. Hodges SD, Eck JC, Humphreys SC. A treatment and outcomes analysis of patients with coccydynia. Spine J. 2004 Mar–Apr;4(2):138–40.
7. Karadimas EJ, Trypsiannis G, Giannoudis PV. Surgical treatment of coccygodynia: an analytic review of the literature. Eur Spine J. 2011 May;20(5):698–705.
8. Patijn J, Janssen M, Hayek S, Nekhail N, Van Zundert J, van Kleef M. Coccygodynia. Pain Pract. 2010 Nov–Dec;10(6):554–9.
9. Cheng YW, Delaney SS, Hopkins LM, Caughey AB. The association between the length of first stage of labour, mode of delivery, and perinatal outcomes in women undergoing induction of labour. Am J Obstet Gynecol. 2009 Nov;201(5):477.e1–e7.
10. National Institute for Health and Care Excellence. Antenatal Care for Uncomplicated Pregnancies. Clinical guideline [CG62], March 2008; https://www.NICE.org.uk.
11. Sutton J, Scott P. *Understanding and Teaching Optimal Foetal Positioning*. Birth Concepts, 1995.
12. Gardberg M, Laakkonen E, Sälevaara M. Intrapartum sonography and persistent occiput posterior position: a study of 408 deliveries. Obstet Gynecol. 1998 May;91 (5 Pt 1):746–9.
13. Gardberg M, Tuppurainen M. Acta Anterior placental location predisposes for occiput posterior presentation near term. Obstet Gynecol Scand. 1994 Feb;73(2):151–2.
14. Stremler R, Hodnett E, Petryshen P, Stevens B, Weston J, Willan AR. Randomized controlled trial of hands-and-knees positioning for occipitoposterior position in labor. Birth. 2005 Dec;32(4):243–51.
15. Burgos J, Melchor JC, Pijoán JI, Cobos P, Fernández-Llebrez L, Martínez-Astorquiza T. A prospective study of the factors associated with the success rate of external cephalic version for breech presentation at term. Int Journal Gynecol Obstet. 2011 Jan;112(1):48–51.

9 Postpartum Issues

It is good practice to encourage your patients to come for a postnatal visit at 6 weeks, after they have been discharged by the obstetrician, GP, or midwife.

Low Back and Pelvic Pain

There is ample evidence to suggest that many women suffer from low back or pelvic pain after their pregnancy. In some cases this is a continuation of the pain that was present during the pregnancy, and in other cases it appears to start after the baby is delivered. The effects can be short- or long-term. In one study the authors state that, although physical problems typically associated with the postpartum period are often regarded as transient or comparatively minor, they are strongly related both to women's functional impairment and to poor emotional health.[1] Careful assessment of the physical, functional, and emotional health status of women in the year after childbirth may improve the quality of postpartum care.[1,2,3]

There are fears among our patients that the use of epidural anesthesia can be responsible for back pain post partum. During a review of the literature, five studies show that, in fact, no correlation has been found. If your patients ask your advice regarding this method of pain relief during labor, you can safely reassure them as to the lack of evidence of postnatal consequences.[4,5,6,7,8]

The effect of relaxin is thought to be negligible within 48 hours of the birth, but there may be a correlation between ligamentous laxity and breast feeding. What is certain is that, as levels of estrogen rise during pregnancy, so do levels of relaxin. Likewise, after delivery, estrogen levels fall rapidly with the absence of the placenta, and serum relaxin levels reduce to zero by 48 hours post partum.[9,10] It is, therefore, unlikely that it is the postpartum effect of relaxin alone that is responsible for back pain.

Psychosocial factors have been deemed to be important in understanding why some women have problems and others do not. As such, these should not be ignored in osteopathic practices.[11]

For a young mother bringing up a new baby, back and neck pain can be common problems because the body is undergoing a program of repair after the trauma of childbirth (though this is quite a natural trauma), and she is more likely to hurt herself because of the extra demand that being a new mother places on her.

The house is a potential minefield for new mothers bringing up a young baby. After the pregnancy, her ligaments will take up to 6 months to regain their pre-pregnancy tone and strength – longer if she continues to breast feed for a year or more. During the previous 40 weeks, her body has been secreting large amounts of estrogen and relaxin, both of which change muscle or ligament tone.

After the birth, the joints are still potentially quite weak and therefore, at this time, the mother lacks the normal protection from lifting traumas that her body normally affords her. In normal circumstances, it is the ligaments which limit the range of movement in our joints and thus prevent us from overstraining or "putting something out." The muscles move one bone on another and also help protect the joints in times of emergency or physical effort. However, if the ligaments are weakened, the muscles can quickly fatigue and become stiff and sore: hence the familiar pattern of back pain and so on after pregnancy.

Commonly, patients report that they were fine during the pregnancy and it was only after having the baby that they developed back pain. In the past, practitioners have looked at the delivery for the etiology of the problem, but if one considers the sorts of activities that a new mother has to cope with, then the potential for trouble becomes clearer.

Firstly, there is bending. She needs to bend in every activity that she has to do with her new infant. Changing the baby, bathing it, putting it to bed, and getting it up all involve lifting, and as the baby grows bigger, so does the risk. Even the position she chooses for (breast) feeding her baby, if badly adopted, will lead to the typical new mother's stoop.

Changing mats or trolleys are all very well, but they are often not at the correct height for everyone, unless they are adjustable. In the house, a baby changing table might be the best place for the task, but when visiting friends new mothers should ask if they can change the baby on a bed, instead of bending to lift it from the floor. The baby lies on its back on a changing mat on the bed, and the person changing the baby kneels to face it. After the baby has been cleaned and changed, there is a minimal bend forwards to pick up the baby, as opposed to bending from a standing position or worse if the baby is on the floor; thus the risk of injury is minimized.

As far as picking up the baby from a cot or putting it to bed is concerned, a cot with drop sides is best so that the new mother can kneel down and again avoid bending from the waist.

It is this author's considered opinion that the type of baby sling that enables a mother to carry her child around strapped to the front of her chest is not very good for a woman who suffers from back pain. It tends to pull her over too far forwards, producing a strain on her neck and shoulders or lumbar spine muscles.

Heavy car seats, combined with the weight of a sleeping baby, can also be a real challenge if the back is sore soon after the birth. The actual weight of a baby car seat can vary, according to the individual manufacturer. On average, an infant carrier (without the base) weighs about 8 pounds, a convertible seat (the kind that are good from birth) and a belt positioning booster seat about 9 pounds. There can be the difference of a pound or two among infant seats, which you carry the most, but put a 10–15-pound baby in there too and they *all* feel heavy! There is no one simple solution to the problem. The best advice is to look around at as many car seats as possible and choose the lightest one available; take a baby along with you, sit it in the seat, and see just how you cope with lifting and carrying it around.

Mothers looking after a new baby can be at risk, then, but women with a new baby and a toddler are probably at the greatest risk of all. Not only do they have the potential problems outlined above, but also there is the added task of bending and attending to a heavy toddler while their back is in a weakened state. A toddler very much needs love and affection at this time, but patients should always go down to the level of the toddler and kneel before attempting to pick them up. They should never bend from the waist. Once they are down, they should encourage the toddler to hug them close, with their arms around the mother's neck; the mother should then hold the child tight, with one hand under them, while using the other hand to lever herself up, holding on to a table or chair for added support.

Advice is essential because of the increased lifting, bending, and carrying that looking after a neonate entails. Sometimes this is available from the midwife or health visitor, but often it is not. As osteopaths, we should have strategies in place that we can share with our patients after they have had their babies, so that they minimize the risks involved at this difficult time.

Problems with Breast Feeding

Osteopaths are often asked their advice about postnatal problems with breast feeding. This author's personal opinion is that "breast is best" if the new mother is capable of feeding and wants to breast feed. It is important not to ignore the fact that some women find breast feeding very difficult, and it can be stressful if the baby does not gain weight or has trouble latching on.

There are, however, many benefits to breast feeding from the point of view of the baby.

Breast milk is the ideal baby food. It has the perfect combination of proteins, fats, carbohydrate, and fluids that newborn babies require.

Breast feeding reduces the risk of developing infection. On average, breast-fed babies have fewer infections in their early life. In particular, they have less diarrhea and vomiting, chest infections, and ear infections compared to babies who are not breast fed. The main reason for this is that antibodies and other proteins are passed in the breast milk from mother to baby. These help to protect against infection.

There is good evidence that sudden infant death syndrome (cot death) is less common in breast fed babies. This is not fully explained, although the fact that breast fed babies have fewer infections is possibly a contributing factor.

One study reported that performance in childhood intelligence tests was better in children who had been breast fed compared to those who had been bottle fed.[12]

It is difficult to assess emotional factors, and no firm conclusions can be drawn. However, it is thought that breast feeding enhances the "bonding" process between baby and mother.

Many studies have looked at the possible long-term health benefits of breast feeding. There is now good evidence that, on average, some health problems in later life are less common in those who breast fed, compared to those who were not (Box 9.1).

Exclusive breastfeeding for the first 6 months of life provides maximum benefit. However, there is still a reduction in the risk of developing these diseases even in partially breast fed babies and in those who breast feed for a shorter time.

BOX 9.1

Potential health risks that are less common in later life for breast feeding women

- Obesity and overweight
- High blood pressure
- High cholesterol level
- Eczema
- Diabetes
- Leukemia
- Asthma

BOX 9.2

Problems that are less common in women who have breast fed one or more children compared to those who never breast fed

- Breast cancer
- Ovarian cancer
- Type 2 diabetes
- Postnatal depression

There are definite advantages for the mother if she can breast feed. Various studies have looked at the possible health benefits and there is now good evidence that, on average, the following health problems are less common in women who have breast fed one or more babies, compared to those who have never breast fed (Box 9.2).

Another health benefit for some mothers is that it is easier to lose weight after giving birth if you are breast feeding.[13,14,15,16,17]

If prolonged, breast feeding can and does have a weakening effect on the ligaments of the spine and pelvis. Once again, it is the action of the mother's hormones on the body tissues that is to blame, and if she has a particular problem that is related to weak ligaments, such as a pre-existing diagnosis of hypermobility, it might even be sensible to suggest that she stop feeding the baby herself after only 3 months.

This author advises new mothers that the age of 6 months is about right to start weaning their children, and after about 10 months they should be off the breast altogether. By this time, the child has all the passive immunity that it needs to protect itself from disease, and psychologically should be well bonded. Any continuation beyond this point can mean that if the mother has a back problem, it might be made worse by continued feeding.

In any case, it is a good idea for any mother who is feeding her child, either by breast or by bottle, to take a really close look at her posture while feeding; if need be, she should make sure that she is well supported by plenty of cushions to prevent ligament overstrain.

The safest position in which to feed your child is lying down on your side, with the neck well supported by pillows. You should avoid looking down and try instead to bring the baby to the breast and not the breast to the baby. If sitting, you should be positioned well back in the chair, with a pillow behind your head and the baby supported on cushions.

Lastly, the decision to breast feed or not is one that should be discussed with the midwife or health visitor, rather than the osteopath. Our role is to be supportive rather than informative per se.

References

1. Mogren I. Perceived health six months after delivery in women who have experienced low back pain and pelvic pain during pregnancy. Scand J Caring Sci. 2007 Dec;21(4):447–55.
2. Gutke A, Ostgaard HC, Oberg B. Predicting persistent pregnancy-related low back pain. Spine (Phila PA 1976). 2008 May;33(12):E386–93.
3. Van de Pol G, Van Brumman HJ, Bruinse HW, Heintz APM, van de Vaart CH. Pregnancy-related pelvic girdle pain in the Netherlands. Acta Obstet Gynecol Scand. 2007 Apr;86(4):416–22.
4. Malevic A, Jatuzis D, Paliulyte V. Epidural analgesia and back pain after labor. Medicina (Kaunas). 2019 Jul;55(7):354.
5. Butler R, Fuller J. Back pain following epidural anaesthesia in labour. Can J Anaesth. 1998 Aug;45(8):724–8.
6. Macarthur AJ, Macarthur C, Weeks SK. Is epidural anesthesia in labor associated with chronic low back pain? A prospective cohort study. Anesth Analg. 1997 Nov;85(5):1066–70.
7. Breen TW, Ransil BJ, Groves PA, Oriol NE. Factors associated with back pain after childbirth. Anesthesiology. 1994 Jul;81(1):29–34.
8. Mogren IM. Does caesarean section negatively influence the post-partum prognosis of low back pain and pelvic pain during pregnancy? Eur Spine J. 2007 Jan;16(1):115–21.
9. Eddie LW, Martinez F, Healy DL, Sutton B, Bell RJ, Tregear GW. Relaxin in sera during the luteal phase of in vitro fertilization cycles. Br J Obstet Gynaecol. 1990 Mar;97(3):215–20.
10. Eddie LW, Sutton B, Fitzgerald S, Bell RJ, Johnston PD, Tregear GW. Relaxin in paired samples of serum and milk from women after term and pre term delivery. Am J Obstet and Gynaecol. 1989;161(4):970–3.
11. Webb DA, Bloch JR, Coyne JC, Chung EK, Bennett IM, Culhane JF. Postpartum physical symptoms in new mothers: their relationship to functional limitations and emotional well-being. Birth. 2008 Sep;35(3):179–87.
12. Isaacs EB, Fischl BR, Quinn BT, Chong WK, Gadian DG, Lucas A. Impact of breast milk on intelligence quotient, brain size, and white matter development. Pediatr Res. 2010 Apr;67(4):357–62.
13. Hoddinott P, Tappin D, Wright C. Breast feeding. BMJ. 2008 Apr;336(7649):881–7.
14. Britton C, McCormick FM, Renfrew MJ, Wade A, King SE. Support for breastfeeding mothers. Cochrane Database Syst Rev. 2007 Jan;(1):CD001141 [abstract].
15. Food Standards Agency. EAT Study: early introduction of allergenic foods to induce tolerance. Study duration January 2008 to August 2015, Kings College, London; https://www.food.gov.uk/research/food-allergy-and-intolerance-research/.
16. Mosca F, Giannì ML. Human milk: composition and health benefits. Pediatr Med Chir. 2017 Jun;39(2):155.
17. Binns C, Lee M, Low WY. The long term public health benefits of breast feeding. Asia Pac J Public Health. 2016 Jan;28(1):7–14.

PERMISSIONS

Figs 3.19, 7.1, 7.3, 7.4, 7.7-7.12, 7.14-7.17, 7.19-7.21 © Informa UK Ltd (trading as Primal Pictures), 2020. Primal Pictures, an informa business www.primalpictures.com www.anatomy.tv

Fig 2.1 Fetal growth chart. © Dr Mark Hill; https://embryology.med.unsw.edu.au/embryology/index.php/Fetal_Development#Growth

Fig 3.5 The heart in the mediastinum. From Gray's Anatomy for Students, 4th edn, Richard Drake, A. Wayne Vogl, Adam Mitchell. Copyright Elsevier, 2019. Reproduced by kind permission of the publishers.

Fig 3.6 The Heart Gross Anatomy. From Gray's Anatomy for Students, 4th edn, Richard Drake, A. Wayne Vogl, Adam Mitchell. Copyright Elsevier, 2019. Reproduced by kind permission of the publishers.

Fig 3.7 and 4.19 The fascial chain/Fascial connections of the pericardium. (After Paoletti.) © Sully Editions.

Fig 3.8 The ligaments of the pericardium. (After Paoletti.) © Sully Editions.

Fig 5.20 The splanchnic nerves. From Gray's Anatomy for Students, 4th edn, Richard Drake, A. Wayne Vogl, Adam Mitchell. Copyright Elsevier, 2019. Reproduced by kind permission of the publishers.

Fig 5.23 The attachments of the gut to the ascending colon. © François Ricard.

Fig 6.39 The hepatic (left) and splenic (right) flexures. © François Ricard.

Fig 6.40 Formation of a visceral adhesion. © François Ricard.

Fig 7.13 Dissection of the pelvic floor to show levator ani. © Stanford Visible Female

Fig 7.18 The gutter or sling-shaped pelvic floor. From Gray's Anatomy for Students, 4th edn, Richard Drake, A. Wayne Vogl, Adam Mitchell. Copyright Elsevier, 2019. Reproduced by kind permission of the publishers.

Fig 8.33 The hand hold showing the hand on one side. © Nicholas Woodhead.

Fig 8.34 As in Figure 8.33 but using the skeleton to show where the hand is applied to the bone. © Nicholas Woodhead.

Fig 8.35 The bimanual hand hold. © Nicholas Woodhead.

INDEX

Note: Page numbers followed by f indicate figure.

Index

R

S

T

U

V